PRACTICE TIPS

FOURTH EDITION

JOHN MURTAGH AM

MBBS, MD, BSc, BEd, FRACGP, DipObstRCOG

Adjunct Professor of General Practice
Department of General Practice,
Monash University, Melbourne

Professorial Fellow, Department of General Practice,
University of Melbourne

Adjunct Professor, Graduate School of Integrative Medicine,
Swinburne University, Melbourne

Adjunct Clinical Professor, Graduate School of Medicine,
University of Notre Dame, Fremantle, Western Australia

The *McGraw·Hill* Companies

Sydney New York San Francisco Auckland
Bangkok Bogotá Caracas Hong Kong
Kuala Lumpur Lisbon London Madrid
Mexico City Milan New Delhi San Juan
Seoul Singapore Taipei Toronto

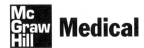

Medical

First edition, 1991
Reprinted 1992 (twice), 1993 (twice), 1994 (twice)
Second edition, 1995
Reprinted 1997, 1999, 2001
Third edition, 2000
Reprinted 2002, 2004
Fourth edition, 2004

National Library of Australia Cataloguing-in-Publication data:

Murtagh, John.
Practice tips.

4th edition
Includes index.
ISBN 0 074 71499 6.

1. Medicine - Practice - Handbooks, manuals, etc. 2.
Medicine, Rural. 3. Surgery, Minor. I. Title.

610

Published in Australia by
McGraw-Hill Australia PTY Ltd
Level 2, 82 Waterloo Road, North Ryde NSW 2113
Acquisitions Editor: Thu Nguyen
Production Editor: Tess Hardman
Editor: Kathy Riley
Proofreader: Lynn Cole
Indexer: Diane Harriman
Designer (cover and interior): Jan Schmoeger/Designpoint
Illustrator: Alan Laver, Shelly Communications
Typeset in Stone Serif 9.5/12 by Midland Typesetters
Printed on 80 gsm woodfree by Pantech Limited, Hong Kong.

Foreword to the fourth edition

Practice Tips continues to be an excellent source of practical advice for the family doctor, emergency physician and health-care professional.

John Murtagh has again produced an outstanding book, with valuable additions covering a wide range of topics and providing information not readily available. Examples include indications and techniques for periarticular injections, physical therapy for cervical and lumbar spine strain, safe times for sun exposure and optimal timing of paediatric surgical procedures.

This book has proved to be invaluable for the newly graduated doctor and community health nurse and I am confident it will remain so for many years to come.

GEOFF QUAIL
Clinical Associate Professor
Department of Surgery
Monash University
Melbourne

Foreword to the first edition

In a recent survey of medical graduates appointed as interns to a major teaching hospital, the question was posed, 'What does the medical course least prepare you for?' Half the respondents selected practical procedures from seven choices.

While we are aware that university courses must have a sound academic basis, it is interesting to note that many newly graduating doctors are apprehensive about their basic practical skills. Fortunately, these inadequacies are usually corrected in the first few months of intern training.

Professor John Murtagh, who has been at the forefront of medical education in Australia for many years, sensed the need for ongoing practical instruction among doctors. When appointed Associate Medical Editor of *Australian Family Physician* in 1980 he was asked to give the journal a more practical orientation, with a wider appeal to general practitioners. He was able to draw on a collection of practical procedures from his 10 years as a country doctor that he had found useful, many of which were not described in journals or textbooks. He began publishing these tips regularly in *Australian Family Physician*, and this encouraged colleagues to contribute their own practical solutions to common

problems. The column has been one of the most popular in the journal, and led to an invitation to Professor Murtagh to assemble these tips in one volume.

The interest in practical procedures is considerable—as witnessed by the popularity of practical skills courses, which are frequently fully booked. These have become a regular part of the Monash University Postgraduate Programme, and some of the material taught is incorporated in this book.

It is particularly pleasing to see doctors carrying out their own practical procedures. Not only is this cost-effective, in many cases obviating the need for referral, but it also broadens the expertise of the doctor and makes practice more enjoyable.

I congratulate Professor Murtagh on the compilation of this book, which I feel certain will find a prominent place on the general practitioner's bookshelf.

GEOFF QUAIL
Past Chairman
Medical Education Committee
Royal Australian College of General Practitioners
(Victorian Faculty)

Contents

Preface

Practice Tips is a collection of basic diagnostic and therapeutic skills that can be used in the offices of general practitioners throughout the world. The application of these simple skills makes the art of our profession more interesting and challenging, in addition to providing rapid relief and cost-effective therapy to our patients.

The art of medicine appears to have been neglected in modern times and, with the advent of super-specialisation, general practice is gradually being deskilled. I have been very concerned about this process, and believe that the advice in this book could add an important dimension to the art of medicine and represent a practical strategy to reverse this trend. The tips have been compiled by drawing on my own experience, often through improvisation, in coping with a country practice for many years, and by requesting contributions from my colleagues. Doctors from all over Australia have contributed freely to this collection, and sharing each other's expertise has been a learning experience for all of us.

I have travelled widely around Australia and overseas running workshops on practical procedures for the general practitioner. Many practitioners have proposed the tips that apparently work very well for them. These were included in the text if they seemed simple, safe and worth trying. The critical evidence base may be lacking but the strategy is to promote 'the art of medicine' by being resourceful and original and thinking laterally.

Most of the tips have previously been published in *Australian Family Physician*, the official journal of the Royal Australian College of General Practitioners, over the past decade or so. The series has proved immensely popular with general practitioners, especially with younger graduates commencing practice. The tips are most suitable for doctors working in accident and emergency departments. There is an emphasis on minor surgical procedures for skin problems and musculoskeletal disorders. A key feature of these tips is that they are simple and safe to perform, requiring minimal equipment and technical knowhow. Regular practice of such skills leads to more creativity in learning techniques to cope with new and unexpected problems in the surgery.

Several different methods to manage a particular problem, such as the treatment of ingrowing toenails and removal of fish hooks, have been submitted. These have been revised and some of the more appropriate methods have been selected. The reader thus has a choice of methods for some conditions. Some specific procedures are more complex and perhaps more relevant to practitioners such as those in remote areas who have acquired a wide variety of skills, often through necessity.

It must be emphasised that some of the procedures are unorthodox but have been found to work in an empirical sense by the author and other practitioners where other treatments failed. The book offers ideas, alternatives and encouragement when faced with the everyday nitty-gritty problems of family practice.

Sterilisation guidelines for office practice

The strict control of infection, especially control of the lethal HIV virus, is fundamental to the surgical procedures outlined in this book.

Summarised guidelines include:

- Use single-use pre-sterilised instruments and injections wherever possible.
- The use of single-use sterile equipment minimises the risk of cross-infection. Items such as suturing needles, injecting needles, syringes, scalpel blades and pins or needles used for neurological sensory testing should be single-use.
- Assume that any patient may be a carrier of hepatitis B and C, HIV and the human papilloma virus.
- Hand-washing is the single most important element of any infection control policy: hands must be washed before and after direct contact with the patient. For non-high-risk procedures, disinfect by washing with soap under a running tap and dry with a paper towel which is discarded.
- Sterile gloves should be worn for any surgical procedure involving penetration of the skin, mucous membrane and/or other tissue.
- Avoid using multi-dose vials of local anaesthetic. The rule is 'one vial—one patient'.
- Safe disposal of sharp articles and instruments such as needles and scalpel blades is necessary. Needles must not be recapped.
- Instruments cannot be sterilised until they have been cleaned. They should be washed as soon after use as possible.
- Autoclaving is the most reliable and preferred way to sterilise instruments and equipment. Bench-top autoclaves should conform to Australian standard AS 2182.
- Chemical disinfection is not a reliable system for routine processing of instruments, although it may be necessary for heat-sensitive apparatus. It should definitely *not* be used for instruments categorised as high risk.
- Boiling is not reliable as it will not kill bacterial spores and, unless timing is strictly monitored, may not be effective against bacteria and viruses.

Note: For skin antisepsis for surgical procedures, swab with povidone-iodine 10% solution in preference to alcoholic preparations.

1 Injection techniques

Basic injections

Painless injection technique

Method 1

The essence of this technique is to ensure good muscle relaxation. The patient should be as comfortable as possible. For injections into the deltoid region, the patient should be sitting down with hand on the hip and with the muscle as relaxed as possible. For deep intramuscular injections the buttock is preferred, but care must be taken to inject in the upper outer quadrant. These patients should be lying face down. The buttock should be exposed and the patient encouraged to relax.

1. *Massage for muscular relaxation:* The injection site should be well massaged for 20–30 seconds. This is a traditional preparation of the injection site, but it is probably more important for achieving relaxation than for ensuring that the skin is cleaned. It is easy to ensure that the underlying muscle is fully relaxed if firm, gentle pressure is applied with the left hand. When the muscle is relaxed, hold the syringe like a dart between the thumb and forefinger of the right or dominant hand.
2. *Sharp tap over site:* Before giving the injection, use the side of the back of the right (or dominant) hand to give a smart tap over the injection site (Fig. 1.1). A sharp flick with a finger can also be effective, but not as much as a tap.
3. *The injection:* Follow this immediately by injecting the needle using the dart technique.

Note: These steps follow in very rapid succession.
   Many patients will tell you with surprise that they did not feel the needle but were conscious of the sting of the injection material going into the tissues.

Method 2: Almost painless injections

A subcutaneous or intramuscular injection is almost always painless if the skin is stretched firmly before inserting the needle. If injecting the arm, for example, the third, fourth and fifth fingers should go medial to the arm while the thumb and index finger stretch the skin on the lateral surface (Fig. 1.2). The needle should be inserted quickly into the stretched skin.

(continues)

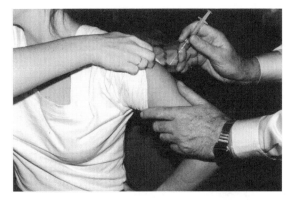

Fig. 1.1 Sharp tap with side of hand

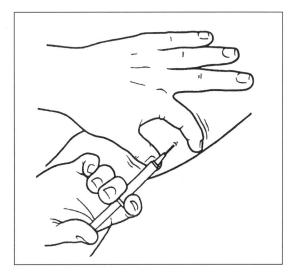

Fig. 1.2 Stretching the skin with thumb and index finger

Method 3: Muscle contraction–relaxation method

Use the muscle energy method by asking the patient to push their elbow against their hip as an isometric contraction for 7 seconds. Then quickly give the injection into the deltoid muscle (now relaxed).

Method 4: Needle gauge

The discomfort from an IM or SC injection can be minimised by using a smaller gauge needle, e.g. 30 gauge, especially for vaccinations in children.

Reducing the sting from an alcohol swab

The sting from alcohol on the skin can be reduced by drying the skin with a piece of sterile gauze or cotton wool after swabbing. Alternatively, one can blow onto the preparation site to achieve drying.

Painless wound suturing

The objective is to administer local anaesthetic (LA) as painlessly as possible when treating a wound that requires suturing. The method applies to non-contaminated wounds only.

Method

1. Irrigate the wound with a small volume of LA.
2. Rather than inserting the needle into the skin, insert it into the subcutaneous tissue through the open wound (Fig. 1.3).
3. Infiltrate for the length of the wound on both sides.

This method is relatively painless.

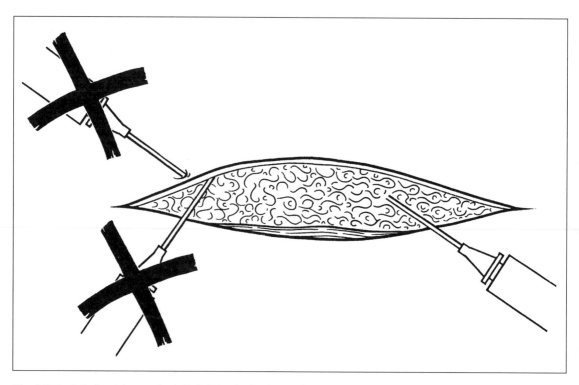

Fig. 1.3 A relatively painless method of administering local anaesthetic at a wound site requiring suturing

Slower anaesthetic injection cuts pain

A study has shown that subcutaneous infiltration of local anaesthetic causes only half the pain if injected slowly over 30 seconds rather than rapidly over 5 seconds.

Disposal of needles

Recapping of used needles should be avoided, to eliminate as far as possible the risk of accidental puncture of the medical practitioner or practice nurse. The risk of contracting such infections as hepatitis B, C and HIV from a sharps injury is ever-present. Needles should be disposed of directly into a sharps container. There are many types of sharps containers available for use in the surgery and even in the doctor's bag.

The 'take it with you' needle disposal unit consists of a plastic bottle 2.5 cm in diameter and 8 cm in depth. The lid has an opening with a plastic flap on the underside. This opening is designed to allow introduction of the needle attached to its syringe and then withdrawal of the syringe to 'trap' the needle in the container. After the needle is introduced into the centre of the opening, it is tilted to the side. The syringe is then pulled sharply upwards to disconnect the needle (Fig. 1.4). (In Australia the unit is available from Go Medical Industries Pty Ltd.)

Recapping of needles

Although the recapping of needles should be avoided, probably the safest way, if it really must be done, is to scoop up the needle guard with the used needle and syringe unit, using the dominant hand only. This reinforces the principle of always staying 'behind the needle', and keeps the thumb and forefinger of the non-dominant hand out of danger.

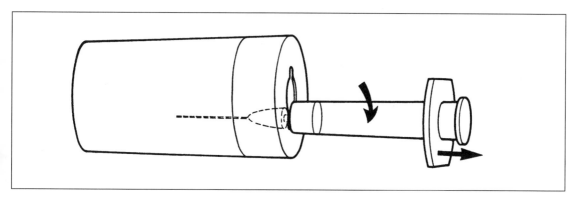

Fig. 1.4 The doctor's bag needle-disposal bottle

Rectal 'injection'

When no veins can readily be found for intravenous injections, in some emergency situations the use of the rectal route is effective.

Diabetic hypoglycaemia

In some unconscious patients it may not be possible to administer the 'difficult' intravenous injection of 50% glucose, due to such factors as vasoconstriction and obesity in the patient.

However, the glucose can be given simply by pressing the nozzle of the syringe (usually a 20 mL syringe) gently but firmly into the rectum and slowly injecting the solution.

Convulsions

In children with a persistent febrile convulsion or in patients with status epilepticus, the rectal route can be used for administering a diazepam or paraldehyde solution with amazing success.

Example

Consider a 2-year-old child (weight 12 kg) with a persistent febrile convulsion. The dose of diazepam injectable is 0.4 mg/kg, so 5 mg (1 mL) of diazepam is diluted with isotonic saline (up to 5–10 mL of solution) and introduced into the rectum, preferably with a plastic fluid-drawing-up nozzle attached to the syringe.

Finger lancing with less pain

A method of minimising the pain of lancing fingers for blood samples, especially for diabetics, is outlined.

Theory

The sides of the fingers are less painful than the pad or the base of the nailbed of the thumb or index finger (as traditionally used for bleeding). The thumb and index finger have heightened sensitivity, as presented in Penfield and Boldrey's homunculus (Fig. 1.5).

Method

- Clean the finger with a non-alcohol swab.
- Insert the lancet into the medial or lateral aspect of the 3rd or 4th finger of either hand.
- Provide firm pressure on the pad of the lanced finger with the opposing thumb on the pad of the finger. This ensures an adequate blood flow for the test strips.

Other viewpoints

Side of thumb

According to a randomised controlled trial published in *The Lancet* (1999, 354, pp. 921–2), the least painful area to lance for blood sugar testing was the side of the thumb. It would be worth conducting our

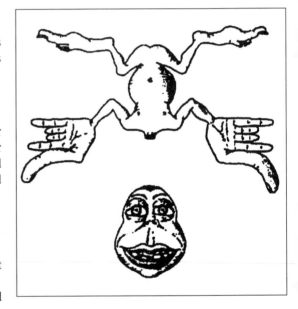

Fig. 1.5 Penfield and Boldrey's homunculus

own trial—the side of the thumb or the 3rd or 4th finger!

Earlobe

A UK study of diabetic patients in 2003 found that the average pain score for finger pricking was 4–5 times higher than pricking the earlobe.

Nerve blocks

Digital nerve block

The digital nerve block is indicated for simple procedures on the fingers and toes. (A more proximal block, such as the brachial plexus block, is indicated for extensive injury.)

Each digit is supplied by four nerve branches, two dorsal and two palmar (or plantar). These nerves run forward adjacent to the respective metacarpal or metatarsal bone. The nerves to the fingers and toes are blocked at the base of the digit.

Method

1. Perform the block at the level of the respective metacarpal or metatarsal from the dorsal aspect.
2. Introduce the 25- or 23-gauge needle proximal to the metacarpal head (for the hand) immediately alongside the bone.
3. Insert at right angles to the skin and proceed as far as the palmar or plantar skin.
4. Inject 1–2 mL of LA on each side of the digit as the needle is slowly being withdrawn, so that the solution is spread evenly superficially and deeply (Fig. 1.6).

Alternatively, a wheal can be raised on the dorsal surface and the needle advanced as the injection is given.

Dosage

This is 2–4 mL of lignocaine or prilocaine 1% without adrenaline.

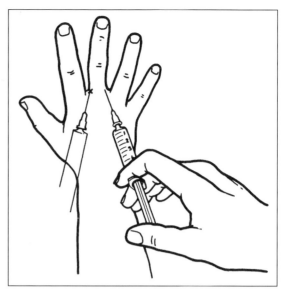

Fig. 1.6 The digital nerve block blocks both palmar (or plantar) and dorsal nerve branches

Note: Never use a vasoconstrictor in the injection. Allow sufficient time for anaesthesia (5–20 minutes).

Adrenaline antidote

If adrenaline is injected into a digit and causes vaso-constriction, inject 1 mL phentolamine (Regitine) directly into the same area.

The thumb

The thumb requires only one injection in the midline of the palmar surface at the base of the thumb.

Regional nerve blocks to nerves to hand

Partial or complete wrist block is very valuable for minor surgery or wound repair of the hand. The distribution of the cutaneous nerves to both surfaces of the hand is shown in Figure 1.7.

Median nerve block

Area supplied

- Palmar surface on radial (lateral) side involving fingers 1, 2, 3 and the radial half of 4.
- Dorsal distal aspect of same fingers.

Technique of block

- Identify palmaris longus (PL) tendon (flex wrist against resistance).
- Insert 25-gauge needle between tendons flexor carpi radialis (FCR) and just lateral to PL.
- Insert at level of proximal skin crease.
- Inject 1 mL 1% lignocaine superficially and 1–2 mL deep, angling the needle at about 60°.

Note: if PL absent, inject midway between the flexor tendons and FCR.

(continues)

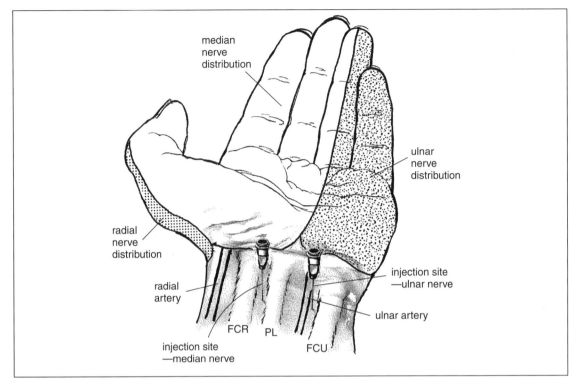

Fig. 1.7 Illustration of median and ulnar nerve blocks

Ulnar nerve block

Area supplied

- Ulnar (medial) aspect of hand (fingers 5 and half 4).

Technique of block

- Identify flexor carpi ulnaris (FCU) tendon and styloid process of ulna.
- Insert 25-gauge needle on radial side FCU just medial to the radial artery at the level of the styloid process of ulna (similar level as for median nerve block).
- Inject 4 mL 1% lignocaine, preferably when paraesthesia has been induced by the needle.

Radial nerve block

Area supplied

- Radial half of dorsal aspect of hand.
- Base of thenar eminence.

Technique

It is preferable to raise a subcutaneous ring of 5 mL 1% lignocaine radially (from level with the FCR tendons), then around the radial border of the wrist dorsally (about 6 cm proximal to the wrist) to just lateral to the styloid process of the ulna.

Tibial nerve block

The tibial (posterior tibial) nerve can be blocked as it passes behind the medial malleolus, in front of the tendoachilles, usually midway between these structures. It innervates most of the sole of the foot (Fig. 1.8).

Indications

- Operations on the foot.
- Removal of plantar warts.
- Injecting the plantar fascia.
- Foreign bodies in sole.

Method

1. Palpate the posterior tibial artery behind the medial malleolus. The tibial nerve lies immediately behind the artery.
2. Insert a fine-gauge needle just posterior to the artery, either at the level of the medial malleolus or just below it, pointing in an anterolateral direction (Fig. 1.9). Alternatively, insert the needle anterior to the artery.
3. At about a depth of 1 cm, paraesthesia may be elicited, indicating the ideal location for injection. The depth of injection varies from 0.5 to 2 cm.
4. Inject 6–10 mL of 1% lignocaine, taking care not to puncture a blood vessel.

The block should induce an area of anaesthesia around the sole of the foot, making it ideal for the procedures listed. It usually does not anaesthetise the most proximal and lateral parts. The anaesthesia develops over 10 minutes and lasts for up to 2 hours.
Note: Avoid bilateral nerve blocks at the same visit. Bilateral anaesthesia may cause falls due to loss of balance. To obtain almost full anaesthesia of the plantar aspect of the foot a sural nerve block is necessary, as well as the tibial block.

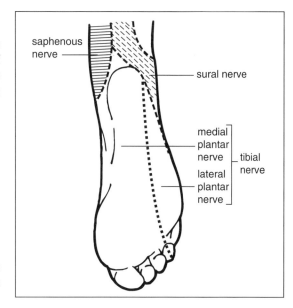

Fig. 1.8 Innervation of the heel and sole of the foot

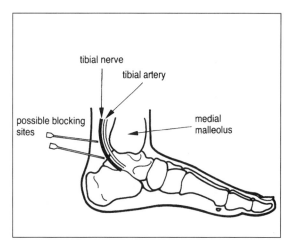

Fig. 1.9 Tibial nerve block

Caution: Ensure that the injection is not given into the nerve.

Sural nerve block

The sural nerve, which innervates most of the back of the heel and the lateral border of the sole, is blocked by a subcutaneous infiltration of up to 5–8 mL of 1% lignocaine in a fanwise fashion from the Achilles tendon to the outer and upper border of the lateral malleolus (Fig. 1.10). This procedure anaesthetises the most proximal and lateral aspects

(continues)

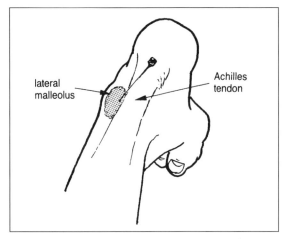

Fig. 1.10 Sural nerve block (infiltrate between Achilles tendon and lateral malleolus)

of the sole of the foot. If combined with a tibial nerve block, most of the heel and sole of the foot will be covered.

Facial nerve blocks

Regional nerve blocks have advantages over infiltration for facial and oral anaesthesia because there is less tissue swelling at the operative site, a wider area is anaesthetised, and they are less painful.

General points

• Use 2% lignocaine with adrenaline.
• Allow 5–10 minutes before commencing the procedure.
• Always aspirate to check for blood before injecting.

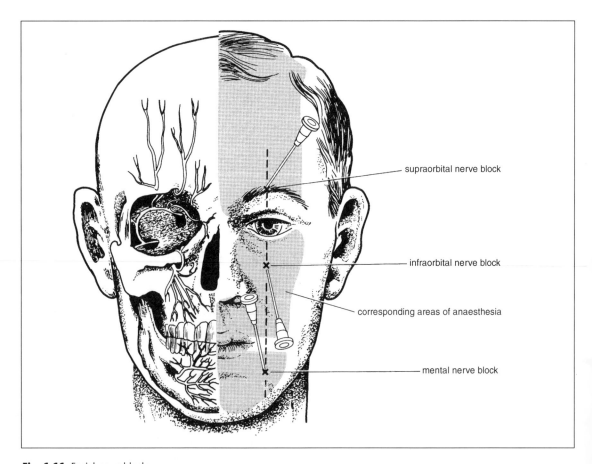

Fig. 1.11 Facial nerve blocks

Supraorbital nerve block

Indications

Surgery to forehead and scalp to vertex.

Method

1. Insert a 23- or 25-gauge 3.5 cm needle over the supraorbital foramen, at the upper border of the orbit, under the eyebrow, 2.5 cm from the midline (Fig. 1.11).
2. Inject 3–4 mL of LA.

Infraorbital nerve block

Indications

Surgery to:

- lower eyelid,
- cheek,
- side of nose and upper lip,
- gingival tissues from midline to first molar.

Method 1: Intraoral approach (preferred to the extraoral route)

The infraorbital foramen lies above and in line with the second premolar, 1 cm below the infraorbital margin.

1. Elevate the upper lip and align the syringe along the long axis of the tooth.
2. Enter the mucosa at its reflection from the gum and advance a 23- or 25-gauge needle to just short of the foramen (until the bone is just contacted).
3. Inject 2–3 mL of LA.

Method 2: Extraoral approach

1. Instruct the patient to look straight ahead.
2. Insert the needle 1 cm below the infraorbital margin in line with the pupil, directing the needle towards the infraorbital foramen. Do not attempt to enter it.
3. Inject 2 mL of LA.

Mental nerve block

Indications

- Excision of oral and skin lesions.
- *Suturing lacerations:* from midline to lower border of mandible (Fig. 1.11) to include lower lip and chin.

Method (intraoral approach)

1. Palpate the mental foramen, which lies at the apex of the lower second premolar tooth.
2. Lift the lip forward and align the syringe with the long axis of this tooth.
3. Penetrate the mucosa and advance the needle to just short of the foramen. This is about half-way between the gum margin and the lower border of the mandible.
4. Aspirate and inject 2 mL of LA.

If the patient is edentulous, use as a reference a vertical line from the midpoint of the pupil.

Specific facial blocks for the external ear

For minor surgery and repair of lesions of the external ear, widespread infiltration can be used (Fig. 1.12). However, more specific blocks using 3 mL of 1% plain lignocaine for each nerve can be used. Care should be used because of the proximity of branches of the carotid artery. The skin of the external ear is mainly supplied by three branches of the trigeminal nerve, namely:

- **Auriculotemporal nerve**—innervates upper anterior quadrant of lateral surface including tragus, crux of helix and adjacent helix.

  Blockage: insert needle immediately posterior-inferior to temporomandibular joint.

- **Greater auricular nerve**—innervates remainder of lateral surface, including anti-helix and ear lobe and most of medial (cranial) surface.

  Blockage: insert needle just behind and inferior to the ear lobe at the anterior border of the sterno-mastoid muscle.

- **Lesser occipital nerve**—innervates upper part of medial (cranial) surface.

  Blockage: insert needle about 1 cm posterior to the ear at its midpoint.

  (continues)

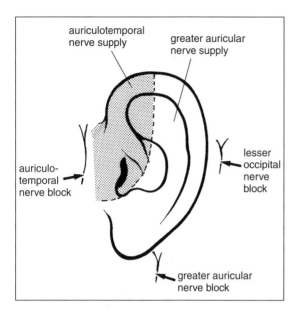

Fig. 1.12 Nerve supply to the ear and sites for the three nerve blocks

Penile nerve block

The penis can be anaesthetised for procedures such as circumcision, wound repair and paraphimosis reduction by injecting local anaesthetic (without adrenaline) into the dorsal and ventral surfaces.

Method

1. Inject a ring of 5 mL of LA subcutaneously around the base of the penis, with the needle resting against the corpus cavernosum (Fig. 1.13a).

2. Inject 2 mL of LA into each of the grooves on the ventral surface (between the corpus cavernosum and spongosium) (Fig. 1.13b).

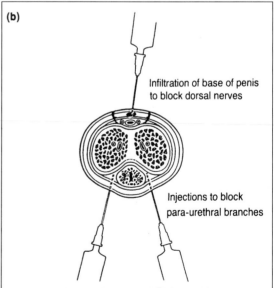

Infiltration of base of penis to block dorsal nerves

Injections to block para-urethral branches

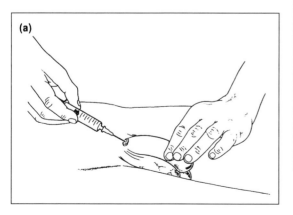

Fig. 1.13 Penile nerve block: **(a)** infiltration of base of penis; **(b)** three injection approaches

Intravenous regional anaesthesia (Bier's block)

This technique uses an intravenous injection of local anaesthetic into an arm or leg that is isolated from the circulation by an arterial tourniquet. It produces excellent anaesthesia, muscle relaxation and (if desired) a bloodless operating field.

Indications

- Minor surgery, especially to upper arm (e.g. release of trigger finger, removal of foreign bodies).
- Reduction of limb fractures (e.g. Colle's fracture).

Precautions

- Exclude patients with unstable epilepsy, second- or third-degree heart block, liver disease, severe vascular disease or allergy to LA agents.
- Obtain informed consent.
- Ensure patient fasting.
- Avoid sudden release of LA (e.g. escaping beneath tourniquet).
- Maintain IV access with a needle in the vein of the opposite arm.
- Check the pressure of the tourniquet throughout.
- Have resuscitation equipment available.
- Maintain inflation for at least 20 minutes.
- Maximum inflation 45–60 minutes.

Method (for arm)

1. Cannulate vein (e.g. plastic IV cannula of IV set) and tape on.
2. Drain blood by simple elevation for 3 minutes or (for bloodless field) by an Esmarch bandage.
3. Apply a sphygmomanometer cuff or (better still) arterial pneumatic tourniquet.
4. Inflate to 100 mmHg above the patient's systolic blood pressure.
5. Slowly inject 2.5 mg/kg of 0.5% lignocaine or prilocaine (preferred) (*without* adrenaline) into the indwelling needle (Fig. 1.14). *Note:* Usual adult dose is 30 mL of 0.5% prilocaine (maximum 40 mL).
6. The onset of anaesthesia is rapid (3–6 minutes). Confirm its adequacy.
7. Watch carefully for side effects, e.g. restlessness, dizziness, tinnitus, seizures, bradycardia or hypotension.
8. Use a second doctor (if available) to perform the procedure.
9. On completion, ensure very slow release of the tourniquet. As soon as it is deflated, pump it up again rapidly then slowly deflate. (Repeat this three times at the rate of once per minute if inflated for only 20–25 minutes.)
10. Observe the patient carefully for at least 15 minutes.

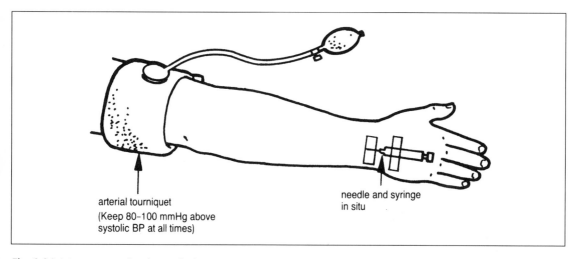

arterial tourniquet
(Keep 80–100 mmHg above systolic BP at all times)

needle and syringe in situ

Fig. 1.14 Intravenous regional anaesthesia

Therapeutic injections

Intercostal nerve block

Indications

- Relief from severe pain of fractured rib.
- Malignant pain.
- Other painful chest conditions, e.g. post-thoracotomy pain.

Method

1. The patient sits up bending slightly forwards, hugging a pillow.
2. Apply antiseptic over the paravertebral area, corresponding to the posterior end of the fractured rib and the two adjacent ribs.
3. Insert a smaller-gauge needle (25 or 23) into the lower border of the neck of the fractured rib about four finger-breadths from the spinous process—that is, at about the angle of the rib or 8–10 cm from the midline (Fig. 1.15a).
4. Advance the needle forward until it reaches the rib and inject a small amount of LA (1% lignocaine).
5. Now 'walk' the needle slowly downward to allow it to slip below the inferior border of the rib (Fig. 1.15b).
6. Advance the needle anteriorly a further 2–3 mm only (take care not to puncture the pleura) and inject 3–5 mL of LA (Fig. 1.15c).

Note: Perform this block with great care. Pleural puncture is indicated by coughing, pleuritic pain or aspiration of air into the syringe.

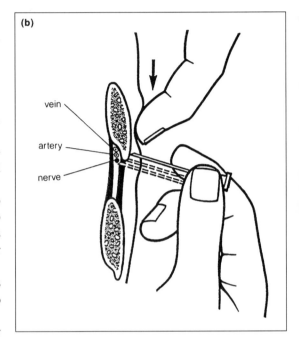

(b)

vein

artery

nerve

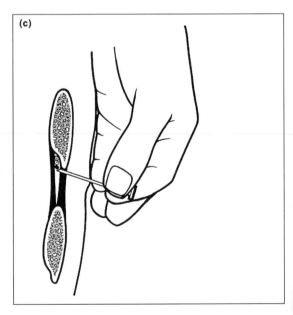

(c)

(a)

X = site(s) of infiltration

Fig. 1.15 **(a)** Shows sites of infiltration (X); **(b)** 'walking' the needle; **(c)** final position

The caudal (trans-sacral) injection

An epidural injection is the appropriate way to treat persistent painful sciatica without neurological signs in a patient who is not a candidate for surgery but is making slow progress.

The lumbar epidural is technically more difficult than the caudal epidural and requires hospital day care. The caudal epidural is safer and within the skill of any medical practitioner. It can be performed in a general practice procedure treatment room with resuscitation facilities. The key to success is to identify the sacral hiatus and insert a needle (usually a 21- or 22-gauge, 36 mm needle is sufficient for most patients) at the appropriate angle in a cranial direction.

Identifying the sacral hiatus

The sacral hiatus can be identified in the following ways:

- Palpate the two sacral cornua and mark the hiatus at the top end of the hollow formed by the cornua.
- It lies directly beneath the upper limit of the intergluteal fold.
- It tends to correspond to the proximal interphalangeal (PIP) joint with the tip of the index finger resting on the tip of the coccyx.
- It lies at the caudal apex of an equilateral triangle drawn with the horizontal base between the posterior superior iliac spines (PSIS) (opposite S2). This apex is usually situated over the sacral hiatus (Fig. 1.16).

Injection procedure

Method

1. Inform the patient that the procedure is surprisingly comfortable but that some heaviness will be felt in the back of the legs and that pain may be initially exacerbated.
2. Mark the sacral hiatus after its identification.
3. Lie the patient prone with a pillow under the symphysis pubis to slightly flex the hips (or with the operating table 'broken').
4. Relax the glutei by inversion of the ankles (feet in pigeon-toe position).

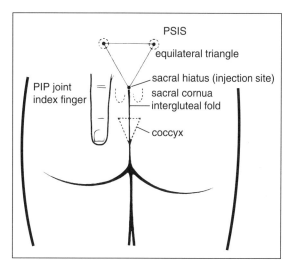

Fig. 1.16 Identify the sacral hiatus by four methods:
1. palpating the sacral cornua
2. noting the upper limit of the intergluteal fold
3. measuring the tip of the coccyx to the PIP of the index finger
4. drawing an equilateral triangle with the base being the line between the postero-superior iliac spines
REPRODUCED FROM C. KENNA & J. MURTAGH, *BACK PAIN AND SPINAL MANIPULATION*, BUTTERWORTHS, SYDNEY, 1989, WITH PERMISSION

5. Clean and drape the area, avoiding spirit running onto the anus. Using a 23- or 25-gauge needle, anaesthetise the skin and subcutaneous tissue.
6. Select a spinal tap cannula: 21-, 22- or 23-gauge 50 mm or a 21-gauge 38 mm standard single-use needle (preferred).
7. Insert the needle upwards (cranially) keeping strictly to the midline. The angle to the skin should be about 25–30 degrees (Fig. 1.17); if too superficial, the needle will pass above the hiatus. When the ligament is pierced there is a sensation of 'giving'.
8. Angle the needle slightly downwards as you insert it for about 2 cm. Avoid proceeding any further because of the risk of piercing the dura.
9. The needle is rotated through 90 degrees twice—check for a back flow of cerebrospinal fluid (CSF) or blood. If blood is obtained, partly withdraw the needle and reinsert it, keeping as far posterior as possible to avoid the greater concentration of veins anteriorly. If CSF is withdrawn, abandon the procedure. *(continues)*

10. Inject the fluid carefully and slowly over a five-minute period (at least) with at least three aspiration checks for blood. The plunger of the syringe should move with relative ease.
11. Ask the patient to report any unusual symptoms such as giddiness or light-headedness, which is reasonably common but indicates a need for caution. Monitor the pulse and blood pressure during the procedure and stop the injection if an adverse reaction develops.

The injection can be repeated if the patient experiences a good, albeit temporary, result.

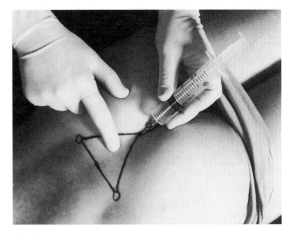

Fig. 1.17 The caudal epidural: the appearance of the procedure

Hormone implants

Suitable sites for the subcutaneous insertion of crystalline pellets of the hormones oestradiol and testosterone into the abdominal wall are shown in Figure 1.18a. The preferred sites are in the anterior abdominal wall above and parallel to the inguinal ligament. A site just superolateral to the pubic hair is ideal.

The procedure is performed under local anaesthesia using a wide-bore trocar and cannula. It is simple and effective, and takes a few minutes only.

Equipment

You will need:

- 2–5 mL of 1% lignocaine with syringe,
- povidone-iodine 10% antiseptic,
- wide-bore trocar and cannula (use an expellor if available),
- scalpel with no. 11 (or similar) blade,
- crystalline pellets (that will fit into the cannula),
- sterile gauze or suitable container, for 'catching' a dropped pellet,
- sterile adhesive strips.

Method

To insert the hormone implants:

1. Choose the implantation site.
2. Infiltrate the sterilised skin with LA so that a small bleb is raised.
3. Make a small incision 5–10 mm long with the scalpel blade.
4. Insert the trocar and cannula through the incised skin at a shallow angle (Fig. 1.18b) for at least 2 cm. The end of the cannula now rests in a pocket in the subcutaneous tissue (care should be taken to avoid the rectus sheath).
5. Remove the trocar.
6. Grasp a pellet with sterile forceps and place it in the cannula. (*Note:* This part of the procedure is the most delicate because the pellet is likely to be accidentally dropped. Have an assistant standing by with a sterile receptacle or gauze to catch it.)

7. Reinsert the trocar or expellor (ideally the expellor should extend 5 mm beyond the end of the cannula) and push the pellet into the sub-cutaneous 'pocket' (Fig. 1.18c).
8. The cannula and trocar (or expellor) are removed while maintaining pressure over the site for 1 minute to minimise bruising.
9. Apply sterile adhesive strips (or a suture) over the wound and then a light dressing.

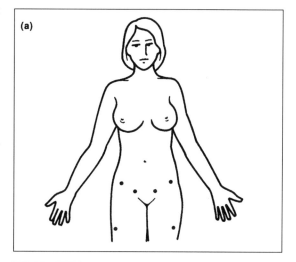

(a)

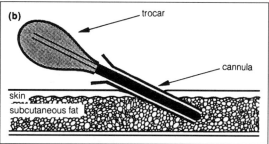

(b)

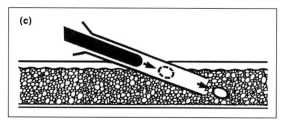

(c)

Fig. 1.18 **(a)** Suitable sites for insertion of pellets; **(b)** trocar and cannula are angulated into subcutaneous tissue after initial, more upright entry; **(c)** shows pellet in cannula pushed gently into place with expellor

Musculoskeletal injections

Musculoskeletal injection guidelines

Conditions that are considerably relieved by injections include:

- rotator cuff tendinitis, especially supraspinatus tendinitus;
- subacromial bursitis;
- bicipital tendinitis;
- lateral and medial epicondylitis;
- trigger finger and thumb;
- trochanteric bursitis and gluteus medius tendinitis;
- tendinitis around the wrist, e.g. de Quervain's tenosynovitis;
- plantar fasciitis;
- knee conditions—-anserinus tendinitis/bursitis, biceps femoris tendinitis

Rules and guidelines

- Use any one of the depot (long acting) corticosteroid formulations: betamethasone (Celestone Chronodose), triamcinolone (Kenocort–A10 or A40) or methyl-prednisolone (Depo-Medrol, Depo-Nisolone).

- Use the more soluble formulation (Celestone Chrondose) for tendon sheath injection.
- Use a mixture of 1 mL of LA corticosteroid (CS) with 1% Xylocaine (0.5 mL–8 mL) for most injections.
- Conditions not very responsive and best avoided include patellar tendinitis and Achilles tendinitis.
- Conditions responsive for about 3 weeks only include epicondylitis and plantar fasciitis.
- Trochanteric bursitis gluteus medius tendinitis is common, misdiagnosed often and responds exceptionally well to 1 mL CS + 8 mL Xylocaine 1%.
- Corticosteroids are not very effective for trigger spots of the back.
- A subacromial space injection (posterior approach) will be effective for most rotator cuff problems.
- Use corticosteroid alone for carpel tunnel injections and small joints.
- Intra-articular injections for arthritic joints have limited use: perhaps 2–3 times for osteoarthritis—best for monarticular rheumatoid arthritis.
- Tendons should never be injected; inject tendon sheaths but with caution because of the danger of rupture.

Injection of trigger points in back

The injecton of painful myofascial trigger points of the back and neck (Fig. 1.19) is relatively easy and may give excellent results. A trigger point is one characterised by:

- circumscribed local tenderness,
- localised twitching with stimulation of juxtaposed muscle,
- pain referred elsewhere when subjected to pressure.

Don't: use large volumes of LA; use corticosteroids; cause bleeding.
Do: use a moderate amount of LA (only).

Method

1. Identify and mark the trigger point, which must be the maximal point of pain.
2. Select a 21-, 22- or 23-gauge needle of a length compatible with the injection site. (A 38 mm needle will cover most areas of the back and neck.)
3. Insert the needle into the point until the patient complains of reproduction of pain, which may be referred distally.
4. At this point, introduce 5–8 mL of LA of your choice. (Lignocaine/lidocaine, procaine or bupivacaine 1% or 0.5% can be used.)
5. Recommend post-injection exercises and local massage for the affected segment.

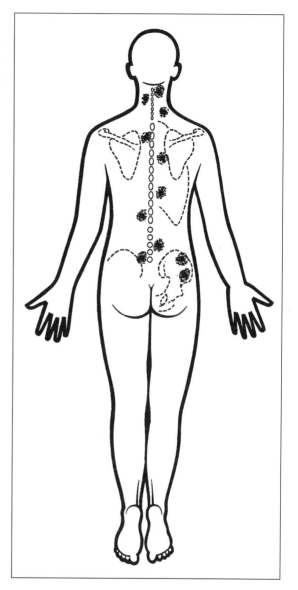

Fig. 1.19 Typical trigger points of the back
REPRODUCED FROM C. KENNA & J. MURTAGH, *BACK PAIN AND SPINAL MANIPULATION*, BUTTERWORTHS, SYDNEY, 1989, WITH PERMISSION

Injection for rotator cuff lesions

Injections of local anaesthetic and corticosteroid produce excellent results for inflammatory disorders around the shoulder joint, especially for supra-spinatus tendinitis. The best results are obtained with precise localisation of the area of inflammation, although injections into the subacromial space are all that is necessary to reach inflammatory lesions of the tendons comprising the rotator cuff and the sub-acromial bursa.

The subacromial space injection for rotator cuff lesions

The recommended approach is from the postero-lateral aspect of the shoulder, with the patient sitting upright.

Method

1. Draw up 1 mL of corticosteroid and 2–3 mL of 1% LA.
2. Sit the patient upright and explain the procedure in general terms.
3. Identify the gap between the acromium and the humeral head with the palpating finger or thumb.
4. Mark this spot.
5. Swab the area with antiseptic.
6. Place the needle (23-gauge, 32 or 38 mm long) into this gap, just inferior to the acromium (Fig. 1.20).
7. Aim the needle slightly medially and anteriorly.
8. Insert for a distance of about 30 mm. The solution should flow into the subacromial space without resistance.

Tip: Place a weight (0.5–1 kg) in the hand nearest to the affected side to facilitate opening the subacromial space. It also distracts the patient!

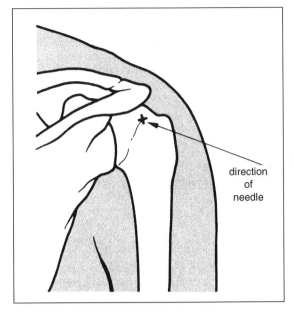

direction of needle

Fig. 1.20 Posterior view of the subacromial bursa injection site

The subacromial space injection for subacromial bursitis

The lateral approach is used for localised bursitis when there is localised tenderness over the sub-acromial space. It is important to angle the needle into the appropriate anatomical plane.

Method

1. Identify the lateral edge of the acromium and select the midpoint.
2. Insert the needle 4–5 mm below the edge of the acromium and angle it between the head of the humerus and the acromium.
3. Inject 1 mL of corticosteriod and 3–5 mL of 1% LA.

Injection for supraspinatus tendinitis

An injection directed onto the inflamed tendon of supraspinatus is so effective that it is preferable to administer a specific injection rather than a general infiltration into the subacromial space.

The tendon can be readily palpated as a tender cord anterolaterally as it emerges from beneath the acromium to attach to the greater tuberosity of the humerus. This identification is assisted by depressing the shoulder via a downward pull on the arm and then externally and internally rotating the humerus. This manoeuvre allows the examiner to locate the tendon readily.

Method

1. Identify and mark the tendon.
2. Place the patient's arm behind the back, with the back of the hand touching the far waistline. This locates the arm in the desired internal rotation and forces the humeral head anteriorly.
3. Insert a 23-gauge 32 mm needle under the acromium along the line of the tendon, and inject around the tendon just under the acromium (Fig. 1.21). If the gritty resistance of the tendon is encountered, slightly withdraw the needle to ensure that it lies in the tendon sheath and not the tendon.
4. The recommended injection is 1 mL of long-acting corticosteroid with 1 mL of LA.

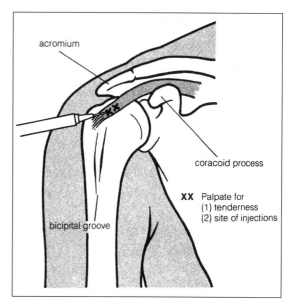

Fig. 1.21 Injection placement for supraspinatus tendinitis

Injection for bicipital tendinitis

Bicipital tendinitis is diagnosed by finding an abnormal tenderness over the tendon when the arm is externally rotated. The usual site is the bicipital groove of the humeral head.

Method

1. The patient sits with the arm hanging by the side and the palm facing forwards.
2. Find and mark the site of maximal tenderness. This is usually in the bicipital groove and more proximal than expected.
3. Insert a 23-gauge needle at the proximal end of the bicipital groove above the tender area.
4. Slide the needle down the groove to reach the tender area (Fig. 1.22).
5. Inject 1 mL of long-acting corticosteroid and 1 mL of LA around this site.

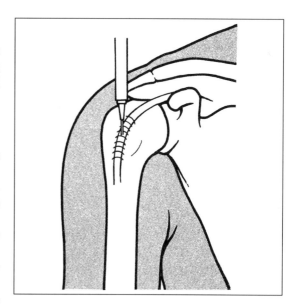

Fig. 1.22 Injection placement for bicipital tendinitis

Injections for epicondylitis

Lateral epicondylitis (tennis elbow)

The key to successful injections is to have the tender lesion pinpointed precisely. The point of maximal tenderness is usually on or just distal to the lateral epicondyle.

Equipment

You will need:

- an antiseptic swab,
- a 25- or 23-gauge needle,
- 1 mL of long-acting corticosteroid and 1 mL of LA (e.g. 1% lignocaine). Use a mixed solution (LA drawn last).

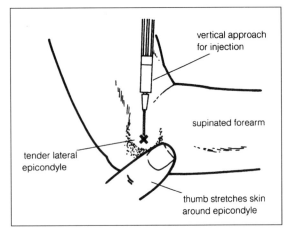

Fig. 1.23 Injection technique for tennis elbow

Method

1. The patient sits with the elbow resting on a table, flexed to a right angle and fully supinated.
2. Using an anterior approach, palpate the tender area and mark it with a pen.
3. With the thumb (of the non-dominant hand) over the patient's lateral epicondyle and the fingers spread out around the elbow to steady it, insert the needle vertically downward to touch the periosteum of the tender point (Fig. 1.23).
4. After introducing about 0.5 mL of the mixed solution, partly withdraw the needle and reinsert it to ensure that the tender area is covered both deeply and superficially.

Post-injection

1. Ask the patient to 'work it in' during the next few hours with repeated extensions of the elbow joint and pronation of the wrist.

2. Warn the patient that the area will be very painful for the next 24 hours and recommend moderately strong analgesics.
3. Repeat the injection in 2–4 weeks unless all the symptoms have been abolished.
4. A maximum of two injections only is recommended.

Medial epicondylitis (golfer's elbow)

A similar method is used to that for lateral epicondylitis. The elbow is flexed and supinated with full external rotation of the shoulder of the affected arm. The anterior approach is used, and the tender area of the medial epicondyle injected as for lateral epicondylitis.

Injection for trigger finger

Treatment of trigger finger or thumb by injection is often very successful, and usually relieves symptoms for a considerable period of time. The injection is made under the tendon sheath and not into the tendon or its nodular swelling. The fourth (ring) finger is commonly affected.

Method

1. The patient sits facing the doctor with the palm of the affected hand facing upward.
2. Draw 1 mL of long-acting corticosteroid solution into a syringe and attach a 25-gauge needle for the injection.

3. Insert the needle at an angle distal to the nodule and direct it proximally within the tendon sheath (Fig. 1.24). This requires tension on the skin with free fingers.
4. By palpating the tendon sheath, you can (usually) feel when the fluid has entered the tendon sheath.
5. Inject 0.5–1 mL of the solution, withdraw the needle and ask the patient to exercise the fingers for 1 minute.

Post-injection

Improvement usually occurs after 48 hours and may be permanent. The injection can be repeated after 3 weeks if the triggering is not completely relieved.

If triggering recurs, surgery is indicated. This involves division of the thickened tendon sheath only.

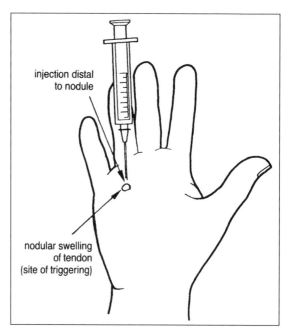

Fig. 1.24 Injection site for trigger finger

Tendon sheath injection

Tenosynovitis of the wrist, especially that of the thumb abductors (de Quervain's disease), is a common problem that can readily be identified by tenderness, swelling and palpable crepitus over the tendon. It may respond to an injection of a long-acting corticosteroid, but care should be taken to inject the suspension into the tendon sheath rather than into the tendon.

Method

1. Identify and mark the most tender site of the tendon and the line of the tendon.
2. Thoroughly cleanse the skin with an antiseptic, such as povidone-iodine 10% solution.
3. Insert the tip of the needle (21-gauge) about 1 cm distal to the point of maximal tenderness (Fig. 1.25).
4. Advance the needle almost parallel to the skin along the line of the tendon.
5. Inject about 0.5 mL of the corticosteroid suspension into the tendon sheath. If the needle is in the sheath, very little resistance to the plunger should be felt and the injection will cause the tendon sheath to billow out.

Alternative method

1. Advance the needle into the tendon, where there will be resistance to the attempted injection in addition to a firm, gritty feel to the needle.
2. Slowly withdraw the needle until the resistance to depressing the plunger disappears.
3. Inject the corticosteroid.

(continues)

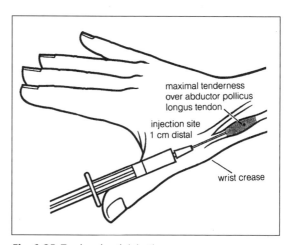

Fig. 1.25 Tendon sheath injection

The ideal site for this injection is into the sheath of the abductor tendons to the thumb just above the radial styloid. It is important, therefore, to avoid injecting into the radial artery, which should always be identified beforehand.

Note: It should be emphasised that the common problem of de Quervain's disease (also known as 'washerwoman's sprain') is best treated by resting and avoiding the causative stresses and strains on the thumb abductors.

Injection for plantar fasciitis

Plantar fasciitis can be treated by injecting local anaesthetic and long-acting corticosteroid into the site of maximal tenderness in the heel. An alternative is to inject the corticosteroid into the anaesthetised heel. On the other hand, to minimise the pain of injecting through the heel, apply liquid nitrogen beforehand and immediately inject through that spot.

Method

1. Perform a tibial nerve block. (The area of maximal tenderness should be marked prior to the nerve block.)

2. When anaesthesia of the heel is present (about 10 minutes after the tibial nerve block), insert a 23-gauge needle with 1 mL of long-acting corticosteroid perpendicular to the sole of the foot at the premarked site (Fig. 1.26). Insert the needle until a 'give' is felt as the plantar fascia is pierced.
3. Inject half the steroid against the periosteum in the space between the fascia and the calcaneus.
4. Reposition the needle to infiltrate into the fascial attachments over a wider area.

Tip for plantar fasciitis: Massage the sole of the foot over a wooden foot massager or glass bottle filled with water for 5 minutes daily to help prevent recurrence.

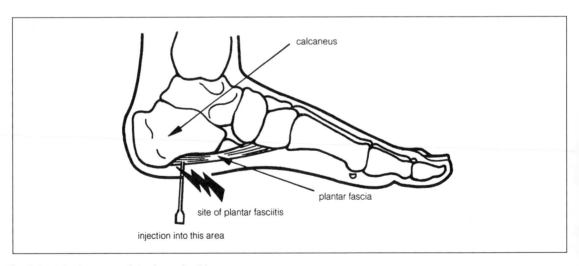

Fig. 1.26 Injection approach in plantar fasciitis

Injection for gluteus medius tendinitis or trochanteric bursitis

Pain around the greater trochanter

Pain around the lateral aspect of the hip is a common disorder, and is usually seen as lateral hip pain radiating down the lateral aspect of the thigh in older people engaged in walking exercises, tennis and similar activities. It is analogous in a way to the shoulder girdle, where supraspinatus tendinitis and subacromial bursitis are common wear-and-tear injuries.

The two common causes are tendinitis of the gluteus medius tendon, where it inserts into the lateral surface of the greater trochanter of the femur, and bursitis of one or both of the trochanteric bursae. Distinction between these two conditions is difficult, and it is possible that, as with the shoulder, both are related. The pain of bursitis tends to occur at night; that of tendinitis occurs with such activity as long walks and gardening.

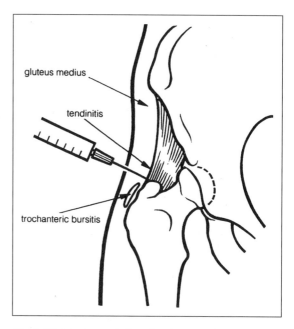

Fig. 1.27 Injection technique for gluteus medius tendinitis (into area of maximal tenderness)

Treatment method

Treatment for both is similar.

1. Determine the points of maximal tenderness over the trochanteric region and mark them. (For tendinitis, this point is immediately above the superior aspect of the greater trochanter; Fig. 1.27.)
2. Inject aliquots of a mixture of 1 mL of long-acting corticosteroid with 5–7 mL of LA into the tender area, which usually occupies an area similar to that of a standard marble.

The injection is invariably very effective. Follow-up management includes sleeping with a small pillow under the involved buttock, and stretching the gluteal muscles with knee–chest exercises. One or two repeat injections over 6 or 12 months may be required. Surgical intervention is rarely necessary.

Extra tips to alleviate gluteus medius tendinitis or bursitis

- Perform straight-leg stretching in dependent adduction (see Fig. 9.56, page 178).
- Develop a 'Charlie Chaplin' gait—legs in external rotation for walking.
- Massage lateral thigh for 2–5 minutes daily using a glass or plastic (preferably grooved) bottle, full of water, as a rolling-pin.

Injection of the carpal tunnel

An injection of long-acting corticosteroid into the carpal tunnel may relieve symptoms permanently or, more commonly, temporarily. It may therefore be useful as a diagnostic test and also to provide symptomatic relief while awaiting surgery.

Note: The injections may be repeated. *Do not* use local anaesthetic in the injection.

Method

1. The patient sits by the side of the doctor with the hand palm upward, the wrist slightly extended.
2. Identify the palmaris longus tendon (best done by flexing the wrist against resistance) and the ulnar artery.
3. Insert the needle (23-gauge) at a point about 2.5–3 cm proximal to the main transverse crease of the wrist and between the palmaris longus tendon and the artery (Fig. 1.28). Take care to avoid the superficial veins.
4. Advance the needle distally, parallel to the tendons and nerve at about 5° to the horizontal. It should pass under the transverse carpal ligament (flexor retinaculum) and come to lie in the carpal tunnel.
5. Inject 1 mL of corticosteroid. This is usually painless and runs freely. Ensure that the patient feels no severe pain or paraesthesia during the injection.
6. Withdraw the needle and ask the patient to flex and extend the fingers for 2 minutes.

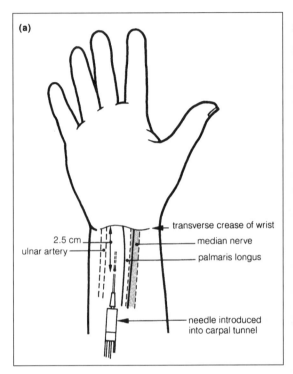

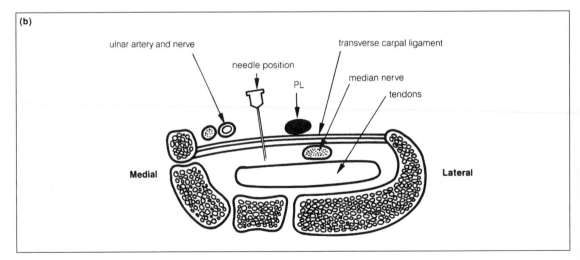

Fig. 1.28 Needle introduced into carpal tunnel: **(a)** anterior view; **(b)** section

Injection near the carpal tunnel

A study reported in the BMJ (1999, 319, pp. 884–6) recommended giving a single injection of corticosteroid, e.g. 40 mg methylprednisolone with lignocaine 1%, close to but not into the tunnel (to avoid potential damage to the median nerve). The results were considered to be as good as giving it into the tunnel.

Injection of the tarsal tunnel

Tarsal tunnel syndrome is caused by an entrapment neuropathy of the posterior tibial nerve in the tarsal tunnel beneath the flexor retinaculum on the medial side of the ankle (Fig. 1.29). The condition, which is uncommon, is due to dislocation or fracture around the ankle or tenosynovitis of tendons in the tunnel from injury, rheumatoid arthritis and other inflammations.

Symptoms and signs

- A burning or tingling pain in the toes and sole of the foot, occasionally the heel.
- Retrograde radiation to the calf.
- Discomfort often in bed at night and worse after standing.
- Removal of the shoe may give relief.
- Sensory nerve loss is variable (may be no loss).
- The Tinel test (finger or reflex hammer tap over the nerve below and behind the medial malleolus) may be positive.
- A tourniquet applied above the ankle may reproduce symptoms.

The diagnosis is confirmed by electrodiagnosis.

Treatment

- Relief of abnormal foot posture with orthotics.
- Corticosteroid injection.
- Decompression surgery if other measures fail.

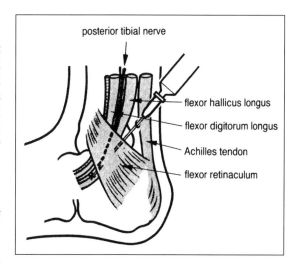

Fig. 1.29 Sites of injection for tarsal tunnel syndrome (above or below the flexor retinaculum that roofs the 'tunnel'). This medial view of the right foot shows the relationship of the posterior tibial nerve to the tendons.

Injection method

Using a 23-gauge 32 mm needle, inject a mixture of corticosteroid in 1% xylocaine or procaine into the tunnel either from above or below the flexor retinaculum. The sites of injection are shown in Figure 1.29. Be careful not to inject the nerve.

Injection for Achilles tendinitis

Management

Inflammation of and around the tendon can be a resistant problem, and conservative measures such as rest, a heel raise and NSAIDs should be adopted. For resistant painful problems, however, an injection of corticosteroid can be helpful. The inflammation must be localised, such as a tender 2 cm area.

Avoid giving the corticosteroid injection in the acute stages and never lodge it in the tendon.

Method

1. Mark the area of peritendinitis, which usually lies immediately anterior and deep to the tendon just above the calcaneus.
2. Infiltrate this tender area adjacent to the tendon with 1 mL of plain local anaesthetic (e.g. 1% lignocaine) and 1 mL of long-acting corticosteroid (Fig. 1.30). The solution should run freely, and care should be taken to avoid the tendon.

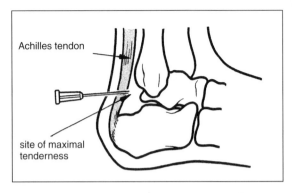

Fig. 1.30 Usual approach for the injection for Achilles tendinitis

Injection for tibialis posterior tendinitis

This is a common and under-diagnosed condition in people presenting with foot and ankle pain, especially on the medial side.

It is usually found in middle-aged females, in ballet dancers, and in those with flat feet with a valgus deformity.

Pain is reproduced on:

- palpitation anterior and inferior to the medial malleolus,
- stretching by passive inversion of the foot,
- resisted inversion of the foot.

Tibialis posterior tendinitis can cause the tarsal tunnel syndrome. The diagnosis can be confirmed by ultrasound imaging.

Method of injection

1. Mark the tender area of the tendon.
2. Use a lower-gauge needle with a syringe containing 0.5–1 mL LA corticosteroid with 0.5–1 mL local anaesthetic.

3. Approach the tendon at a very shallow angle, either proximally or distally, and inject into the sheath, taking care to avoid injecting the tendon (Fig. 1.31).

Note: the tibialis posterior tendon is prone to rupture.

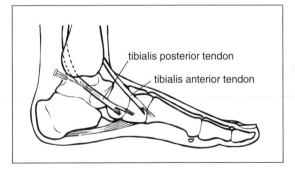

Fig. 1.31 Method of injecting the tendon sheath of tibialis posterior

Injections into joints

Intra-articular injections of corticosteroids can be very therapeutic for some acute inflammatory conditions, particularly severe synovitis caused by rheumatoid arthritis (especially monarticular rheumatoid arthritis). This use is limited in osteoarthritis but can be very effective for a particularly severe flare-up of osteoarthritis such as in the knee or the acromioclavicular joint. (Corticosteroids can cause degeneration of articular cartilage and hence restricted usage is important.) Strict asepsis is essential, using disposable equipment.

Acromioclavicular joint

Method

1. The patient sits with the arm hanging loosely by the side and externally rotated. The joint space is palpable just distal (lateral) to the bony enlargement of the clavicle. It is about 2 cm medial to the lateral edge of the acromion.
2. Palpate the 'gap' for maximal tenderness.
3. Insert a 25-gauge needle, which should be angled according to the different surfaces encountered. (Fig. 1.32). It should reach a depth of about 2 cm when it is certainly intra-articule.
4. Inject a mixture of 0.25–0.5 mL of corticosteroid with 0.25–0.5 mL of 1% lignocaine.

Shoulder joint

Method

1. The patient sits in the same position as for the acromioclavicular joint injection.
2. Use an anterior approach and insert a 21- to 23-gauge needle just medial to the head of the humerus. Feel for the space between the head of the humerus and the glenoid cap. (If in doubt, feel for it by rotating the humerus externally.)
3. This insertion should also be 1 cm below and just lateral to the coracoid process (Fig. 1.32).
4. Inject a mixture of 1 mL of corticosteroid and 1 mL of 1% lignocaine.

Hip joint

Method

1. The patient lies supine with the hip in extension and internal rotation.

2. Use an anterior approach, with the insertion point being 2.5 cm below the inguinal ligament and 2 cm lateral to the femoral artery.
3. Use a 20-gauge 6–7 cm needle and insert it at about 60° to the skin.
4. Introduce the needle downwards and medially until bone is reached (Fig. 1.33).
5. Withdraw it slightly and inject the mixture of 1 mL of corticosteroid and 2 mL of 1% lignocaine.

(continues)

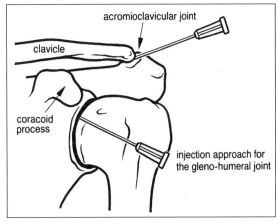

Fig. 1.32 Approaches for injections into the acromio-clavicular joint and the gleno-humeral joint of the shoulder

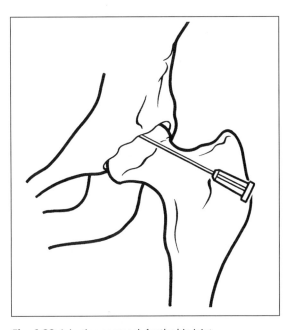

Fig. 1.33 Injection approach for the hip joint

(continues)

Knee joint

Method for infrapatellar route

1. The patient flexes the knee to a right angle. (The patient can sit on the couch with the leg over the side.) Alternatively, the knee can be extended with the quadriceps relaxed.
2. A 21-gauge needle can be inserted either medially (preferably) or laterally.
3. Insert the needle in the triangular space bounded by the femoral condyle, the tibial condyle and the patellar ligament (Fig. 1.34).
4. Direct the needle inwards and slightly posteriorly in a plane pointing slightly upwards to the horizontal (to avoid the infrapatellar fat pad).
5. Inject 1 mL of LA corticosteroid (an anaesthetic agent isn't necessary).

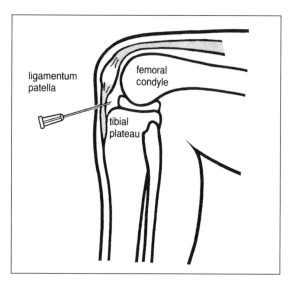

Fig. 1.34 Injection of the knee joint (note the needle angled into the triangular space)

Wrist joint

Method

Inject on the dorsal surface in the space just distal to the ulnar head at its midpoint.

1. Palpate the space between the ulnar head and the lunate.
2. Insert the needle at right angles to the skin between the extensor tendons of the 4th and 5th fingers.
3. Insert to a depth of about 1 cm.
4. Inject 0.5 mL of corticosteroid and 0.5 mL of 1% lignocaine.

First carpometacarpal joint of thumb

Method

1. Palpate the proximal margin of the first metacarpal in the anatomical snuffbox.
2. Insert the needle to a depth of about 1 cm between the long extensor and long abductor tendons into the joint space.
3. Inject 0.5 mL of corticosteroid.

Finger joint

The technique for injections of the metacarpophalangeal and interphalangeal joints is similar.

Method

It is important to have an assistant for this injection.

1. The joint is flexed to an angle of 30°, and this position is maintained by the assistant who simultaneously applies longitudinal traction to 'gap' the dorsal aspect of the joint.
2. Insert the needle, which is kept at right angles to the base of the more distal phalanx, from the dorsal aspect in the midline.
3. Direct the needle through the tendon of extensor digitorum just distal to the head of the more proximal bone (phalanx or metacarpal) to a depth of 3–5 mm (Fig. 1.35).

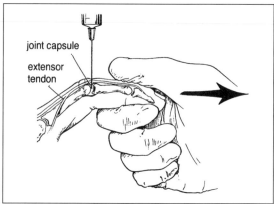

Fig. 1.35 Injection of the proximal interphalangeal joint

Temporomandibular joint

This injection is useful in the treatment of painful rheumatoid arthritis, osteoarthritis or temporomandibular joint dysfunction that is not responding to conservative measures.

Method

1. The patient sits on a chair, facing away from the doctor. The mouth is opened to at least 4 cm.
2. Palpate the joint line anterior to the tragus of the ear. This is confirmed by opening and closing the jaw.
3. Insert a 25-gauge needle into the depression above the condyle of the mandible, below the zygomatic arch and one finger breadth (2 cm) anterior to the tragus.
4. Direct the needle inwards and slightly upwards so that it is free within the joint cavity (Fig. 1.36).
5. Inject the 1 mL solution containing 0.5 mL of local anaesthetic and 0.5 mL of corticosteroid, which should flow freely.

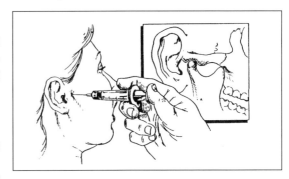

Fig. 1.36 Injection of the temporomandibular joint

Acute gout in the great toe

Injection technique

Acute gouty arthritis invariably presents with exquisite pain in the great toe and the diagnosis and relief of pain is a special challenge to the general practitioner.

An effective and caring, albeit invasive, treatment is as follows:

- Perform a modified digital block using 1% plain local anaesthetic to the affected toe.
- When anaesthesia has been obtained, use a 19-gauge needle to aspirate fluid from the joint or the periarticular region.
- Examine the fluid under polarised light microscopy. The presence of long, needle-shaped urate crystalis is diagnostic.
- If sepsis is eliminated, inject corticosteroids, e.g. 0.5–1.0 mL of triamcinolone, into the joint (Fig. 1.37).

Drug treatment

Two NSAIDs options are usually employed, one a heavier dosage than the other. Indomethacin is the preferred one but others can be used.

Conventional method

Indomethacin 50 mg (o) 8 hourly for 24 hours, then 25 mg (o) 6 hourly until resolution.

'Shock' method

Indomethacin 100 mg (o) statim, 75 mg 2 hours later, then 50 mg (o) 8 hourly (relief is usual within 48 hours)

plus

Metoclopramide (Maxolon) 10 mg (o) 8 hourly (or other anti-emetic).

(*continues*)

Other corticosteroids

- Prednisolone 40 mg/day for 3–5 days
  then taper by 5 mg over 10 days
  or
  Corticotrophin (ACTH) IM

- Colchicine
  Consider if NSAIDs are not tolerated.
  0.5–1.0 mg statim, then 0.5 mg every 2 hours until
  pain disappears or GIT side effects develop.

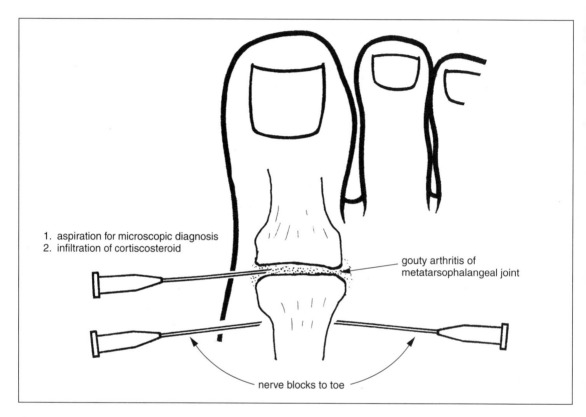

1. aspiration for microscopic diagnosis
2. infiltration of cortiscosteroid

gouty arthritis of
metatarsophalangeal joint

nerve blocks to toe

Fig. 1.37 Management of acute gout of the great toe, illustrating nerve blocks and joint injection

2 Skin repair and minor plastic surgery

Principles of repair of excisional wounds

It is important to keep the following in mind:

1. Plan all excisions carefully.
2. Check previous scars for healing properties.
3. Aim to keep incision lines parallel to natural skin lines.
4. Take care in poor healing areas, such as backs, calves and knees; and in areas prone to hypertrophic scarring, such as over the sternum of the chest, and the shoulder.
5. Use atraumatic tissue-handling techniques.
6. Practise minimal handling of wound edges.
7. Use Steri-strips after the sutures are removed.

Common mistakes for excisional surgery

- Skimping (inadequate margins).
- Tension on skin edges.
- Knots too strongly tied.
- Stitches too thick.
- Too large a bite.
- Stitches in too long.
- Inadequate early compression.

Minimising bleeding in the elderly

Stop anticoagulants (if possible) before a significant procedure. Examples:

- warfarin—3 days
- aspirin—10 days
- NSAIDs—2–5 days (check half life)

Suture material (Table 2.1)

- Monofilament nylon sutures are generally preferred for skin repair.
- Use the smallest calibre compatible with required strains.
- The synthetic, absorbable polyglycolic acid or polyglactin sutures (Dexon, Vicryl) are stronger than catgut of the same gauge, but do not use these (use catgut instead) on the face or subcuticularly.

Table 2.1 Selection of suture material (guidelines)

Skin	nylon 6/0	face
	nylon 3/0	back, scalp
	nylon 5/0	elsewhere
Deeper tissue	catgut 4/0	face
(dead space)	Dexon/Vicryl 3/0 or 4/0	elsewhere
Subcuticular	catgut 4/0	
Small-vessel ties	plain catgut 4/0	
Large-vessel ties	chromic catgut 4/0	

Instruments

Examples of good-quality instruments:

- locking needle holder (e.g. Crile-Wood 12 cm),
- skin hooks,
- iris scissors.

Holding the needle

The needle should be held in its middle because this will help to avoid breakage and distortion, which tends to occur if the needle is held near its end (Fig. 2.1a).

Incisions

Incisions should be made perpendicular to the skin (*not* angled) (Fig. 2.1b).

Dead space

Dead space should be eliminated, to reduce tension on skin sutures. Use buried absorbable sutures to approximate underlying tissue. This is done by starting suture insertion from the fat to pick up the fat/dermis interface so as to bury the knot (Fig. 2.2).

Everted wounds

Eversion is achieved by making the 'bite' in the dermis wider than the bite in the epidermis (skin surface) and making the suture deeper than it is wide.

(continues)

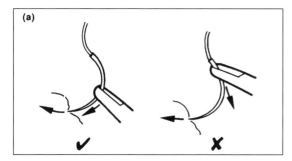

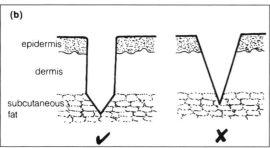

Fig. 2.1 Correct and incorrect methods of: **(a)** holding the needle; **(b)** making incisions

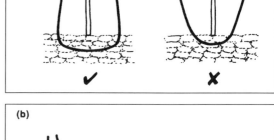

Fig. 2.2 Eliminating dead space

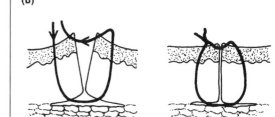

Fig. 2.3 Everted wounds: **(a)** correct and incorrect methods of making a simple suture; **(b)** making a vertical mattress suture

Shown is:

- a simple suture (Fig. 2.3a),
- a vertical mattress suture (Fig. 2.3b).

The mattress suture is the ideal way to evert a wound.

Number of sutures

Aim to use a minimum number of sutures to achieve closure without gaps, but sufficient sutures to avoid tension. Place the sutures as close to the wound edge as possible.

Debridement and dermabrasion for wound debris

If grit and other foreign material such as oil is left in the wound, an unacceptable tattoo effect will occur in the healed wound. This can be avoided by meticulous exploration of the wound to remove debris and dermabrasion for superficial grit.

Continuous sutures

Continuous subcuticular (intradermal) suture

This is ideal for the repair of episiotomy wounds with catgut after the dead space has been closed. It does have a limited place in skin repair where monofilament nylon material is best, especially for removal of the suture. Supplementary interrupted skin sutures may be necessary for accurate skin-edge apposition.

Method

This suture picks up dermis only (picking up the epidermis and fat is not acceptable), and should be inserted uniformly at the same level without gaps in the linear direction (Fig. 2.4a).

'Over-and-over' suture

This is a useful time-saver, especially where a meticulous cosmetic result is not required. One disadvantage is the tendency to bunch the wound up. The suturing should not be too tight nor too widely spaced (Fig. 2.4b).

Blanket stitch

This stitch does not tend to bunch the wound up. A double turn at each stitch converts it into a locked suture (Fig. 2.4c).

The pulley suture

The pulley suture, also called the 'near–far, far–near' suture, is a very useful technique for the closure of difficult wounds, especially those on the lower leg. It permits approximation of the wound when an extra 2–3 mm of space needs closing and the normal method falls short of adequate closure.

Method

1. Introduce the needle 3–4 mm from the edge of the wound.
2. Let the needle emerge about 8–10 mm from the wound edge on the opposite side.
3. Reintroduce the needle at 8–10 mm on the original side.
4. Finally, let the needle emerge at 3–4 mm on the opposite side (Fig. 2.4d).

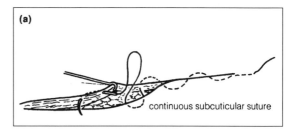

(a) continuous subcuticular suture

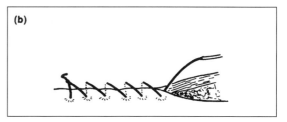

(b)

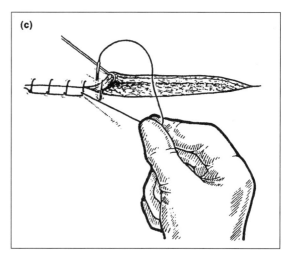

(c)

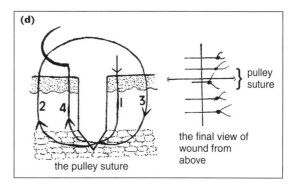

(d)

the final view of wound from above

the pulley suture

Fig. 2.4 (a) Subcuticular suture; **(b)** 'over-and-over' suture; **(c)** blanket stitch; **(d)** pulley suture (a), (b) and (c)
REPRODUCED FROM I. McGREGOR, *FUNDAMENTAL TECHNIQUES OF PLASTIC SURGERY*, CHURCHILL LIVINGSTONE, EDINBURGH, 1989, WITH PERMISSION

(continues)

After the suture is in place, normal interrupted sutures can close the wound. However, the pulley suture may create too much tension and, if it does, should be removed and replaced with a simple suture.

The cross-stitch

The cross-stitch, which is a type of pulley suture, is an excellent method for closing difficult wounds where there is likely to be some tension across the wound.

The cross-stitch is ideal for small circular wounds left after a 3–5 mm punch biopsy. It will shorten the scar and avoid the placement of two sutures. It gives a neater result than the vertical mattress or the horizontal mattress. Circular wounds up to 10 mm in diameter in areas of thicker skin can be closed with one such figure-of-eight suture.

Method

Consider a punch biopsy wound of 5 mm in diameter. Using a 5/0 or 6/0 nylon atraumatic suture insert the needle from right of centre across the wound to left of centre, then from left of centre to right of centre on the next pass (or the other way, i.e. from left to right and back). Thus four strands cross the wound and when tied create a pulley effect (Fig. 2.5).

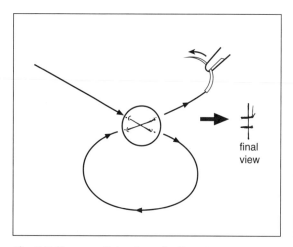

Fig. 2.5 The cross-stitch: a type of pulley suture

Planning excisions on the face

It is important to select optimal sites for elliptical excisions of tumours of the face. As a rule, it is best for incisions to follow wrinkle lines and the direction of hair follicles in the beard area. Therefore, follow the natural wrinkles in the glabella area, the 'crows feet' around the eye, and the nasolabial folds (Fig. 2.6). To determine non-obvious wrinkles, gently compress the relaxed skin in different directions to demonstrate the lines.

For tumours of the forehead, make horizontal incisions, although vertical incisions may be used for large tumours of the forehead. Ensure that you keep your incisions in the temporal area quite superficial, as the frontal branch of the facial nerve is easily cut.

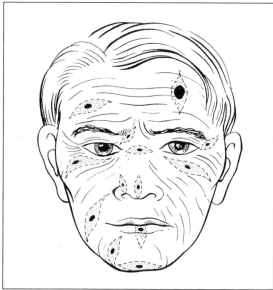

Fig. 2.6 Recommended lines for excisions on the face
ADAPTED FROM J.S. BROWN, *MINOR SURGERY, A TEXT AND ATLAS,* CHAPMAN AND HALL, LONDON, 1986

Elliptical excisions

Small lesions are best excised as an ellipse. Generally, the long axis of the ellipse should be along the skin tension lines identified by natural wrinkles.

The intended ellipse should be drawn on the skin (Fig. 2.7). The placement will depend on such factors as the size and shape of the lesion, the margin required (usually 2–3 mm) and the skin tension lines.

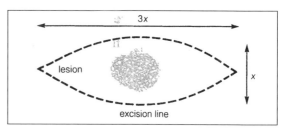

Fig. 2.7 Elliptical excision

Excision margin rules

- 1–2 mm: moles and benign lesions
- 3–5 mm: BCCs
- 5–10 mm: SCCs

General points

- The length of the ellipse should be three times the width (usually for head and neck).

- This length should be increased (say, to four times) in areas with little subcutaneous tissue (dorsum of hand) and high skin tension (upper back).
- Incisions should meet, rather than overlap, at the ends of the ellipse.
- A good rule is to obtain an angle at the end of 30° or less.
- These rules should achieve closure without 'dog ears'.

Prevention and removal of 'dog ears'

'Dog ears' are best avoided by using a long axis (at least 3 to 1) for an elliptical excision.

The fish-tail cut

However, if this axis turns out too short after excision, performing a fish-tail cut (Fig. 2.8a) will avoid the necessity of later correction.

Correction of 'dog ear'

If a 'dog ear' results in the suture line after elliptical defect closure, it can be dealt with by limited further excision and closure.

Method

1. Place a hook in the end of the wound, which is elevated; this defines the extent of the 'dog ear' (Fig. 2.8b).
2. Incise the skin around the base (1).
3. Stretch the resultant flap across the wound so that excess skin is defined and removed (2).
4. Complete the suturing of the wound, which will have a slight curve (3).

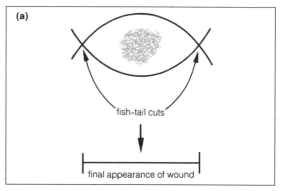

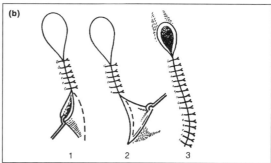

Fig. 2.8 Prevention of 'dog ears': **(a)** the fish-tail cut; **(b)** correction of defect   2.7(b) REPRODUCED FROM I. MCGREGOR, *FUNDAMENTAL TECHNIQUES OF PLASTIC SURGERY*, CHURCHILL LIVINGSTONE, EDINBURGH, 1989, WITH PERMISSION

The three-point suture

In wounds with a triangular flap component, it is often difficult to place the apex of the flap accurately. The three-point suture is the best way to achieve this while minimising the chance of strangulation necrosis at the tip of the flap.

Method

1. Pass the needle through the skin of the non-flap side of the wound.
2. Pass it then through the subcuticular layer of the flap tip at exactly the same level as the reception side.
3. Finally, pass the needle back through the reception side so that it emerges well back from the V flap (Fig. 2.9).

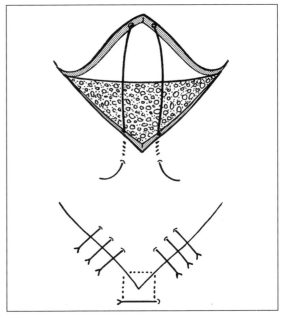

Fig. 2.9 The three-point suture

Inverted mattress suture for perineal skin

This method of repair of the perineum is suitable either for an episiotomy or a simple tear, and uses a technique of inverted vertical mattress sutures.

It is a simple method that provides a sound and comfortable repair. Because it is an interrupted suture wound, drainage is not sacrificed for the sake of comfort.

Method

1. Suture the vaginal tissue with a normal, continuous absorbable suture tied subcutaneously.
2. If the wound is very deep, a second internal layer of sutures should be inserted initially.
3. Close the perineal skin with the inverted mattress sutures (Fig. 2.10) using an absorbable suture. It is preferable to commence anteriorly, as this provides accurate opposition of the skin edges.

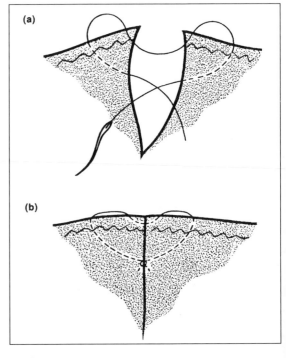

Fig. 2.10 Inverted mattress suture

Triangular flap wounds on the lower leg

Triangular flap wounds below the knee are a common injury and are often treated incorrectly. Similar wounds in the upper limb heal rapidly when sutured properly, but lower limb injury usually will not heal by first intention unless the apex of the flap is excised and a small donor graft implanted. Also think twice about suturing a pretibial laceration in an elderly person.

Proximally based flap

A fall through a gap in flooring boards will produce a proximally based flap; a heavy object (such as the tailboard of a trailer) striking the shin will result in a distally based flap.

Usually the apex of the flap is crushed and poorly vascularised; it will not survive to heal after suture.

Treatment method

1. Infiltrate a wide area around the wound with LA.
2. Excise the apex of the skin flap back to healthy tissue.
3. Loosely suture the angles at the base of the flap.
4. With a no. 24 scalpel, shave a small, split-thickness graft from the anaesthetised area proximal to the wound; place it on the raw area (Fig. 2.11).
5. Cover both the wound and donor site with petroleum jelly gauze, a non-stick dressing and a combine pad; strap firmly with a crêpe bandage.

The patient should rest with the leg elevated for 3 days. Re-dress the wound on the fourth day.

Alternative (preferred) method

It may be possible to save the distal avascular flap, especially in younger patients, by scraping away the subcutaneous tissue on the flap and using it as a full-thickness graft.

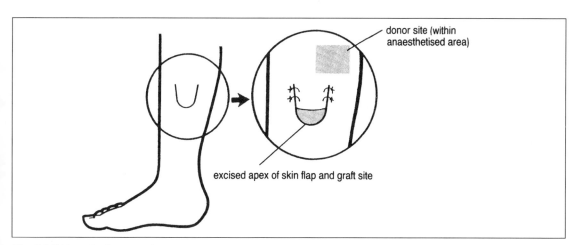

Fig. 2.11 Triangular flap wound suture

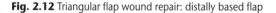

Distally based flap

This flap, which is quite avascular, has a poorer prognosis. The same methods as for the proximally based flap can be used (Fig. 2.12).

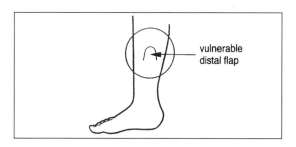

Fig. 2.12 Triangular flap wound repair: distally based flap

Excision of skin tumours with sliding flaps

General practitioners, in both city and country, not uncommonly excise small skin tumours under local anaesthesia using an elliptical incision. Where the skin is tight, as on the trunk or thigh, suture of an elliptical wound creates tension at the centre. A split skin graft or Wolfe graft will solve the problem but all too often leaves a depressed, unsightly scar. A rotation flap will cover the deficiency nicely but requires the undermining of a large area of skin and time-consuming suturing.

Double Y on V advancement flap method

Tumours up to 2.5 cm in diameter can be excised and the deficiency repaired without tension by means of a double advancement flap fashioned from the 'wings' of the ellipse after the lesion has been excised. As the viability of the flaps relies on a blood supply from the subcutaneous tissue, do not undermine the flaps. Incise the skin and subcutaneous tissue vertically to the fascia. The elasticity of the subcutaneous tissues will permit the flaps to be advanced to the midline to be united by sutures (Fig. 2.13).

Alternative flap technique

More flexibility of the flaps can be obtained by undermining the flaps above and below the incision lines (Fig. 2.14). Viability of the flaps is not a problem.

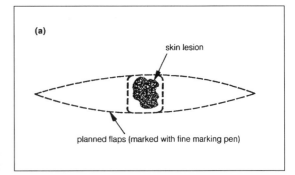

(a)

skin lesion

planned flaps (marked with fine marking pen)

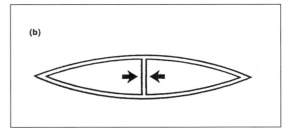

(b)

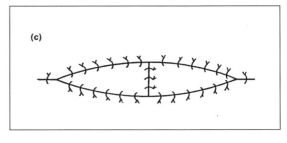

(c)

Fig. 2.13 Method of excising skin tumour: **(a)** planned flaps marked; **(b)** triangular flaps advanced to midline; **(c)** flaps sutured to repair defect

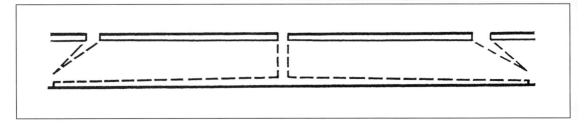

Fig. 2.14 Undermining of subcutaneous tissue (alternative variation)

The Y on V (or Island) advancement flap

This flap, which maintains a good blood supply, is ideal to close the end of an amputated finger tip in a child, or to use as an excision procedure on the face in the area of the nasolabial fold and lip where it conforms to skin creases.

Method

1. Mark the excision lines carefully before excising (Fig. 2.15a).
2. Excise the lesion as a square or rectangle.
3. Fashion the flap as a triangle about 2–2$^1/_2$ times the length of the defect. Carefully free the flap so that the skin remains on its subcutaneous tissue pedicle. This flap is referred to as an 'island'.
4. Using skin hooks, advance the base of the flap to the far edge of the defect with the help of blunt dissection and avoiding excessive tension (Fig. 2.15b).
5. Use three-point sutures at the two edges and at the apex.

6. Suture the sides of the wound (Fig. 2.15c).

    Thus the V 'Island' is converted to a Y-shaped scar.

H double advancement flap

Like the double Y on V flap this is suitable for areas with a good pad of subcutaneous tissue (e.g. re-excision of a melanoma on the arm). It is useful in places such as the forehead where the scars conform to skin creases. It is used where skin closure is impossible for a large ellipse. It can be tested, aborted or grafted.

Method

1. Excise the tumour with a square excision.
2. Extend the excision lines to about 1$^1/_2$ times the length of the defect (Fig. 2.16a).
3. Excise the skin and subcutaneous tissue with care vertically to the fascia.
4. Dissect the skin flaps from the subcutaneous tissue and advance them towards each other (preferably with skin hooks) to meet in the middle (Fig. 2.16b).
5. Use three-point sutures to anchor the corners of the flaps and then suture the wound as shown in Figure 2.16c.

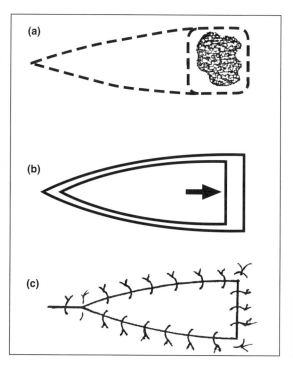

Fig. 2.15 The single Y on V method: **(a)** planned flaps marked; **(b)** 'Island' flap advanced to midline; **(c)** flaps sutured to repair defect

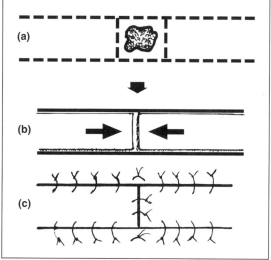

Fig. 2.16 The H double advancement flap: **(a)** excision of tumour with planned flaps; **(b)** pulling the flaps together; **(c)** flaps sutured to repair defect

Primary suture before excision of a small tumour

Before excising a small tumour, such as a dermatofibroma, skin tag or similar benign tumour, a primary suture can be inserted.

The advantages include better initial haemostasis and ability to operate singlehandedly.

Method

1. Infiltrate around the lesion with local anaesthetic.
2. Insert an appropriate suture (you may choose to insert more than one) to straddle the tumour (Fig. 2.17).
3. Excise the tumour. (Take care not to cut the suture.)
4. Secure the suture.
5. Add more sutures if necessary.

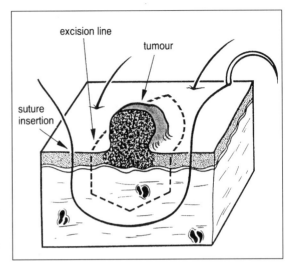

Fig. 2.17 Insertion of primary suture before excision of small tumour

Multiple ragged lacerations

Lacerations in a cosmetically important place such as the face, that have ragged edges or multiple components should be trimmed and/or excised (Fig. 2.18). This will provide vertical edges and an organised wound which can then be sutured meticulously. For the face, use 6/0 nylon. Sacrifice of small amounts of facial skin is justified in the interest of a linear and less obvious scar. Sometimes Z-plasty is required.

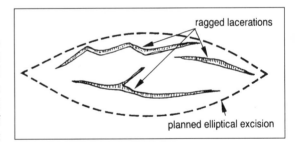

Fig. 2.18 Example of managing a group of multiple lacerations

Avoiding skin tears

Avoid using adhesive tapes on friable skin or dehydrated skin. Instead, use a cohesive bandage such as Easifix or Tubigrip.

The rotation flap

The local rotation flap is a most useful procedure in general practice for the excision of skin lesions such as basal cell carcinomas (BCCs). This method is favoured for the excision of BCCs greater than 5 mm and other tumours, especially on shoulders and backs.

Method

1. Excise the tumour using a triangular excision which, ideally, should be equilateral. Extend the excision beyond subcutaneous fat to the deep fascia-covering muscle (Fig. 2.19a).
2. Extend the excision in a curve to a length about three times that of the length of a side of the original triangular excision.
3. Now undercut the skin flap to the line AD (Fig. 2.19b).
4. Rotate this flap so that AC corresponds to AB without excessive tension.
5. Use simple sutures to close the wound (Fig. 2.19c).

Note: Blood is supplied to the skin on the back by the lateral cutaneous branch of each posterior intercostal artery and hence follows the line of the ribs. Make sure that the extended incision allows a blood supply to the flap—that is, that AD faces medially and not laterally.

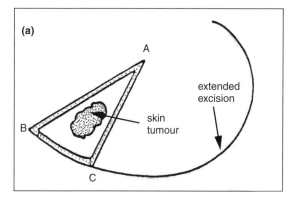

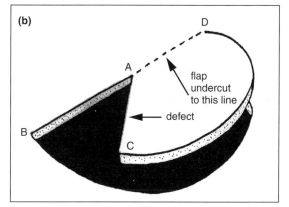

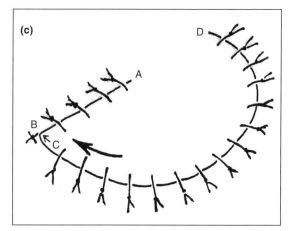

Fig. 2.19 Rotation flap: **(a)** triangular area of excision with extended excision; **(b)** resultant skin defect; **(c)** appearance after suturing

The rhomboid (Limberg) flap

The rhomboid flap is very useful for repairing defects that are difficult to suture directly or where the tension is in the wrong direction. It is most useful for removing lesions on the forehead, temple and scalp.

Method

1. Draw out the rhomboid and the relief extensions, making sure that the angles, lengths and directions are correct. The short diagonal of the rhomboid equals the length of the sides, giving the appearance of two equilateral triangles placed side by side. The direction of the relief extensions (theoretically four options) depends on the availability of skin.
2. Extend the diagonal for an equal distance in the desired direction and then draw a back line parallel to one of the sides of the rhomboid (Fig. 2.20a).
3. Remove the lesion and free the flaps by back-cutting.
4. Ensure that the 'x' lengths are equal.
5. Rotate the flap so that A moves to A_1, B to B_1 and C to B. This should fill the defect perfectly (Fig. 2.20b).
6. Care is required in suturing the corners—especially A and B, where subcutaneous three-point sutures are appropriate (Fig. 2.20c).
7. The resultant tension from the example illustrated is transverse ($\leftarrow \rightarrow$). This contrasts with long-itudinal tension if sutured directly.

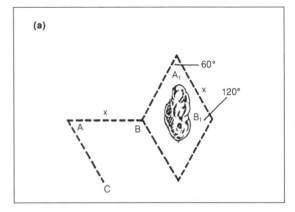

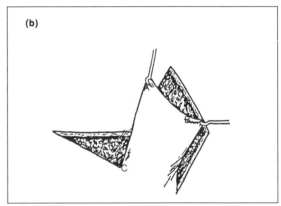

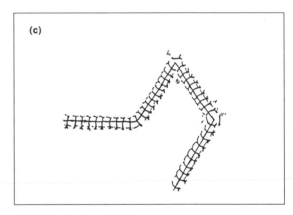

Fig. 2.20 The rhomboid flap   REPRODUCED FROM I. McGREGOR, *FUNDAMENTAL TECHNIQUES OF PLASTIC SURGERY*, CHURCHILL LIVINGSTONE, EDINBURGH, 1989, WITH PERMISSION

The 'crown' excision for facial skin lesions

When the standard elliptical skin excision is unworkable or inappropriate, a crown-shaped excision provides an excellent alternative. This applies particularly to skin lesions adjacent to key facial structures such as the nose, lips, ears and eyes. The shape of the crown excision can vary—it does not always have to be curved.

Method

(Using a basal cell carcinoma adjacent to the nose as an example.)

1. Mark out the lines of excision around the lesion in a circle.
2. Extend the axis of the excision in the free skin (Fig. 2.21a).
3. On the 'obstacle' side, excise two small curved flaps as illustrated.
4. Suture the defect so that a Y-shaped wound is eventually produced (Fig. 2.21b).

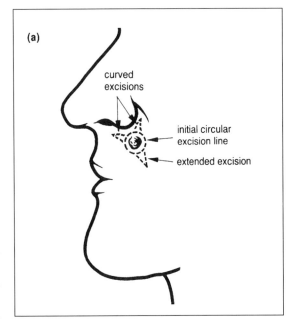

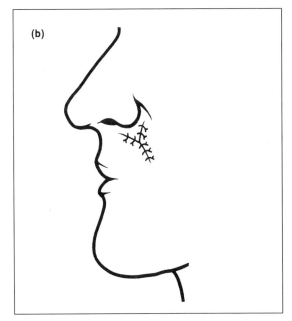

Fig. 2.21 **(a)** The 'crown' excision; **(b)** final appearance

Z-plasty

The Z-plasty is a procedure that redistributes wound tension by transposing two interdigitating triangular flaps. It brings in tissue from the sides to lengthen the wound and break up the tension across it. All arms of the Z are equal in length.

Indications

- Treatment of contractures (to lengthen).
- Facial scars (to change direction).

Method (scheme for a longitudinal contracture)

1. Mark out the Z so that the angles are 60° and the arms are of equal length.
2. Incise along the lines to produce two flaps and free the flaps by dissection.
3. Transpose the flaps and suture (Fig. 2.22).

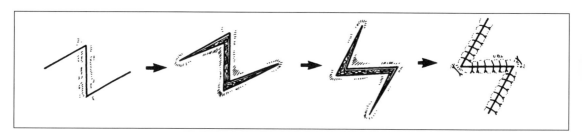

Fig. 2.22 Z-plasty

Repair of cut lip

While small lacerations of the buccal mucosa of the lip can be left safely, more extensive cuts require careful repair. Local anaesthetic infiltration may be adequate, although a mental nerve block is ideal for larger lacerations of the lower lip.

For wounds that cross the vermilion border, meticulous alignment is essential. It may be advisable to premark the vermilion border with gentian violet or a marker pen. It is desirable to have an assistant.

Method

1. Close the deeper muscular layer of the wound using 4/0 CCG. The first suture should carefully appose the mucosal area of the lip, followed by one or two sutures in the remaining layer (Fig. 2.23).
2. Next, insert a 6/0 monofilament nylon suture to bring both ends of the vermilion border together. The slightest step is unacceptable.
3. Close the inner buccal mucosa with interrupted 4/0 plain catgut sutures.

4. Close the outer skin of the lip (above and below the vermilion border) with interrupted nylon sutures.

Post-repair

1. Apply a moisturising lotion along the lines of the wound.
2. Remove nylon sutures in 3–4 days (in a young person) and 5–6 days (in an older person).

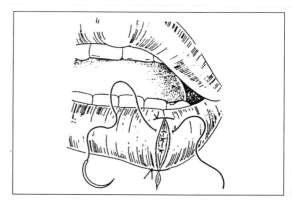

Fig. 2.23 Repair of cut lip

Wedge excision and direct suture of lip

Indications

Small, invasive squamous cell carcinomas leading to a defect on less than one-third of the lip. Alternative procedures are required for larger defects and for tumours close to the angles of the mouth.

An assistant is necessary to help achieve haemostasis, due to the copious bleeding from the inferior labial artery in the posterior third of the lip.

Method

1. Provide anaesthesia with a mental nerve block.
2. Carefully mark the excision outline, with special attention to the vermilion border (allow a 2–3 mm margin from the lesion). A small marker 'nick' or a stay suture at the border can be used as a guide.
3. Have the assistant hold the lip firmly on either side of the excision lines with gauze for a good grip, and slightly evert the lip.
4. Excise a clean, full-thickness wedge, with the apex extending almost to the mental fold (Fig. 2.24a).
5. Identify the labial arteries and either use diathermy or clamp and tie these bleeders.
6. Close the dead space of the muscular layer with interrupted 4/0 CCG sutures, starting with accurate apposition of the main lip area (Fig. 2.24b).
7. Insert a 6/0 nylon suture precisely at the vermilion border (the slightest step is unacceptable) and one at the apex of the wound.
8. Close the buccal mucosa with interrupted plain catgut sutures.
9. Finally, insert nylon sutures to the vermilion border and skin.

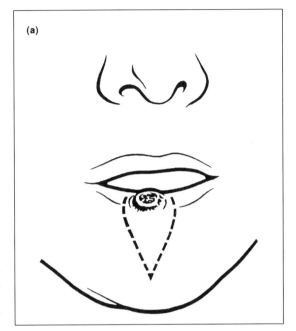

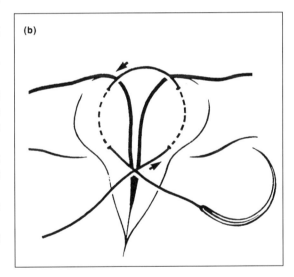

Fig. 2.24 Wedge excision of lip: **(a)** wedge of lip removed; **(b)** precise initial suture

Wedge resection of ear

This procedure is ideal for small tumours on the superior surface of the helix. The requirements are the same as for wedge excision of the lip.

Method

1. Provide LA by infiltrating subcutaneously around the appropriate margin of the ear. The area for infiltration (to cover all the ear) is shown in Figure 2.25a. This V infiltration method is the simplest way to block the ear completely. Specific nerve blocks are outlined on page 9.
2. Cleanse with antiseptic.
3. Mark an outline of the area of excision with the back of the scalpel and, with a marker, the margins for the first suture (e.g. the rim of the helix).
4. With tension applied by the assistant, excise a wedge, cutting cleanly through the skin and cartilage (Fig. 2.25b).
5. Brisk bleeding should soon cease with direct pressure.
6. Place the first suture to achieve meticulous alignment.
7. Suture the skin on the anterior surface with 6/0 nylon.
8. When the assistant folds the ear over, place and bury a few interrupted CCG sutures in the cartilage (Fig. 2.25c). This step is optional, as granuloma formation may complicate buried sutures.
9. Suture the skin of the posterior surface with nylon.

The dressing

A single layer of paraffin gauze is used, then a double layer of gauze folded around the ear, so that it sits back in its normal position. The dressing is firmly fastened with tape.

The dressing is changed in 3 days and the sutures removed in 6 days.

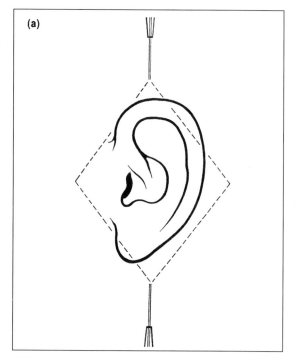

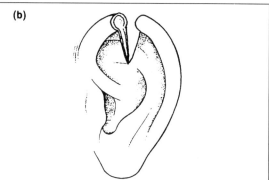

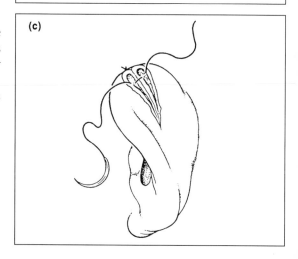

Fig. 2.25 Wedge resection of ear: **(a)** method of ear block with local anaesthesia infiltrated subcutaneously; **(b)** wedge of ear removed; **(c)** suturing in layers

Repair of lacerated eyelid

General points

- Ensure that the tear duct is not involved.
- Preserve as much tissue as possible.
- Do not shave the eyebrow.
- Do not invert hair-bearing skin into the wound.
- Ensure precise alignment of the wound margins.
- Tie suture knots away from the eyeball.

Method

1. Place an intermarginal suture behind the eye lashes if the margin is involved (Fig. 2.26a).
2. Repair conjunctiva and tarsus with 6/0 catgut (Fig. 2.26b).
3. Then repair the skin and muscle (orbicularis oculi) with 6/0 nylon (Fig. 2.26c).

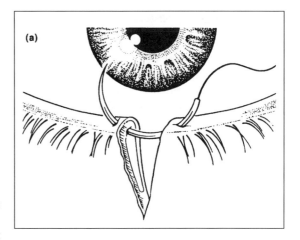

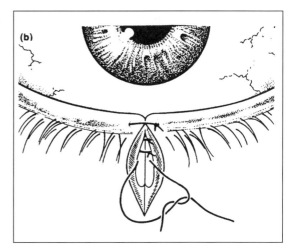

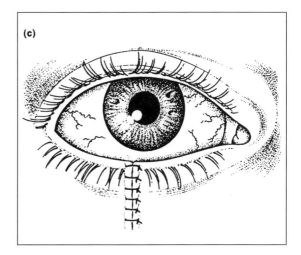

Fig. 2.26 Repair of lacerated eyelid: **(a)** initial suture; **(b)** repair of deeper layer; **(c)** outer skin sutured last

Repair of tongue wound

Wherever possible, it is best to avoid repair to wounds of the tongue because these heal rapidly. However, large flap wounds to the tongue on the dorsum or the lateral border may require suturing. The best method is to use buried catgut sutures.

Method

1. Infiltrate with 1% lignocaine LA and leave for 5–10 minutes. (Sucking ice may provide adequate analgesia.)
2. Use 4/0 or 3/0 catgut sutures to suture the flap to its bed, and bury the sutures (Fig. 2.27).

It should not be necessary to use surface sutures. If so, 4/0 silk sutures will suffice.

The patient should be instructed to rinse the mouth regularly with salt water until healing is satisfactory.

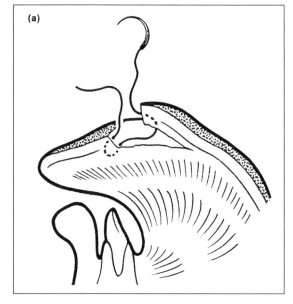

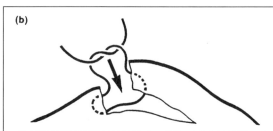

Fig. 2.27 Repair of tongue wound

Avascular field in digit

A bloodless field in the anaesthetised digit (after a digital block) can be achieved by using a rubber band as a simple tourniquet.

Method

1. Elevate the hand vertically (or the leg) for 2 minutes and wrap tape from the tip of the digit to its base.
2. Wrap a rubber band around the base of the digit to block circulation, and unwrap the tape.
3. Now place the limb on the table and complete the procedure (e.g. removing a foreign body or repairing a wound).
4. When completed, apply a dressing and snip the rubber band with a scalpel or scissors.

Wedge resection of axillary sweat glands

Indication

Profuse sweating of axillary hyperhydrosis especially with body odour, unresponsive to antiperspirants.

Method

1. Shave the axilla.
2. Apply iodine starch powder to the axilla. This produces a dark blue/purple response in the area of highest sweat production.
3. Mark the area requiring wedge resection, which is usually elliptical.
4. Swab with antiseptic and infiltrate with local anaesthetic.
5. Perform a wedge resection to remove the sweat glands which lie in the layer immediately below the dermis. Clearing the undersurface of the flap of subcutaneous fat will remove these sweat glands.
6. Close the wound, which may be sutured directly or by employing a flap if extensive.

Removal of skin sutures

Suture marks are related to the time of retention of the suture, its tension and position. The objective is to remove the sutures as early as possible, as soon as their purpose is achieved. The timing of removal is based on commonsense and individual cases. Nylon sutures are less reactive and can be left for longer periods. After suture removal it is advisable to support the wound with micropore skin tape (e.g. Steri-strips) for 1–2 weeks, especially in areas of skin tension.

Method

1. Use good light and have the patient lying comfortably.
2. Use fine, sharp scissors which cut to the point or the tip of a scalpel blade, and a pair of fine, non-toothed dissecting forceps that grip firmly.
3. Cut the suture close to the skin below the knot with scissors or a scalpel tip (Fig. 2.28a).
4. Gently pull the suture out towards the side on which it was divided—that is, *always towards the wound* (Fig. 2.28b).

Note: In children, cut all sutures before removal.

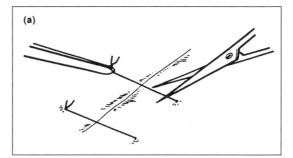
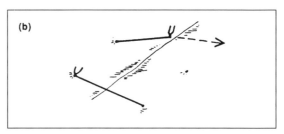

Fig. 2.28 Removal of skin sutures: **(a)** cutting suture; **(b)** removal by pulling towards wound

Pitfalls for excision of non-melanoma skin cancer

There are several anatomical pitfalls awaiting surgical excision. The following summarises potential or real problem areas.

- The face—for cosmetic reasons.
- The face—for potential nerve damage, e.g. temporal branch of facial nerve (Fig. 2.29).
- The lips and helix of the ear—because of malignant potential.
- The eyelids.
- The inner-canthus of the eye with close proximity to the nasolacrimal duct.
- Mid-sternomastoid muscle areas where the accessory nerve is superficial.
- Fingers where functional impairment may be a concern.
- Lower limb below the knee where healing, especially in the elderly, will be a problem.

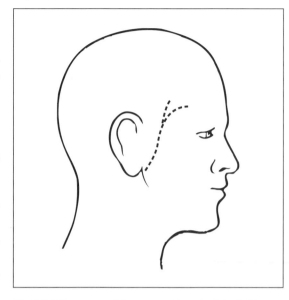

Fig 2.29 The course of the temporal branch of the facial nerve

Referral to a specialist

Referral should be considered when one or more of the following is involved:

- uncertainty of diagnosis,
- any doubts about appropriate treatment,
- tumours larger than 1 cm,
- multiple tumours,
- recurrent tumours, despite treatment,
- incompletely excised tumours, especially when complete excision may be difficult,
- recommended treatment beyond the skills of the practitioner,
- anticipation of difficulty with technique or anatomy where an appropriate specialist should be consulted,

- squamous cell carcinomas on the lips and ears,
- infiltrating or scar-like morphoeic BCCs—particularly those on the nose or around the nasal labial fold, as there may be a problem in determining the tumour's extent and depth,
- cosmetic concerns such as lesions of the upper chest and upper arms where keloid scarring is a potential problem,
- areas where palpable regional lymph nodes suggestive of metastatic spread of squamous cell carcinoma exist, namely head and neck, axilla and groin.

W-plasty for ragged lacerations

Jagged lacerations are usually best debrided with a small elliptical excision following wrinkle lines, when possible.

As a rule it is better to close a ragged wound without tension than to trim it and close it with considerable tension.

There is no rule that dictates that a laceration has to be closed as a straight line.

One procedure that debrides the sides of a ragged wound (too large for simple elliptical debridement) in a saw-toothed fashion is W-plasty. The sides of the wound have to match each other (Fig. 2.30a). With W-plasty, care should be taken to ensure that adequate blood supply is maintained. Select the pattern of debridement and, using a scalpel with a no. 15 blade, make the initial incisions through the dermis, avoiding full-length incisions which tend to result in rolled skin edges.

Apply simple sutures using three-point sutures at the apices of the triangular components (Fig. 2.30b).

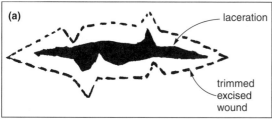

(a) laceration / trimmed excised wound

(b) final 'saw-tooth' appearance

Fig. 2.30 Technique of W-plasty

Debridement of skin in a hairy area

When debriding skin in a hairy area, it is important to realise that hair shafts grow obliquely to the skin. In order to avoid creating a hairless path along the length of the scar, try to debride the skin edges at the same angle as the hair shafts (Fig. 2.31). This avoids damage to the hair follicles.

Natural lacerations (such as from a blunt blow) to hairy areas such as the eyebrow do not leave a hairless patch of scar when sutured correctly.

Keeping hairs out of wounds for suturing

While suturing in a hair-bearing area such as the scalp, it is important to keep hair out of the wound. This can be done by smoothing the hair down with K-Y gel, hair gel such as Brylcream, or adhesive tape.

Clearing shaved areas

An effective way to clean up a shaved area such as a scalp prior to surgical repair is to use strips of adhesive tape such a Micropore to pick up loose hairs.

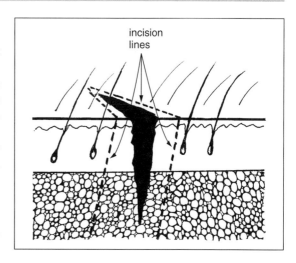

incision lines

Fig. 2.31 Direction of trimmed incision lines in a hair-bearing area

Wound management tips

Dressings

Table 2.2 indicates examples of the most appropriate dressing materials for the exudate level of the wound being treated.

Post-operative wound care

Useful guidelines are:

- Use non-adherent dressings over excision wounds. Leave for 24–48 hours. Place an occlusive dressing over this for protection and when showering.
- After removal of dressing clean daily with saline to remove crusting and to minimise infection.
- If concerned about infection use thin application of chloramphenicol (or similar ointment).

For healing by secondary intention (such as after curette or diathermy):

- Use hydrocolloidal dressings (e.g. Intrasite, Duoderm, Rapid Healing Band Aids).
- Leave in situ for up to seven days.

Healing cavities of incised cysts and abscesses

This practice tip outlines a simple method of promoting the healing of cavities resulting from drained abscesses or removed sebaceous cysts, especially infected cysts. The concept originally came from veterinary management of cysts in animals.

Table 2.2 Appropriate dressing materials for various exudate levels

Dressing type	Exudate level
Film dressings e.g. Tegaderm	Nil/minimal
Hydrocolloid e.g. Duoderm	Low/moderate
Alginate e.g. Algisite	Moderate/high
Foam e.g. Allevyn	Moderate/high
Hydrogel e.g. Solosite	Dry/sloughy

Method

1. For deep cavities resulting from surgical incision it is best to pack them first with sterile non-adherent gauze while the patient is anaesthetised. This controls haemostasis and maintains drainage.
2. The following day infiltrate the cavity with intrasite gel.
3. Cover the wound with opsite or appropriate waterproof dressing.
4. Change this every day or every second day until the wound heals.

Advantages

- The gel infuses to all recesses of the cavity that packing cannot reach.
- Patients can continue management themselves.
- More convenient for patients who have a considerable distance to travel.
- Less pain and discomfort compared with other dressings.
- Rapid healing.

When to remove non-absorbable sutures

For removal of sutures after non-complicated wound closure in adults, see Table 2.3. *Note:* Decisions need to be individualised according to the nature of the wound and health of the patient and healing. In general, remove sutures as soon as possible. One way of achieving this is to remove alternate sutures a day or two earlier and remove the rest at the usual time. Steri-strips can then be used to maintain closure and healing.

Additional aspects

In children, usually remove 1–2 days earlier. Allow additional time for backs and legs, especially the calf. Nylon sutures can be left longer because they are less reactive. Alternate sutures may be removed earlier (e.g. from the face in women).

Table 2.3 Time after insertion for removal of sutures

	Days later
Scalp	6
Face	3 (or alternate at 2, rest 3–4)
Ear	5
Neck	4 (or alternate at 3, rest 4)
Chest	8
Arm (including hand and fingers)	8–10
Abdomen	8–10 (tension 12–14)
Back	12
Inguinal and scrotal	7
Perineum	2
Legs	10
Knees and calf	12
Foot (including toes)	10–12

3 Treatment of lumps and bumps

Removal of skin tags

Skin tags (fibroepithelial polyps) are very benign tumours, and can safely be left. However, patients often request their removal for cosmetic reasons. There are several ways to remove skin tags. These include:

- simple excision (see also *Perianal skin tags* for elliptical excision),
- cutting with scissors,
- electrocautery (to base); a very effective method,
- tying a fine thread around the base,
- crushing with bone forceps,
- liquid nitrogen therapy.

Liquid nitrogen therapy

1. Use a pair of forceps (dissecting or artery) to grasp the skin tag, preferably on the base or stalk.
2. Holding the skin tag upright and taut, apply a liquid-nitrogen-soaked cotton bud to the forceps close to the tumour (Fig. 3.1).
3. Apply for several seconds to freeze the tumour. It can be left or cut off with scissors.

A variation

The tips of the forceps can be dipped directly into the liquid nitrogen and then clamped onto the base of the skin tag. Multiple tags can be frozen rapidly in this way.

Bone forceps method

A simple procedure is to crush the base of the skin tag flush with the skin using bone forceps (Fig. 3.2a). The advantages are that:

- no local anaesthetic is required,
- the procedure is relatively painless,
- the procedure is very quick,
- immediate haemostasis is achieved (Fig. 3.2b).

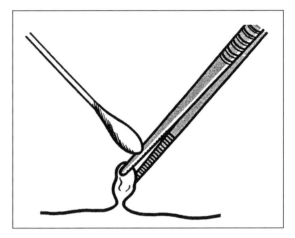

Fig. 3.1 Removal of skin tag by liquid nitrogen

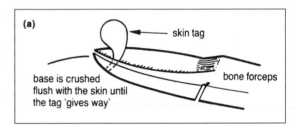

(a) skin tag

base is crushed flush with the skin until the tag 'gives way'

bone forceps

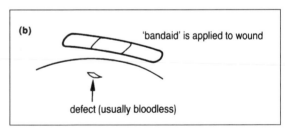

(b) 'bandaid' is applied to wound

defect (usually bloodless)

Fig. 3.2 Removal of skin tag using bone forceps method

Removal of epidermoid (sebaceous) cysts

There are several methods for removal of sebaceous cysts after infiltration of local anaesthetic over and around the cyst. These include the following methods.

Incision into cyst

Make an incision into the cyst to bisect it, squeeze the contents out with a gauze swab and then avulse the lining of the cyst with a pair of artery forceps or remove with a small curette.

Punch biopsy method

Use a 5 mm punch biopsy to punch a hole into the apex of the cyst. Squeeze vigorously to express the contents. Look for the cyst wall, grasp it with forceps and *carefully* enucleate it. A suture is not necessary.

Incision over cyst and blunt dissection

Make a careful skin incision over the cyst, taking care not to puncture its wall. Free the skin carefully from the cyst by blunt dissection. When it is free from adherent subcutaneous tissue, digital pressure will cause the cyst to 'pop out'.

Standard dissection

Incise a small ellipse of skin to include the central punctum over the cyst (Fig. 3.3a). Apply forceps to this skin to provide traction for dissection of the cyst from the adherent dermis and subcutaneous tissue. Ideally, forceps should be applied at either end. The objective is to avoid rupture of the cyst. Insert curved scissors (e.g. McIndoe's scissors) and free the cyst by gently opening and closing the blades (Fig. 3.3b). Bleeding is not usually a problem. When the cyst is removed, obliterate the space with subcutaneous catgut. The skin is sutured with a vertical mattress suture to avoid a tendency to inversion of the skin edges into the slack wound. Send the cyst for histopathology.

Electrocautery method

On the *first visit*, inject LA into the overlying skin. Insert a heated electrocautery needle in the cyst and cauterise the contents for several seconds (Fig. 3.4).

On the *second visit*, 7–10 days later, inject LA, then make a small incision in the cyst and express the contents.

Treatment of infected cysts

Incise the cyst to drain purulent material. When the inflammation has resolved completely, the cyst should be excised as outlined above.

(continues)

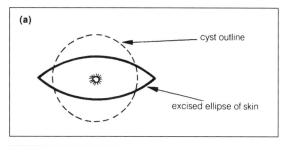

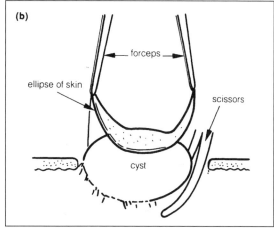

Fig. 3.3 Standard dissection of sebaceous cyst

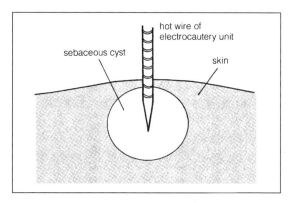

Fig. 3.4 Electrocautery to sebaceous cyst

Simple deroofing method

This method simply unroofs the cyst and allows healing by dressings over an open area. It should be avoided on the face or other areas where a puckered scar is unacceptable. It is very useful for an infected cyst.

Method

1. Infiltrate the skin over the cyst with local anaesthetic.
2. Unroof the cyst by removing a disc of skin with scalpel or scissors. This disc should be slightly smaller than the diameter of the cyst (Fig. 3.5).
3. Evacuate the contents of the cyst and pack with paraffin gauze.
4. Apply pressure if bleeding is a problem.
5. Apply non-adherent dressings daily.

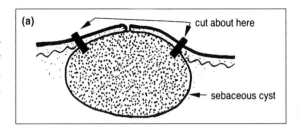

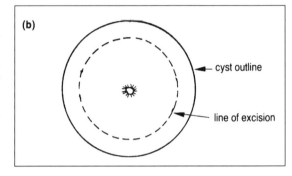

Fig. 3.5 A simple deroofing method: **(a)** cross-sectional view; **(b)** surface view

The infected sebaceous cyst

When an infected cyst is encountered, it is appropriate to open it and drain the pus through a cruciate incision or a 4–6 mm punch biopsy (under local anaesthetic). Evacuate the contents with sterile gauze and determine if it is possible to avulse the cyst wall. Usually it heals, often definitively, through open healing.

Sebaceous hyperplasia

Sebaceous hyperplasia presents as a single or multiple nodules on the face, especially in older persons. The nodules are small, yellow-pink, slightly umbilicated and are found in a similar distribution to basal cell carcinoma, for which they may be mistaken. There is no need for surgical excision.

Acne cysts

Acne cysts can be treated by an injection of a long-acting corticosteroid preparation in such a way as to flush out the follicular contents and subdue the sterile inflammation. The treatment is suitable for small numbers of cysts.

Equipment

You will need:

- 25-gauge needles,
- small syringe,
- 1 mL long-acting corticosteroid (e.g. triamcinalone acetonide, methylprednisolone acetate).

Method

1. Introduce a 25-gauge needle into one side of the cyst and inject a small quantity of steroid. Remove the needle (Fig. 3.6a).
2. Introduce a needle into the opposite side of the cyst. Inject steroid so that material is flushed out through the initial entry point (Fig. 3.6b). This removes the follicular material and leaves residual amounts of steroids in a depot form.

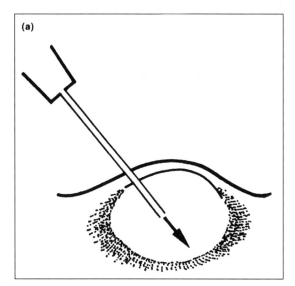

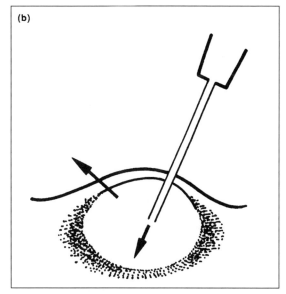

Fig. 3.6 Treatment of acne cyst

Biopsies

There are various methods for taking biopsies from skin lesions. These include scraping, shaving and punch biopsies, which are useful but not as effective or safe as excisional biopsies.

Shave biopsies

This simple technique is generally used for the tissue diagnosis of premalignant lesions and some malignant tumours, but not melanoma.

Method

1. Infiltrate with LA.
2. Holding a no. 10 or 15 scalpel blade horizontally, shave off the tumour just into the dermis (Fig. 3.7).
3. Diathermy may be required for haemostasis.

The biopsy site usually heals with minimal scarring.

Punch biopsy

This biopsy has considerable use in general practice, where full-thickness skin specimens are required for histological diagnosis. (Good-quality disposable punch biopsies are available from Dermatech.)

Method

1. Clean the skin.
2. Infiltrate with LA.
3. Gently stretch the skin between the finger and thumb to limit rotational movement.
4. Select the punch (4 mm is the most useful size) and hold it vertically to the skin.
5. Rotate (in a clockwise, screwing motion) with firm pressure to cut a plug about 3 mm in depth (Fig. 3.8). Remove the punch.
6. Use fine-toothed forceps or a tissue hook to grip the outer rim of the plug.
7. Exert gentle traction and undercut the base of the plug parallel to the skin surface using fine-pointed scissors or a scalpel.
8. Place the specimen in fixative.
9. Secure haemostasis by firm pressure or by diathermy.
10. Apply a dry dressing or a single suture to the defect.

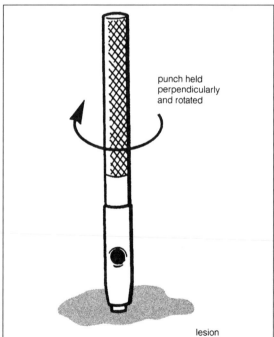

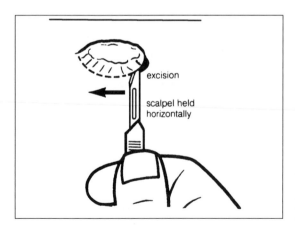

Fig. 3.7 Shave biopsy

Fig. 3.8 Punch biopsy

Treatment of ganglions

Ganglions have a high recurrence rate after treatment, with a relapse of 30% after surgery.

A simple, relatively painless and more effective method is to use intralesional injections of long-acting corticosteroid, such as methylprednisolone acetate.

Method 1

1. Insert a 21-gauge needle attached to a 2 mL or 5 mL syringe into the cavity of the ganglion.
2. Aspirate some (not all) of its jelly-like contents, mainly to ensure that the needle is in situ.
3. Keeping the needle exactly in place, swap the syringe for an insulin syringe containing up to 0.5 mL of steroid.
4. Inject 0.25–0.5 mL (Fig. 3.9).
5. Rapidly withdraw the needle, pinch the overlying skin for several seconds and then apply a light dressing.
6. Review in 7 days and, if still present, repeat the injection using 0.25 mL of steroid.

Up to six injections can be given over a period of time, but 70% of ganglions will disperse with only one or two injections.

Method 2

Insert a larger gauge catgut suture through the middle of the ganglion and firmly tie it over the ganglion. Side pressure may express the contents through the needle holes. Remove the knot 12 days later.

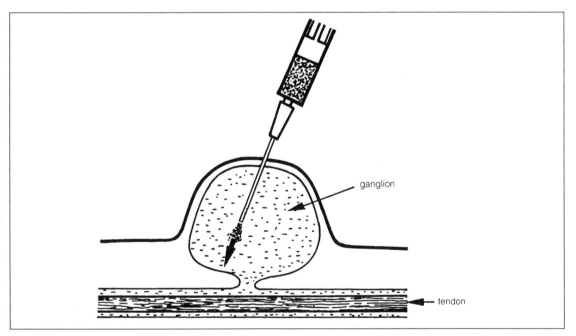

Fig. 3.9 Injection treatment of ganglion

Olecranon and pre-patellar bursitis

Simple aspiration–injection technique

Chronic recurrent traumatic olecranon or pre-patellar bursitis with a synovial effusion may require surgery, but most cases can resolve with partial aspiration of the fluid and then injection of LA corticosteroid through the same needle.

Excision of lipomas

Lipomas are benign fatty tumours situated in sub-cutaneous tissue. They are common on the back, but can occur anywhere.

Lipomas rarely require removal, but removal may be desired for cosmetic reasons or to relieve discomfort from pressure. Many lipomas can be simply enucleated using a gloved finger, but there are a few traps: some are deeper than anticipated, and some are adjacent to important structures such as large nerves and blood vessels. Others are tethered by fibrous bands, and recurrence can occur if excision is incomplete.

Larger lipomas may require referral.

Method

1. Outline the extent of the lipoma and mark it with a ball-point pen. Note its anatomical relationships.
2. Infiltrate the area with 1% lignocaine with adrenaline. (Include the deepest part of the lipoma.)
3. Make a linear incision (Fig. 3.10a) in the overlying skin, preferably in a natural crease line, for about three-quarters of its length. The lipoma should bulge through the wound. For large lipomas, incise an ellipse of skin (Fig. 3.10b).
4. Deepen the incision until the lipoma can be seen.

5. Insert a gloved finger between the skin and fatty tumour to find a plane of dissection and to determine whether it will shell out.
6. It is important to seek the outer edge of each lobule, dissect it and bring it to the wound surface (Fig. 3.10c). If necessary, insert curved scissors and use a blunt opening action to free any fibrous bands tethering the lipoma (Fig. 3.10d).

   Note: The best way to prevent bleeding is not to dissect around the fatty tissue but to incise it, invert the tumour through the wound and then remove it.
7. Ensure that all the fatty tissue is removed. Send it for histological examination. Clipping and ligation of persistent bleeding vessels may be required.
8. Use a gauze swab to control bleeding and remove debris from the dead space.
9. Close the dead space with interrupted catgut sutures.
10. Close the skin with interrupted or subcuticular sutures.

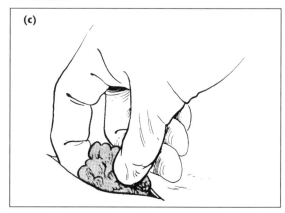

(c)

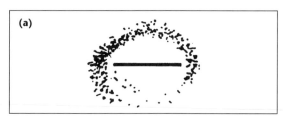

(a)

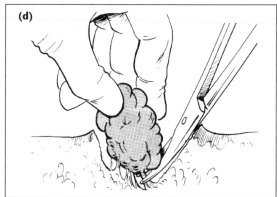

(d)

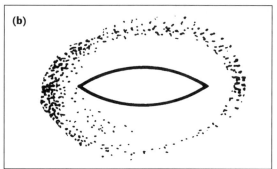

(b)

Fig. 3.10 **(a)** Linear incision for small lipomas; **(b)** elliptical incision for large lipomas; **(c)** gloved finger dissection to bring lipoma to the surface; **(d)** blunt scissors dissection to free lipoma from tethering fibrous bands

Keratoacanthoma

Most keratoacanthomas (KAs) occur singly on light-exposed areas. The major problem is differentiation from squamous cell carcinoma (SCC), especially if on the lip or ear.

Although KAs can be treated by curettage and cautery, the recommended treatment is surgical excision and histological examination. Ensure a 2–3 mm margin for excision. Most patients will not tolerate a tumour on an exposed area such as the face for 6 months while waiting for a spontaneous remission to confirm the clinical diagnosis. Also, if it is an SCC, a potentially lethal cancer has remained in situ for an unnecessarily long period.

Note: SCCs on the ear metastasise 15 times more rapidly than elsewhere. The relative growth rates of SCC, KAs and basal cell carcinomas (BCCs) are shown in Figure 3.11.

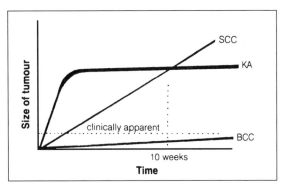

Fig. 3.11 Relative growth rates of three types of skin tumours

Basal cell carcinoma (BCC)

BCCs are the most common type of skin cancer. They can occur on any part of the body, but the most common site is on the face, especially next to the eyes or nose. It is useful to think of it as the area covered by an eye mask (Fig. 3.12). Another common area is the neck, and the upper back and chest are becoming more common sites.

Increased risk occurs with:

- age over 50 years,
- exposure to excessive sunlight,
- fair complexion,
- lack of sun protection.

Treatment guidelines

- Surgery is the primary treatment: use a simple ellipse (where possible) under local anaesthetic with a 3 mm margin (in most cases).
- Cryotherapy is suitable for primary, well-defined, histologically confirmed superficial tumours, at sites away from the head and neck.
- Superficial X-ray therapy is an option in larger tumours in older people.

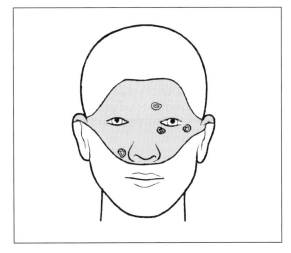

Fig. 3.12 Typical sites of basal cell carcinoma: the 'mask' area of the face

Squamous cell carcinoma (SCC)

SCCs usually develop in skin exposed to the sun, in particular the face (especially the lower lip), ears, neck, forearm, back of the hands and lower legs (Fig. 3.13). A special trap is on the scalps of men who are bald or have thin scalp hair.

Increased risk occurs with:

* age over 60 years,
* fair complexion,
* outdoor occupations,
* development of sunspots (solar keratoses).

Treatment guidelines

* Surgery is the treatment of choice—use a simple ellipse under LA with a 4 mm margin (in most cases).
* Superficial X-ray therapy is an option in a primary untreated tumour when surgery is not feasible.

Cryotherapy and curettage are not treatments of choice.

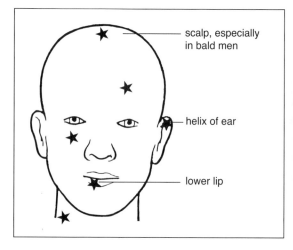

Fig. 3.13 Important common sites of squamous cell carcinoma on the head and face

scalp, especially in bald men

helix of ear

lower lip

Pyogenic granuloma

These solitary, raised, bright red tumours (granuloma telangiectaticum) tend to bleed profusely. The most effective treatment is curettage and electrocautery under local anaesthesia.

However, it must be stressed that histological confirmation of the diagnosis is essential to exclude anaplastic squamous cell carcinoma or amelanotic melanoma. Thus, after the tumour has been shaved off or curetted it should be sent for examination.

Seborrhoeic keratoses

Regular applications of liquid nitrogen may remove these benign skin tumours, or at least decolourise them.

Immediately after freezing you can use a scalpel (e.g. size 15 blade) to scrape off the lesion at skin level.

Another method is to apply carefully concentrated phenol solution. Repeat in 3 weeks if necessary.

Yet another method is to apply trichloroacetic acid to the surface and instil it in gently by multiple pricks with a fine gauge needle. Perform twice weekly for 2 weeks.

Stucco keratoses

This subtype of seborrhoeic keratoses are multiple non-pigmented small friable keratoses over the lower legs. They can be treated with a topical keratolytic such as 3–5% salicyclic acid in sorbolene.

Orf

Rapid healing of the skin lesion orf can be achieved by injecting corticosteroids into the pustular nodule.

Precautions

- Ensure that the diagnosis of orf is correct.
- Warn the patient of likely increased discomfort for 24 hours.

Method

1. Mix 0.5 mL of 1% plain lignocaine with 0.5 mL of long-acting corticosteroid, e.g. triamcinolone. Use more solution for a larger lesion.
2. Infiltrate the solution into the lesion, around its margins and into its base.
3. The lesion is left to heal without dressings.

   Rapid healing occurs within 5–10 days. Otherwise it takes 3–4 weeks.

Milker's nodules

These nodules can heal more rapidly if the same intralesional corticosteroid injection is given as for orf.

Haemangioma of the lip

Attempted excision of these common lesions should be avoided because of bleeding. Perform a mental nerve block (preferable to local infiltration) and insert the needle of the electrocautery or hyfrecator into the centre of the haemangioma. More than one treatment may be necessary.

Molluscum contagiosum

Individual lesions usually involute spontaneously over several months. There are several simple treatments available for this viral tumour of the skin, the choice being influenced by the person's age. Treatment choices are:

- liquid nitrogen (a few seconds),
- pricking the lesion with a pointed stick soaked in 1% or 3% phenol,
- application of 15% podophyllin in friar's balsam (compound benzoin tincture),
- application of 30% trichloroacetic acid,
- destruction by electrocautery or diathermy,
- ether soap and friction method,
- lifting open the tip with a sterile needle inserted from the side (parallel to the skin) and applying 10% povidone-iodine (Betadine) solution or 2.5% benzoyl peroxide (parents can be shown this method and continue it at home for multiple tumours),
- paint with clear nail polish,
- cover with a piece of Micropore (or similar paper-based tape) and change every day (may take a few months),
- inject a larger single lesion with corticosteroid, e.g. triamcinolone 10 mg/mL solution.

Most effective method

Extract the core with a curette or large needle, then apply 10% povidone-iodine solution.

Ether soap method

Soak the tumour or tumours for 1–2 nights in ether soap (now difficult to obtain), with a plastic covering over the soap-soaked swab. The tumours are then obliterated by rubbing with another damp swab.

For large areas of multiple molluscum contagiosum

Apply aluminum acetate (Burrow's solution 1:30) twice a day.

New alternative treatments

- Extract of the Cantharis beetle (prepared as Canthrone),
- Imiquimod (Aldara) cream.

Aspiration of Baker's cyst

A distended tender popliteal cyst (Baker's cyst) of the knee is really a bursa that communicates with the knee joint. It may be associated with rheumatoid arthritis, osteoarthritis, traumatic knee disruption or a normal joint.

Aspiration and injection may alleviate the symptoms of swelling and tenderness.

Method

1. The patient should be prone, with a small pillow under the knee to produce slight hyperextension of the joint and obvious distension of the bursa.
2. Using a sterile, no-touch technique, insert a 21-gauge 38 mm needle attached to a 20 mL syringe into the bursa.
3. Completely aspirate the fluid, which is usually a clear yellow.
4. Leave the needle in situ and exchange the 20 mL syringe for a 2 mL syringe containing 1 mL of long-acting corticosteroid, which is then injected (Fig. 3.14).

5. Recurrence is common. An alternative treatment is to inject 5 mL of 2.5–3% aqueous phenol or 3% STD (sodium tetradecyl sulfate) solution instead of corticosteroid.

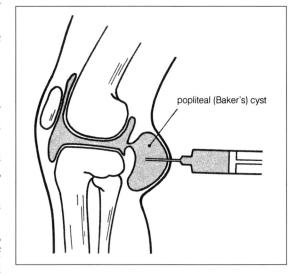

Fig. 3.14 Aspiration of Baker's cyst

Aspiration and injection of hydrocele

Aspiration, followed by an injection of dilute aqueous phenol or STD, can be a very useful treatment technique for primary hydroceles—especially where definitive surgery is inappropriate. Aspiration alone rarely corrects a hydrocele, but the aspiration/injection combination performed two or three times can often cure the problem.

Method

1. Inject LA into the scrotal skin down to the sac.
2. Insert an 18- or 19-gauge intravenous cannula through this site into the sac and remove the stilette, leaving the soft cannula in the sac (Fig. 3.15).
3. Remove the serous fluid initially by free drainage, possibly aided by manual compression on the sac and then by aspiration with a 20 mL syringe.
4. Record the volume.
5. Inject 2.5–3% sterile aqueous phenol into the empty sac (10 mL for 200 mL of fluid removed,

15 mL for 200–400 mL and 20 mL for over 400 mL). An alternative and simpler solution is to use 3% STD. Use 2–5 mL.

The procedure can be repeated after 6 weeks.

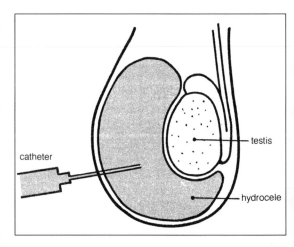

Fig. 3.15 Aspiration of hydrocele

Epididymal cysts

The same method as for hydroceles can be used. Aspirate and then inject sclerosant.

Steroid injections into skin lesions

Indications

Suitable lesions for steroid injections are:

- granuloma annulare,
- hypertrophic scars (early development),
- keloid scars (early development),
- alopecia areata,
- lichen simplex chronicus,
- necrobiosis lipoidica,
- hypertrophic lichen planus,
- plaque psoriasis.

Triamcinolone is the appropriate long-acting corticosteroid (10 mg/mL). It may be diluted in equal quantities of saline.

Method

1. The steroid should be injected into the lesion (not below it).
2. Insert a 25- or (preferably) 27-gauge needle, firmly locked to a small insulin-type 1 mL syringe, into the lesion at the level of the middle of the dermis (Fig. 3.16).
3. High pressure is required with some lesions (e.g. keloid).
4. Inject sufficient steroid to make the lesion blanch.
5. Several sites will be needed for larger lesions, so preceding LA may be required in some instances. Avoid infiltration of steroid in larger lesions: use multiple injections.

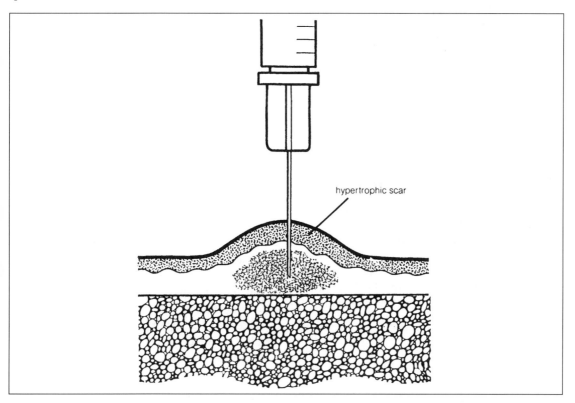

Fig. 3.16 Injection of corticosteroid into mid-dermis

Steroid injections for plaques of psoriasis

An excellent method of effective treatment of small to moderate sized plaques of psoriasis is by intralesional infiltration using a long-acting corticosteroid.

Requirements

- Triamcinolone 10 mg/mL solution (or other corticosteroid).
- 1% (plain) lignocaine (or similar local anaesthetic).
- 25-gauge needle (or 23-gauge if larger plaque).

Method

1. Mix equal parts of corticosteroid and local anaesthetic.
2. Swab the lesion.
3. Insert the needle at the margin of the plaque and infiltrate the lesion at an intradermal level, avoiding going deep into the subcutaneous tissue.
4. Infiltrate the whole plaque.
5. A larger plaque may require needle insertion at two sites (Fig. 3.17).

This treatment, which is ideal for a persistent elbow or knee plaque, is rapidly effective and tends to induce a long remission.

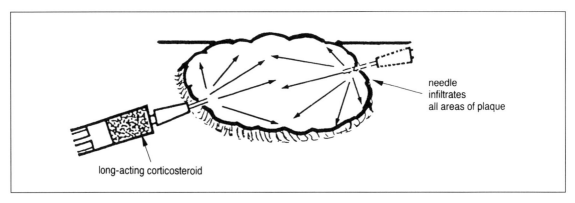

Fig. 3.17 Intralesional corticosteroid injection technique for psoriatic plaque (requiring double injection; smaller plaques cope with one infiltration)

Hypertrophic scars: Multiple puncture method

Hypertrophic scars are usually treated by multiple intradermal injections of long-acting corticosteroids. The injections are not normally painful, but the procedure can be distressing, particularly to children.

It is possible to achieve the same results without 'an injection', delivering the steroid by the multiple-pressure technique used for smallpox vaccinations.

Method

1. The patient is positioned so that the scar to be treated is in the horizontal plane.
2. Cleanse the skin thoroughly with an alcohol swab and allow it to dry.
3. Draw injectable corticosteroid up into a syringe, preferably before the patient enters the treatment room.
4. Spread a film or layer of the steroid aseptically over the scar.
5. Make multiple pressures through the solution into the scar, using a 21-gauge needle held tangentially to the skin. The point of the needle should just penetrate the epidermis and not be deep enough to cause bleeding.
6. There should be approximately 20 pressures per cm².
7. Allow the steroid to dry and cover the area with a dressing if desired.

Treatment can be repeated every 6 weeks if necessary; most simple hypertrophic scars, however, settle after one treatment.

Silicon adhesive gel/dressings

Silicon sheet dressings (e.g. Cica-Care) worn continuously over a wound may prevent hypertrophy of the wound. An adhesive gel sheet can be purchased and a piece cut out to fit the wound. The gel sheet should be re-applied daily for 12 weeks.

Alternatively, silicon gels massaged firmly into the wound each day after the wound has re-epithelialised may help.

Elastoplast™ Scar Reduction Patch

These patches can be used to treat or prevent hypertrophic scars. The patch is applied over the scar and changed every 24 hours. It should not be applied to open wounds or burns.

Keloids

Methods

- Multiple puncture method (on p. 66).
- Inject long-acting corticosteroid, e.g. triamcinolone 10 mg/mL (usually 3 treatments, 6 weeks apart).
- Apply liquid nitrogen, then inject with corticosteroid about 5–15 minutes later—the softer oedematous tissue is easier to inject.
- Radiotherapy.

Prevention of keloids (in susceptible patients)

- Apply high potency topical corticosteroid with occlusive dressing for 2–3 days.
- Inject long-acting corticosteroid into the recess of the wound immediately following suture of the wound (Fig. 3.18).
- Inject long-acting corticosteroid immediately following suture removal.

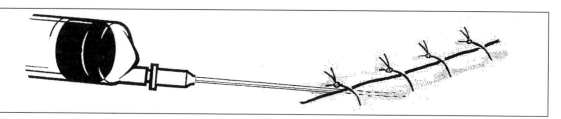

Fig. 3.18 Injecting corticosteroid into wound

Drainage of breast abscess

Acute bacterial mastitis

Resolution without progression to an abscess will usually be prevented by antibiotics (e.g. flucloxacillin 500 mg four times a day orally or erythromycin 500 mg four times a day orally). In addition, therapeutic ultrasound (2 W/cm^2 for 6 minutes) daily for 2–3 days will assist resolution.

The breast abscess

An abscess should be drained surgically under general anaesthesia.

Method

1. Make an incision over the point of maximal tenderness, preferably in a dependent area of the breast. A curvilinear transverse incision which does not continue into breast tissue, following Langer's lines, is optimal (Fig. 3.19a).
2. Use artery forceps to separate breast tissue to reach the pus.
3. Take a swab for culture.
4. Introduce a gloved finger to break down the septa that separate the cavity into loculations (Fig. 3.19b).
5. Insert a corrugated drainage tube into the cavity. Fix it to the skin edge with a single suture (Fig. 3.19c).

Remove the tube 2 days after the operation. Change the dressings daily until the wound has healed. Continue antibiotics until resolution of the inflammation.

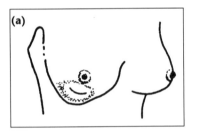 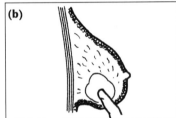 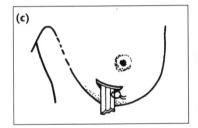

Fig. 3.19 Drainage of breast abscess: **(a)** transverse incision; **(b)** exploring abscess cavity; **(c)** drainage tube in situ

Aspiration of breast lump

This simple technique is very helpful, especially if the lump is a cyst, and will have no adverse effects if the lump is malignant. If so, the needle biopsy will help with the pre-operative cytological diagnosis.

Clues to diagnosis of breast cysts

- Sudden onset; past history at surgery.
- Discrete breast mass, firm, rarely fluctuant, relatively mobile.

Method of aspiration and needle biopsy

1. Avoid LA; use an aqueous skin preparation.
2. Use a 21-gauge needle and a 5 mL sterile syringe.
3. Identify the mass accurately and fix it by placing three fingers of the dominant hand firmly on three sides of the mass (Fig. 3.20a).
4. Introduce the needle directly into the area of the swelling, and once in subcutaneous tissue apply gentle suction as the needle is being advanced (Fig. 3.20b).
5. If fluid is obtained (usually yellowish green), aspirate as much as possible.
6. If no fluid is obtained, try and get a core of cells from several areas of the lump in the bore of the needle.
7. Make several passes through the lump at different angles, without exit from the skin and maintaining suction.
8. Release suction before exit from the skin so as to keep the cells in the needle (not in the syringe).
9. After withdrawal, remove the syringe from the needle, fill with 2 mL of air, reattach the needle and produce a fine spray on two prepared slides.
10. Fix one slide (in Cytofix) and allow one to air-dry, and forward to a reputable pathology laboratory.

Indications for biopsy of lump

- The cyst fluid is bloodstained.
- The lump does not disappear completely with aspiration.
- The swelling recurs within 1 month.

Recurrent cysts

After aspiration, leave the needle in situ and inject 2–5 mL of air. This method reduces the recurrence rate.

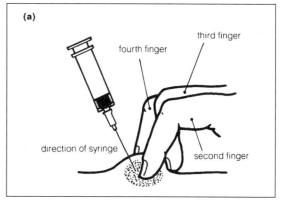

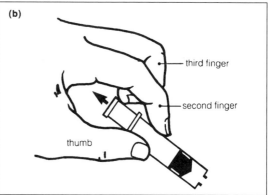

Fig. 3.20 Fixation of the cyst: **(a)** lateral view; **(b)** position of other hand: second (index) finger and thumb steady the syringe while the third (middle) finger slides out the plunger to create suction

Marsupialisation technique for Bartholin's cyst

Bartholin's cyst presents as a swelling at the posterior end of the labium majus, close to the fourchette. The correct treatment of both cyst and abscess is marsupialisation, not excision (which is difficult, bloody and leads to scarring) or incision (which is usually followed by recurrence).

The procedure can be carried out on an outpatient, preferably using local anaesthesia.

Method

1. With the patient in the lithotomy position, swab and drape the vulva.
2. Infiltrate the skin over the medial part of the cyst with 1% lignocaine with adrenaline, using a fine needle and a slow injection.
3. Make a narrow elliptical incision over the medial part of the cyst, at least 3 cm in length (Fig. 3.21a). (As this ostium later contracts, it is a fault to make it too small.)
4. Excise the ellipse of skin, then open the wall of the cyst in the same line, and carefully grasp its edges with mosquito forceps.
5. After the contents of the cyst escape, wash out the cavity with saline, and inspect it then dry it carefully. Any deep loculi must be opened widely. On the postero-inferior cyst wall it is usual to find a punctum leading into the proximal remnant of the duct.
6. Suture the cyst wall to the skin edge at four points using fine catgut, thus creating a pouch (Fig. 3.21b). No dressing is applied and the patient is instructed to take a sitting bath twice a day for a week. Healing is rapid, without pain, and the result is a permanent ostium close to the hymen which delivers free-draining secretion close to the normal site (Fig. 3.21c). If this ostium is too lateral, the woman may complain of discharge and wetness of the skin.

With this technique, even the inexperienced operator will have no difficulty achieving good results with Bartholin's cysts. Abscesses can be more difficult if the lining is friable or necrotic. For this reason, early operation should be advised in the presence of inflammation.

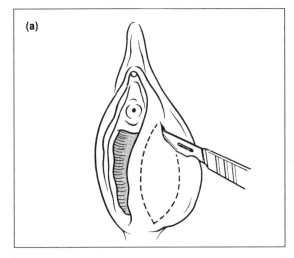

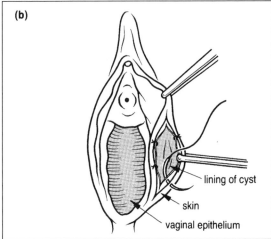

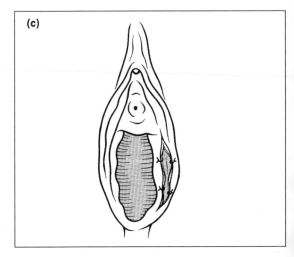

Fig. 3.21 Marsupialisation technique: **(a)** start of operation; **(b)** final suture; **(c)** post-operative appearance

Cervical polyps

Women presenting with small cervical polyps can be readily and simply treated in the office with sponge-holding forceps and a silver nitrate stick. Patients with large polyps require a different approach and referral may be appropriate.

Method

1. Grasp the polyp with sponge-holding forceps and gently twist the polyp until it separates (Fig. 3.22a).
2. Place the polyp in a specimen bottle and send it for histological examination.
3. Cauterise the base of the polyp at the cervical os (Fig. 3.22b) with silver nitrate or by electrocautery.

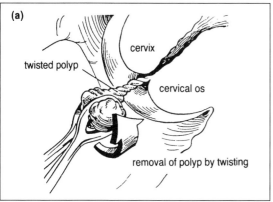
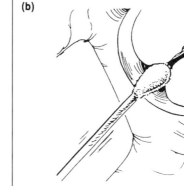

Fig. 3.22 Cervical polyp excision: (**a**) removal by twisting; (**b**) cauterising base with silver nitrate

Liquid nitrogen therapy

Ideally, liquid nitrogen is stored in a special, large container and decanted when required into a small thermos flask or a spray device. The temperature is –193°C.

The easiest method of application to superficial skin tumours (see Table 3.1) is via a ball of cotton wool rolled rather loosely on the tip of a wooden applicator stick. This should be slightly smaller than the lesion, to prevent freezing of the surrounding skin.

Beware of application to the following:

- dark skin,
- upper lips,
- nerves,
- eyelids,
- nails (do not freeze over nail matrix).

Cotton wool application method (basic steps)

1. Inform the patient what to expect.
2. Pare excess keratin with a scalpel.

Table 3.1 Superficial skin tumours suitable for cryotherapy

Warts (plane, periungual, plantar, anogenital)
Skin tags
Seborrhoeic keratoses
Molluscum contagiosum
Solar keratoses

3. Use a cotton wool applicator slightly smaller (*not* larger—see Fig. 3.23a) than the lesion.
4. Immerse it in nitrogen until bubbling ceases.
5. Gently tap it on the side of the container to remove excess liquid.
6. Hold the lesion firmly between thumb and forefinger.
7. Place the applicator vertically (Fig. 3.23b,c) on the tumour surface.
8. Apply with firm pressure: *do not dab.*
9. Redip the applicator every 5–10 seconds.
10. Freeze until a 2–5 mm white halo appears around the lesion.

(continues)

The appropriate length of application varies (see Table 3.2).

Explain likely reactions to the patient, such as the appearance of blisters (possibly blood blisters). The optimal time for retreatment of warts is at or soon after 3 weeks.

Table 3.2 Recommended treatment times for cryotherapy

Solar keratoses, solar lentigos	< 3 seconds
seborrhoeic keratoses	single cycle 5–10 seconds
skin tags	5–10 seconds
warts—hands	single cycle 30 seconds
warts—feet	two cycles 30 seconds with complete thaw in between
molluscum contagiosum	5 seconds

Spray 'gun' method

Spraying liquid nitrogen under high pressure is by far quicker and more effective than the topical method. It produces sufficient intense cold to treat deeper lesions. Spray until the white halo forms. If the spray is too diffuse for the lesion, you can place the opening of an otoscope earpiece over the lesion—then spray into the opening of the earpiece, but wear thick gloves for this manoeuvre. Another strategy is to apply a thick film of petroleum jelly or spray 'plastic skin' such as Op Site to protect the surrounding skin.

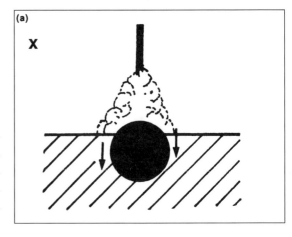

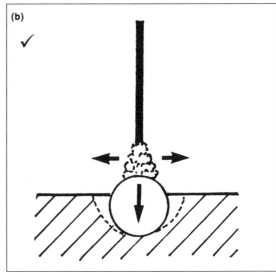

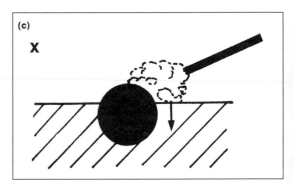

Fig. 3.23 Shows **(a)** applicator too large; **(b)** correct size and approach of applicator; **(c)** correct size but wrong position of applicator

Carbon dioxide slush for skin lesions

Carbon dioxide (CO_2), also known as dry ice, is an effective cryotherapy (freezing) agent for the treatment of warts and keratoses. The CO_2 snow is obtained by the rapid release of CO_2 gas from a cylinder.

Equipment

You will need:

- one sparklet cylinder of CO_2,
- a chamois bag with a purse string around the edge,
- a bottle of acetone,
- a cotton wool bud (preferably on a long stick).

Method

1. Invert the cylinder and connect the chamois bag around the nozzle to collect a small amount of dry ice (snow). The CO_2 snow can be made into a slush by adding a few drops of acetone immediately before use. Alternatively, the cotton bud can be dipped in acetone and then introduced into the snow.
2. Roll the cotton wool bud firmly in this slush to collect an 'ice ball', which must be used immediately as it melts very rapidly. The 'ice ball' should be marginally smaller than the lesion to be treated.
3. Apply this 'ice ball' to the skin lesion for 10–15 seconds.

Simple removal of xanthoma

General practitioners receive many requests to remove cosmetically unacceptable xanthomas of the eyelid. A simple method of removal is described. It is suitable for most sizes, but works best for smaller xanthomas that are bulging and 'ripe' for removal.

Equipment

- A 21-gauge sterile disposable needle.
- Manicure tweezers (flat or slanted, not pointed).

Method

1. Explain the method to the patient, indicating that there is slight discomfort only.
2. Although it is not necessary for all patients, apply some ice or other surface 'anaesthetic' to the xanthoma to lessen the discomfort.
3. Stretch the overlying skin and make a small incision in the skin with the tip of the needle (or a fine scalpel) (Fig. 3.24a).
4. Compress the xanthoma along its axis with the tweezers. It is invariably easily expelled (Fig. 3.24b).

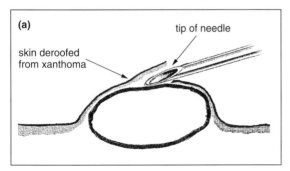
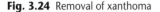
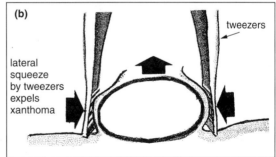

Fig. 3.24 Removal of xanthoma

4 Treatment of ano-rectal problems

Perianal haematoma

This painful condition usually develops with straining to pass stool. Surgical intervention is recommended, especially in the presence of severe discomfort. The treatment depends on the time of presentation after appearance of the haematoma.

Stage 1 treatment:
Within 24 hours of onset

While the haematoma is still fluid, the treatment is by simple aspiration of the blood (Fig. 4.1). No local anaesthetic is necessary. If this is unsuccessful, surgical drainage is recommended.

Equipment

You will need:

- a 2 mL or 5 mL syringe,
- a 19-gauge needle.

Stage 2 treatment:
Within 24 hours to 5 days of onset

By now the blood has clotted, and a simple incision over the haematoma to remove the thrombosis followed by deroofing is the most appropriate treatment.

Equipment

You will need:

- 1% lignocaine with adrenaline (1–2 mL),
- a 25-gauge needle and 2 mL syringe,
- a no. 15 scalpel blade,
- 1 plain-toothed dissecting forceps (not essential).

Method

1. Swab the perianal area with povidone iodine, then inject 1–2 mL of LA into the skin around the base of the haematoma (Fig. 4.2a).
2. Make a stab incision with the scalpel blade into the skin over the haematoma.
3. Extend the incision along the main axis of the haematoma (Fig. 4.2b).
4. Evacuate the thrombus with gentle, lateral pressure (Fig. 4.2c) or lift out with forceps.
5. Deroof the haematoma by a small elliptical skin excision.
6. Apply pressure to the incised area with a plain gauze swab to achieve haemostasis.
7. When bleeding has stopped, apply a small dressing of gauze, then a combine (5 cm × 5 cm) folded in half.

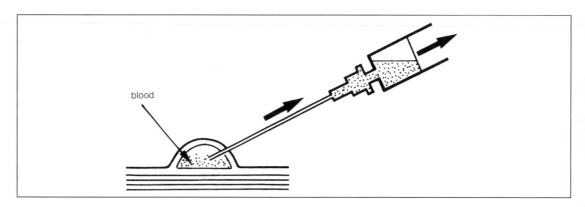

Fig. 4.1 Aspiration of blood for perianal haematoma

8. Retain the dressing with well-fitting underpants (not adhesive) and remove the next day.
9. No stitch is required unless haemostasis is a problem.

Stage 3 treatment:
Day 6 onwards

The haematoma is best left alone unless it is very painful or (rarely) infected. Resolution is evidenced by the appearance of wrinkles in the previously stretched skin. The haematoma will ultimately become a skin tag.

Note: A gangrenous haematoma or a very large thrombosed pile should be surgically excised. The patient should have analgesics and Sitz baths.

Follow-up

The patient should be reviewed in 4 weeks for rectal examination and proctoscopy, to examine for any underlying internal haemorrhoid that may predispose to further recurrence. Prevention includes an increased intake of dietary fibre and avoidance of straining at stool.

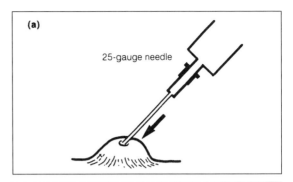

(a)

25-gauge needle

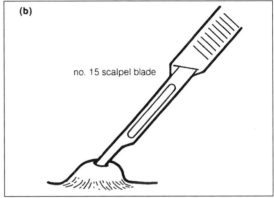

(b)

no. 15 scalpel blade

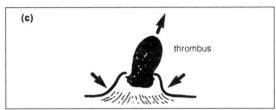

(c)

thrombus

Fig. 4.2 Treatment of perianal haematoma: **(a)** local anaesthetic; **(b)** incision over haematoma; **(c)** thrombus expressed by digital pressure

Perianal skin tags

The skin tag is usually the legacy of an untreated perianal haematoma. It may require excision for aesthetic reasons, for hygiene, or because it is a source of pruritus ani or irritation.

Method

1. Make a simple elliptical excision at the base of the skin under LA (Fig. 4.3). Suturing of the defect is usually not necessary.

2. Apply a light gauze dressing for about 24 hours. The patient is advised to have twice-daily salt baths until healing is complete.

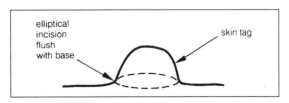

elliptical incision flush with base

skin tag

Fig. 4.3 Excision of perianal skin tag

Rubber band ligation of haemorrhoids

Rubber band ligation of haemorrhoids (best for stages 2 and 3) is a simple technique performed through a lubricated proctoscope which can be held by the patient after insertion (Fig. 4.4a). One or two rubber bands are stretched over the loading cone onto the metal drum of the banding instrument.

Method

1. Thread the long grasping forceps through the drum of the banding instrument and grasp the haemorrhoid about 1 cm above the dentate line (Fig. 4.4b).
2. Apply gentle traction to the haemorrhoid to indent its base.
3. Snap the band or bands onto the haemorrhoid by pushing the trigger mechanism (Fig. 4.4c).

Post-procedure

- If possible, avoid a bowel action on day 1.
- Take simple analgesics as necessary.

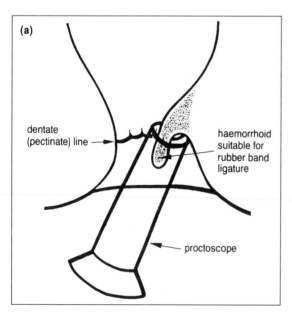

(a)

dentate (pectinate) line

haemorrhoid suitable for rubber band ligature

proctoscope

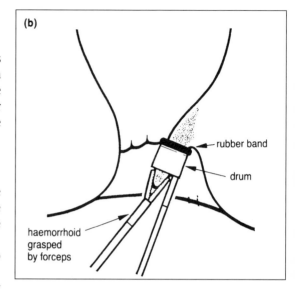

(b)

rubber band

drum

haemorrhoid grasped by forceps

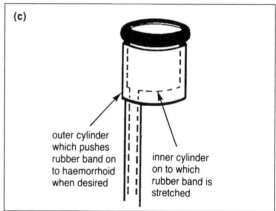

(c)

outer cylinder which pushes rubber band on to haemorrhoid when desired

inner cylinder on to which rubber band is stretched

Fig. 4.4 Rubber band ligation of haemorrhoids: **(a)** proctoscope; **(b)** haemorrhoid grasped by forceps; **(c)** operational end of applicator

Injection of haemorrhoids

Aims

- To exclude associated tumours (? colonoscopy).
- To produce fibrosis in the submucous layer.
- To avoid injection into haemorrhoidal vessels.

The procedure is best for small haemorrhoids that bleed frequently.

Equipment

You will need:

- a proctoscope with illumination and lubricant,
- a haemorrhoid (Gabriel) injection syringe and needle, or a 10 mL disposable syringe with a 21-gauge needle,
- a 5 mL ampoule of 5% phenol in almond oil,
- a 19-gauge drawing-up needle,
- forceps and cotton wool to wipe away faeces.

Method

1. The patient lies in the left lateral position.
2. Insert the lubricated proctoscope to visualise the haemorrhoids.
3. Draw up 5 mL of oily phenol.
4. Aim the injection at the upper end (base) of the haemorrhoid, which should be above the ano-rectal ring (injections given below this are very painful). Pierce the mucosa with a quick stab.
5. Inject up to 3 mL into the submucous plane. The bevel of the needle should be directed towards the mucosa rather than towards the lumen of the rectum. The injection should be painless (Fig. 4.5). Inject the phenol slowly until an opalescent swelling (blanching) is seen, displaying the vessels in the mucosa more superficially (the 'striate' sign).
6. The amount of phenol injected varies from 1 mL to 5 mL (usually 3 mL).

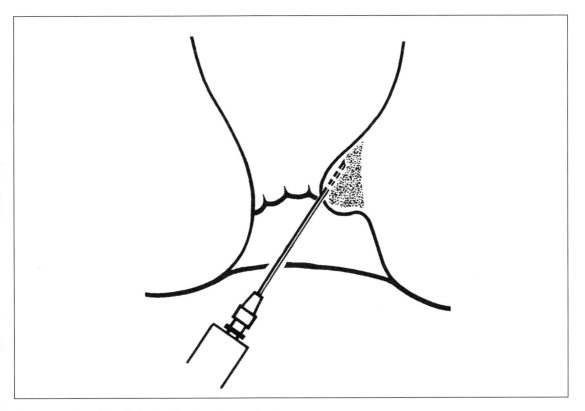

Fig. 4.5 Position of needle for the injection of haemorrhoids

Anal fissure

The acute fissure

Treatment is with warm saline Sitz baths, analgesics and 15 g bran or psyllium fibre orally each day for 3 months.

Milder cases

In a milder case of anal fissure the discomfort is slight, anal spasm is a minor feature and the onset is acute.

Conservative management

- Xyloproct suppositories or ointment.
- High-residue diet (consider the addition of unprocessed bran).
- Avoidance of constipation with hard stools (aim for soft bulky stools).
- Glyceryl trinitrate ointment (Nitro-bid 2%) diluted 1 part with 9 parts white soft paraffin applied to the lower anal canal 2–3 times daily. A commercial preparation is Rectogesic ointment— apply 3 times daily for 4 weeks or until healed.

More severe chronic fissures

The feature here is a hyperactive anal sphincter, and a practical procedure is necessary to solve this painful problem.

Method 1: Digital anal dilatation

Under general anaesthesia (or even adequate local anaesthesia), undertake four-finger (maximum) anal dilatation for 4 minutes. This is effective, but is usually followed by a brief period of incontinence.

Anal dilatation under general anaesthesia is a most appropriate treatment for children with anal fissures.

Method 2: Inject botulinum toxin into the sphincter

Some studies indicate excellent results when botulinum toxin is injected into the fissure and surrounding sphincter. Its availability and cost are limiting factors.

Method 3: Lateral sphincterotomy

The anal sphincter mechanism comprises internal and external sphincters. The spasm of the internal sphincter that occurs because of an anal fissure is relieved by the procedure of lateral sphincterotomy, allowing the fissure to heal in about 2 weeks. The procedure gives dramatic relief; however, the rare complication of permanent faecal incontinence has to be considered.

Procedure under local anaesthetic

1. The patient lies on the side.
2. Palpate the ridge between the internal and external sphincter, and infiltrate local anaesthetic (1% lignocaine with adrenaline) (Fig. 4.6a).
3. Introduce a no. 11 scalpel blade (or fine cataract knife) on a handle through the skin at a tangent to the internal sphincter fibres.
4. Rotate the blade through 90° to face the fibres, with the examining finger in the anal canal.
5. Careful, slow advancement and withdrawal of the blade will cut through the sphincter muscles, the sensation akin to cutting through many rubber bands around a finger (Fig. 4.6b).
6. When the spasm is felt to subside, cease cutting.
7. Rotate the blade 90° again and withdraw. Firm pressure on the wound will stop any bleeding.

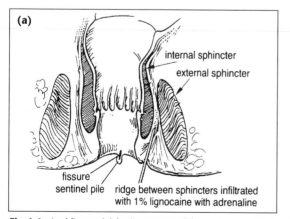

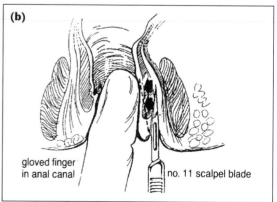

Fig 4.6. Anal fissure: **(a)** basic anatomy of the anal canal; **(b)** direction of cutting through the internal sphincter with a scalpel blade

Procedure under general anaesthetic

A qualified surgeon performs an open lateral sphincterotomy.

Post-procedure

The patient is instructed to take 20 mL of Agarol at night or 12-hourly to achieve loose bowel motions for the next five days.

Proctalgia fugax

Main features

- fleeting rectal pain in adults,
- varies from mild discomfort to severe spasm,
- lasts 3–30 minutes,
- often wakes patient at night,
- a functional bowel disorder.

Management

- explanation and reassurance,
- salbutamol inhaler (2 puffs statim) worth a trial.

Alternatives include glyceryl trinitrate spray for the symptom or prophylactic quinine bisulphate at night.

Perianal abscess

Clinical features

- severe, constant throbbing pain,
- fever and toxicity,
- hot, red, tender swelling adjacent to anal margin,
- non-fluctuant swelling

Careful examination is necessary to make the diagnosis. Look for evidence of a fistula-in-ano.

Treatment

Drainage via a cruciate incision over the point of maximal induration (Fig. 4.7a).

Method

1. Infiltrate 10 mL of 1% lignocaine with adrenaline in the skin overlying the abscess (in some people a general anaesthetic may be preferable).
2. Make a cruciate incision.
3. Insert artery forceps to open the abscess cavity and evacuate the pus.
4. Excise the corners of the cruciate incision to produce a circular skin defect (about 2 cm in diameter) (Fig. 4.7b).
5. Dress the wound with gauze soaked in a mild antiseptic.

Post-procedure

- Change gauze dressings twice daily.

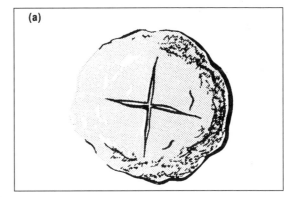

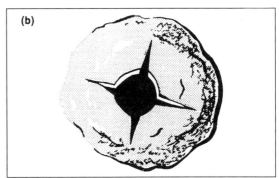

Fig. 4.7 Perianal abscess: **(a)** cruciate incision over abscess; **(b)** extension of cruciate incision

- Have warm saline Sitz baths prior to new dressing.
- If undue bleeding occurs, pack the cavity for 24 hours and add covering dressings.

Perianal warts

It is important to distinguish the common viral warts from the condylomata lata of secondary syphilis. Counselling and support are necessary. Not all warts are sexually transmitted.

Treatment

The warts may be removed by chemical or physical means. The simplest and most effective treatment for readily accessible warts is:

- podophyllotoxin 0.5% paint (a more stable preparation)
  —Apply bd with plastic applicator for 3 days.
  —Repeat in 4 days if necessary (may need four treatments).
  or
- podophyllin 25% solution in tinct benz co
  —Apply with a cotton wool swab to each wart.
  —Wash off in 4 hours, then dust with talcum powder.
  —Repeat once weekly until warts disappear.
  or
- imiquimod (Aldara) cream.

Anal fibro-epithelial polyps

These polyps are usually overgrown anal papillae which present as an irritating prolapse. They are removed by infiltrating the base with local anaesthetic, crushing it with artery forceps and applying a ligature. They are benign but the removed lesion should undergo histological examination if there is any doubt.

Pruritus ani

In addition to the usual measures, consider cleaning the anus (after defaecation) with cotton wool dampened in warm water. Cotton wool is less abrasive than paper, and soap also irritates the problem.

General measures

- Stop scratching.
- Bathe carefully: avoid hot water, excessive scrubbing and soaps.
- Use bland aqueous cream, Cetaphil lotion or Neutrogena soap.
- Keep the area dry and cool.
- Keep bowels regular and wipe with cotton wool soaked in water.
- Wear loose-fitting clothing and underwear.
- Avoid local anaesthetics and antiseptics.

If still problematic and a dermatosis is probably involved, use:

- hydrocortisone 1% cream, or
- hydrocortisone 1% cream with clioquinol 0.5–3% (most effective).

If an isolated area and resistant, infiltrate 0.5 mL of triamcinolone intradermally.

If desperate, use fractionated X-ray therapy.

5 Foot problems

Calluses, corns and warts

The diagnosis of localised, tender lumps on the sole of the foot can be difficult. The differential diagnosis of callus, corn and wart is aided by an understanding of their morphology and the effect of paring these lumps (Table 5.1).

A callus (Fig. 5.1) is simply a localised area of hyperkeratosis related to some form of pressure and friction.

A corn (Fig. 5.2) is a small, localised, conical thickening, which may resemble a plantar wart but which gives a different appearance on paring.

A wart (Fig. 5.3) is more invasive, and paring reveals multiple small, pinpoint bleeding spots.

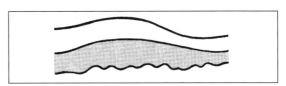

Fig. 5.1 Callus

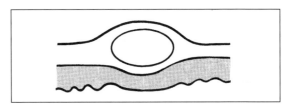

Fig. 5.2 Corn

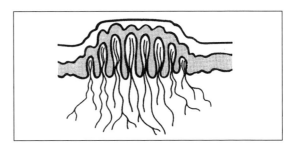

Fig. 5.3 Wart

Table 5.1 Comparison of the main causes of a lump on the sole of the foot

	Typical site	Nature	Effect of paring
Callus	where skin is normally thick: beneath heads of metatarsals, heels, inframedial side of great toe	hard, thickened skin	normal skin
Corn	where skin is normally thin: on soles, fifth toe, dorsal projections of hammer toes	white, conical mass of keratin, flattened by pressure	exposes white, avascular corn with concave surface
Wart	anywhere, mainly over metatarsal heads, base of toes and heels; has bleeding points	viral infection, with abrupt change from skin at edge	exposes bleeding points

Treatment of plantar warts

There are many treatments for this common and at times frustrating problem. A good rule is to avoid scalpel excision, diathermy or electrocautery because of the problem of scarring. One of the problems with the removal of plantar warts is the 'iceberg' configuration (Fig. 5.4) and not all may be removed.

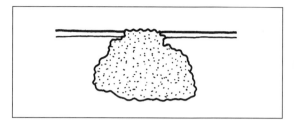

Fig. 5.4 'Iceberg' configuration of plantar wart

Liquid nitrogen

1. Pare wart.
2. Apply liquid nitrogen.
3. Repeat weekly.

Can be painful and results are often disappointing.

Topical chemotherapy

1. Pare wart (particularly in children).
2. Apply Upton's paste to wart each night and cover.
3. Review as necessary.

(Upton's paste comprises trichloroacetic acid 1 part, salicylic acid 6 parts, glycerine to a stiff paste.)

Topical chemotherapy and liquid nitrogen

1. Pare wart (a 21-gauge blade is recommended).
2. Apply paste of 70% salicylic acid in raw linseed oil.
3. Occlude for 1 week.
4. Pare on review, then apply liquid nitrogen and review.

Curettage under local anaesthetic

1. Pare the wart vigorously to reveal the extent of the wart.
2. Thoroughly curette the entire wart with a dermal curette.
3. Hold the foot dependent over a kidney dish until the bleeding stops (this always stops spontaneously and avoids a bleed later on the way home).
4. Apply 50% trichloroacetic acid to the base.

Occlusion with topical chemotherapy

A method of using salicylic acid in a paste for the treatment of plantar warts is described here.

Equipment

You will need:

- 2.5 cm (width) elastic adhesive tape,
- 30% salicylic acid in Lassar's paste. (Ask the chemist to prepare a thick paste, like plasticine.)

(Lassar's paste comprises zinc oxide, starch and salicylic acid, dispersed in white petrolatum.)

Method

1. Cut two lengths of adhesive tape, one about 5 cm and the other shorter.
2. Fold the shorter length in half, sticky side out (Fig. 5.5a).
3. Cut a half circle at the folded edge to accommodate the wart.
4. Press this tape down so that the hole is over the wart.
5. Roll a small ball of the paste in the palm of the hand and then press it into the wart.
6. Cover the tape, paste and wart with the longer strip of tape (Fig. 5.5b).
7. This paste should be reapplied twice daily for 2–3 weeks.
8. The reapplication is achieved by peeling back the longer strip to expose the wart, adding a fresh ball of paste to the wart and then recovering with the upper tape.

The plantar wart invariably crumbles and vanishes. If the wart is particularly stubborn, 50% salicylic acid can be used. For finger warts use 20% salicylic acid. This method should not be used for vaginal, penile or eyelid warts.

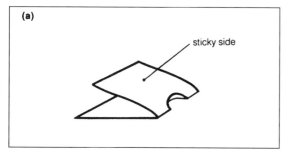

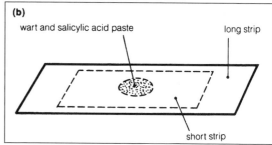

Fig. 5.5 **(a)** 'Window' to fit the wart is cut out of shoulder strip of elastic adhesive tape; **(b)** larger strip covers the wart and shoulder strip

Alternative chemicals

- Salicylic acid 17%, lactic acid 17% in collodion (Dermatech Wart Treatment).
- Paste of trichloroacetic acid 1 part, salicylic acid 6 parts, glycerine 20 gm.
- Salicylic acid, lactic acid in collodion (Duofilm).

Poultice of aspirin and tea tree oil

Method

1. Place a non-effervescent 125–300 mg soluble aspirin tablet on the centre of the wart and dampen it with 15% tea tree oil in alcohol.
2. Cover with a cotton pad and tape firmly with Micropore. Allow it to get wet to encourage dissolution.
3. After one week remove the dressing and debride or curette the friable slough.

4. Repeat if necessary.

Simple (and unusual) treatments

The banana skin method

1. Cut a small disk of banana skin to cover the wart.
2. Apply the inner soft surface of the banana skin to the wart and cover with tape.
3. Perform this daily for a few weeks or as long as necessary.

The citric and acetic acid method

Soak pieces of lemon rind in vinegar for 3–4 days and then apply a small piece to the wart each day and cover with tape. The crumbling slough can usually be curetted out after 2–3 weeks.

Treatment of calluses

- No treatment is required if asymptomatic.
- Remove the cause.
- Proper footwear is essential—wide shoes and cushioned pads over the ball of the foot.
- Provide paring with a scalpel blade (the most effective) or file with callus files.
- If severe, daily applications of 10% salicylic acid in soft paraffin or Eulactol Heel Balm with regular paring.

Paring method

Hold a no. 10 scalpel blade with the bevel almost parallel to the skin and shave the lines of any cracks

with small, swift strokes (Fig. 5.6). Scrape along the lines of any cracks, not into them. Be careful not to draw blood.

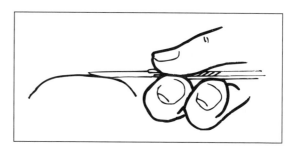

Fig 5.6 Method of using a scalpel or similar knife to shave off a callus

Treatment of corns

- Remove the cause of friction and use wide shoes.
- Soften the corn with a few applications of 15% salicylic acid in collodion and then pare.

An alternative is to apply commercial medicated disks on a daily basis for about 4 days, then pare.

For soft corns between the toes (usually the last toe-web), keep the toe-webs separated with lamb's wool at all times and dust with a foot powder.

'Cracked' heels

- Soak the feet for 30 minutes in warm water containing an oil such as Alpha-Keri or Derma Oil.
- Pat dry, then apply a cream such as Nutraplus (10% urea) or Eulactol Heel Balm.

Plantar fasciitis

Plantar fasciitis is a very common and surprisingly debilitating condition that may take 12–36 months (typically 2 years) to resolve spontaneously.

Features

- Pain:
  —under the heel (about 5 cm from end of heel);
  —can be diffuse over heel;
  —when first step out of bed;
  —relieved by walking around after shower;
  —increasing towards the end of the day;
  —worse after sitting;
  —felt as a severe throbbing while sitting.
- Minimal signs.
- X-ray may reveal a calcaneal spur.

Patient advice

- Avoid standing for long periods if possible.
- Rest from long walks and running.
- Try to cope without injections.
- Keep the heel 'cushioned' by wearing comfortable shoes and/or inserts in shoes.
- Surgery is rarely required and is not usually recommended. Excision of the calcaneal spur is advised against.

Footwear and insoles

Obtain good, comfortable shoes with a cushioned sole (e.g. Florsheim 'comfortech'; sporting 'runners').

Examples of orthotic pads:

- Viscospot orthotic (sold by Melbourne Orthotics),
- Rose insole,
- an insole tailored by your podiatrist,
- a pad made from sponge or sorbo rubber placed inside the shoe to raise the heel about 1 cm. A hole corresponding to the tender area can be cut out of the pad to avoid direct contact with the sole (Fig. 5.7).

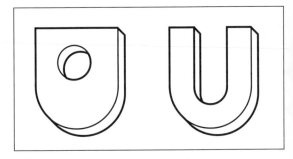

Fig. 5.7 Types of insole heel pads made from sponge or sorbo rubber

Hydrotherapy

The following tips have proved very useful for patients.

Hot and cold water treatment

The patient places the affected foot in a small bath of very hot water and then a small bath of cold water for 20–30 seconds each time. This is continued on an alternating basis for 15 minutes—preferably twice a day and best before retiring at night.

Therapeutic foot massage

Commercial electrical foot hydro-massagers are available at low cost and are recommended for patients with plantar fasciitis.

Exercises

Most foot surgeons now recommend regular stretching exercises as the basis of effective treatment. The aim is to allow the plantar fascia to heal at its 'natural length'. Stretching should be performed at least three times a day with each stretching exercise lasting 10 minutes.

The following exercises are provided courtesy of Andrew Beischer, orthopaedic surgeon.

Exercise 1

1. Stand with the balls of your feet on a step and keep your knees straight.

2. Let your heels gently drop as you count to 20. Do not bounce (Fig. 5.8a).
3. Lift your heels and count to ten.
4. Repeat the cycle twice. You will feel tightness both in the sole or heel of the foot, and at the back of the leg (as the tendo-achilles is also stretched).

Exercise 2

1. Stand against a solid wall with your painful foot behind you and the other foot closer to the wall (Fig. 5.8b).
2. Point the toes of the affected foot towards the heel of the front foot. Keep the knee of the painful foot straight and the painful heel on the floor.
3. Bend the front knee forward—you will feel the Achilles tendon in the painful foot grow tight.
4. Count to 20, then relax for a count of 10.
5. Repeat the cycle twice.
6. Change over the position of each foot and repeat the program to stretch the opposite Achilles tendon.

Exercise 3

You must be wearing flexible sole shoes for this exercise.

1. Stand against the wall with your good foot behind you and the painful foot jammed into the juncture of the wall and floor. (Fig. 5.8c).

(*continues*)

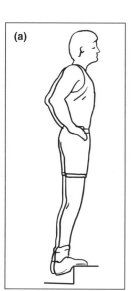
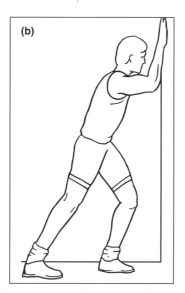
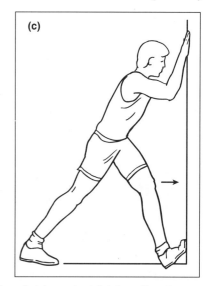

Fig. 5.8 Exercises for plantar fasciitis: **(a)** exercise 1; **(b)** exercise 2 (right foot affected); **(c)** exercise 3 (left foot affected)

2. Bend the knee of the front leg, which will bring it towards the wall. You will feel that both the Achilles tendon and the tissue on the sole of the foot (plantar fascia) are being stretched by this exercise.
3. Count to 20, then relax for a count of 10.
4. Repeat the cycle twice.
5. Change over the position of each foot and repeat the program to stretch the opposite side.

Strapping for plantar fasciitis

Strapping of the affected foot can bring symptomatic relief for the pain of plantar fasciitis. A few strapping techniques can be used but the principle is to prevent excessive pronation, create a degree of inversion and reduce tension on the origin of the plantar fascia by compressing the heel. Use non-stretch sticking tape about 3–4 cm wide.

Method
- Start with the tape on the lateral side of the dorsum of the foot (Fig. 5.9a).
- Run the tape in a figure-of-eight configuration to include the sides of the heel but squeeze the heel from the sides to make a 'pad' immediately before applying and fixing the tape.
- Repeat twice (Fig. 5.9b).

If reinforcement is desired, a U-shaped strip of tape can be applied to the sides of the foot—from the neck of the metatarsals on one side to the other. Also, a strip of holding tape can encircle the foot.

Other tips

Manual massage

Massage the sole of the foot over a wooden foot massager, a glass bottle filled with water, or even a golf ball for 5 minutes, preferably three times daily.

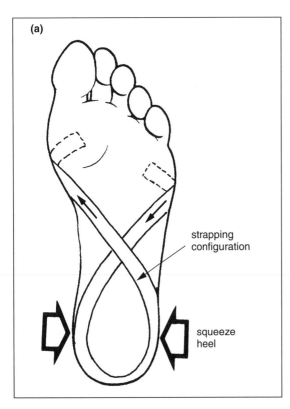
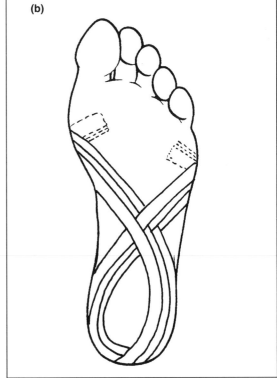

Fig. 5.9 (a) First application; **(b)** final appearance

Course of NSAIDS

It is worthwhile to conduct a trial of a 3-week course of NSAIDS during the time when there is most pain (about 4–7 weeks after the problem commences). It can be continued if there is a good response.

Injection

An injection of corticosteroid mixed with local anaesthetic can be very effective during the period of severe discomfort. (See Fig. 1.26, page 22). The relief usually lasts for 2–4 weeks during this difficult period. However, injections are generally avoided.

6 Nail problems

Splinters under nails

Foreign bodies, mostly wooden splinters, often become deeply wedged under fingernails and toenails (Fig. 6.1a). Efforts by patients to remove the splinters often aggravate the problem. A method of effective removal is outlined here.

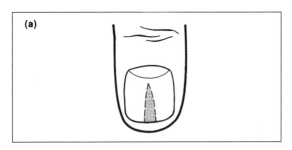

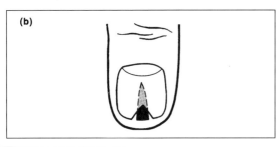

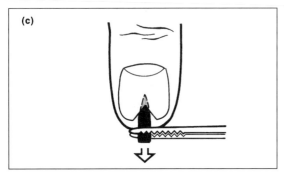

Fig. 6.1 Shows: **(a)** splinter under nail; **(b)** V-shaped incision; **(c)** tug with forceps

The V-cut out method

Equipment

You will need:

- needle, syringe and 1% lignocaine,
- small scissors,
- splinter forceps or small-artery forceps.

Method

1. Perform a digital nerve block to anaesthetise the involved digit (may not be necessary in rugged individuals).
2. Using small but strong scissors, cut a V-shaped piece of nail from over the end of the splinter (Fig. 6.1b). It is important to leave sufficient splinter exposed so that a good grip can be obtained. (A poor grip can result in fragmentation of the splinter.)
3. Obtain a good grip on the end of the splinter with the splinter or small-artery forceps, and remove with a sharp tug in the axis of the finger (Fig. 6.1c).

The 'paring' method

Use a no. 15 scalpel blade to gradually pare the nail overlying the splinter to create a window so that the splinter can be lifted out (Fig. 6.2). This is painless since the nail itself has no innervation.

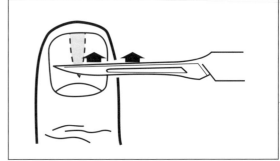

Fig. 6.2 Method of paring over a nail splinter using light shaving strokes

Onychogryphosis

Onychogryphosis, or irregular thickening and overgrowth of the nail, is commonly seen in the big toenails of the elderly (Fig. 6.3). It is really a permanent condition. Simple removal of the nail by avulsion is followed by recurrence some months later. Softening and burring of the nail gives only temporary relief, although burring sometimes provides a good result. The powder from burring can be used as culture for fungal organisms.

Permanent cure requires ablation of the nail bed after removal of the nail. Two methods of nail bed ablation are:

- total surgical excision,
- cauterisation with pure phenol.

Cauterisation method

1. Apply a tourniquet to the toe after administering ring block.
2. Remove the nail by lifting it away from the nail bed and then grasping the total nail or two halves (after it is cut down the middle) with strong artery forceps and using a combination of rotation and traction.
3. Paint the nail bed and germinal layer with pure phenol on a cotton bud, with special attention to the groove containing the nail matrix. Leave the phenol on for 2–3 minutes, flush it with alcohol to neutralise it, mop dry and apply a dressing. Pack a small piece of chlorhexidine (Bactigras) tulle into the wound and then cover with sterile gauze and a bandage.

Caution: Avoid spilling pure phenol onto normal skin.

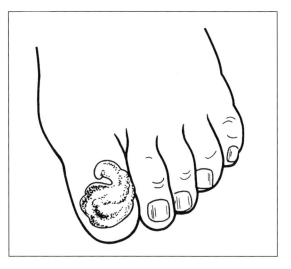

Fig. 6.3 Onychogryphosis ADAPTED FROM A. FORREST ET AL., *PRINCIPLES AND PRACTICE OF SURGERY*, CHURCHILL LIVINGSTONE, EDINBURGH, 1985, WITH PERMISSION

Subungual haematoma

The small, localised haematoma

There are several methods of decompressing a small, localised haematoma under the fingernail or toenail that causes considerable pain. The objective is to release the blood by drilling a hole in the overlying nail with a hot wire or a drill/needle.

Method 1: The sterile needle

Simply drill a hole by twisting a standard disposable hypodermic needle (21- or 23-gauge) into the selected site. Some practitioners prefer drilling two holes to facilitate the release of blood.

Method 2: The hot paper clip

Take a standard, large paper clip (Fig. 6.4a) and straighten it. Heat one end (until it is red hot) in the flame of a spirit lamp (Fig. 6.4b). Immediately transfer the hot wire to the nail, and press the point lightly on the nail at the centre of the haematoma. After a small puff of smoke, an acrid odour and a spurt of blood, the patient will experience immediate relief (Fig. 6.4c).

Method 3: Electrocautery

This is the best method. Simply apply the hot wire of the electrocautery unit to the selected site (Fig. 6.5). It is very important to keep the wire hot at all times and to be prepared to withdraw it quickly, as soon as the nail is pierced. It should be painless.

Important precautions

- Reassure patients that the process will not cause pain; they may be alarmed by the preparations.
- The hot point must quickly penetrate, and go no deeper than the nail. The blood under the nail insulates the underlying tissues from the heat and, therefore, from pain.
- The procedure is effective for a recent traumatic haematoma under tension. Do not attempt this procedure on an old, dried haematoma, as it will be painful and ineffective.

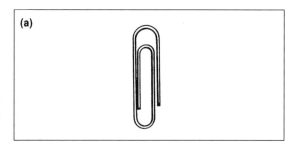

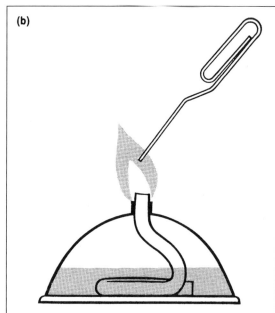

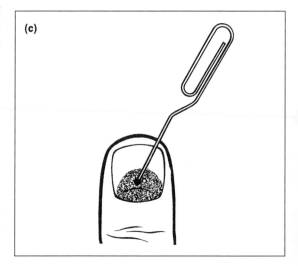

Fig. 6.4 (a) A standard paper clip; **(b)** the end of the paper clip is heated in the flame of a spirit lamp; **(c)** the point of the clip is pressed lightly on the nail at the centre of the haematoma

- Advise the patient to clean the nail with spirit or an antiseptic and cover with an adhesive strip to prevent contamination and infection.
- Advise the patient that the nail will eventually separate and a normal nail will appear in 4–6 months.

The large haematoma

Where blood occupies the total nail area, a relatively large laceration is present in the nail bed. To permit a good, long-term functional and cosmetic result it is imperative to remove the nail and repair the laceration (Fig. 6.6).

Method

1. Apply digital nerve block to the digit.
2. Remove the nail.
3. Repair the laceration with 4/0 plain catgut.
4. Replace the fingernail, which acts as a splint, and hold this in place with a suture for 10 days.

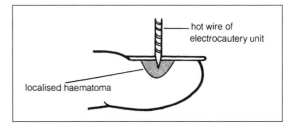

Fig. 6.5 Electrocautery to subungual haematoma

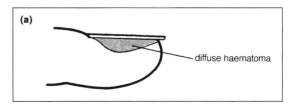

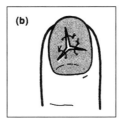 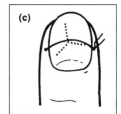

Fig. 6.6 Shows: **(a)** diffuse haematomas; **(b)** sutures to laceration; **(c)** fingernail as splint

Ingrowing toenails

There are myriad methods to treat ingrowing toenails. Some very helpful ones are presented here.

Cautionary note

Treatment of ingrowing toenails is a potential legal 'minefield', especially with wedge resection.
Keep in mind the following:

- Full and detailed discussion with the patient about the procedure used and its risks is recommended.
- Avoid adrenaline with the local anaesthetic—use plain lignocaine or bupivacaine.
- Avoid prolonged use of a tourniquet and do not forget to remove a rubber band if used.
- Avoid tight circumferential dressings.
- Be careful with diabetics and those with peripheral vascular diseases.

- Avoid excessive use of phenol for nail bed cautery.
- Give clear post-operative instructions.

Prevention

It is important to fashion the toenails so that the corners project beyond the skin (Fig. 6.7). Then each day, after a shower or bath, use the pads of both thumbs to pull the nail folds as indicated.

Central thinning method

An interesting method for the prevention and treatment of ingrowing toenails is to thin out a central strip of the nail plate. This is usually performed with the blade of a stitch remover or a no. 15 scalpel blade.

The central strip is about 5 mm wide and is thinned out on a regular basis (Fig. 6.8).

(continues)

Excision of ellipse of skin

Figure 6.9 shows the toe in extremis. The procedure transposes the skinfold away from the nail. The skin heals, the nail grows normally and the toe retains its normal anatomy.

Method

1. An elliptical excision is made after a digital block (Fig. 6.10a). The width of the excision depends on the amount of movement of the skinfold required to fully expose the nail edge.
2. The skinfold is forced off the nail (Fig. 6.10b). Any blunt instrument can be used for this purpose. The wound closure holds the fold in its new position.
3. Any granulation tissue and debris should be removed with a curette. The toe heals well, and there are usually no recurrences of ingrowing.

Electrocautery

If the nail is severely ingrown, causing granulation tissue or infection of the skin or both, a most effective method is to use electrocautery to remove a large wedge of skin and granulation tissue so that the ingrown nail stands free of skin (Fig. 6.11).

This is performed under digital block. The toe heals surprisingly quickly and well (with minimal pain). The long-term result is excellent, because the nail that is not cut in this procedure can grow (and be trimmed) free of flesh.

Phenolisation

This method uses 80% phenol (pure solution) to treat the nail bed after simply removing the wedge of nail. It is not necessary to perform a standard wedge resection of the ingrown nail and nail bed. The success rate is almost 100%.

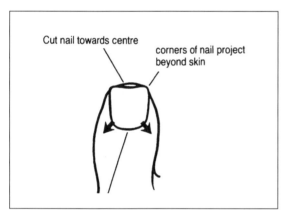

Fig. 6.7 Stretch nail folds with thumbs daily

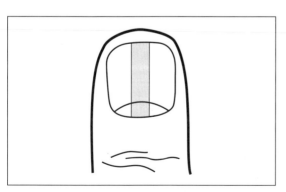

Fig. 6.8 Illustrating strip of nail plate to thin out

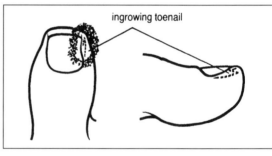

Fig. 6.9 Ingrowing toenail

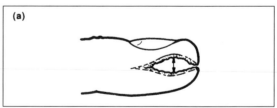

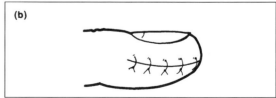

Fig. 6.10 Excision of ellipse of skin

Method

1. Perform a ring block with plain local anaesthetic.
2. Apply a tourniquet so that a bloodless field is obtained.
3. Using scissors, mobilise the nail on the affected side and excise the nail sliver for about one quarter of its width.
4. Curette the nail sulcus to remove any debris from the area.
5. Lift the nail fold and insert a cotton bud soaked (not saturated) in 80% phenol onto the corresponding nail bed (Fig. 6.12).
6. Leave the bud in place for $1^1/_2$ –2 minutes.
7. Remove and wash out the nail fold area with an alcohol swab.
8. Apply a dressing and review as necessary.

Cautionary tale

Pure phenol is a cytotoxic agent that causes a chemical burn and can be destructive to skin, causing a nasty slough. Several doctors using this excellent method claim that its value has been spoilt by causing severe burns to the surrounding skin. This has occurred because the swab had excess phenol that spilt onto the surrounding skin. This must be avoided with carefully controlled application, and if spillage occurs it must be washed off immediately with alcohol.

Wedge resection of nail with delayed nail fold excision

This method works very well where there is infection with swollen tissue.

Method

1. Perform a digital block.
2. Cut a standard wedge of ingrown nail (as for previous method). No further tissue is removed (Fig. 6.13a).
3. Dress and leave for 2–3 months.
4. After this time, perform a linear elliptical excision of the nail fold skin for the length of the nail extending to almost the tip of the toe. This should be about 3–4 mm from the nail margin to ensure skin necrosis does not occur. Suture and allow to heal (Fig. 6.13b).

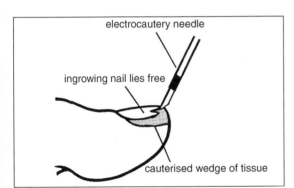

Fig. 6.11 Electrocautery to wedge of tissue

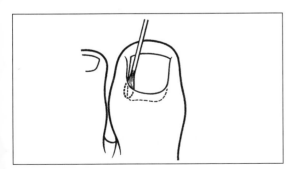

Fig. 6.12 Phenolisation method: lift the nail fold and apply the phenol on a stick

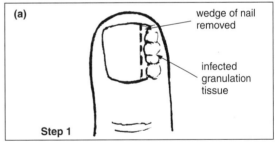

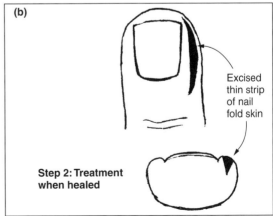

Fig. 6.13 Wedge resection of nail with delayed nail fold excision

The elliptical block dissection open method

This method, described by Chapeski, is claimed to cure all cases of ingrown toenails and the wound, if performed aseptically and dressed properly, will not get infected. The wound heals in about 4 weeks.

Method

1. Perform a digital block.
2. Place an elastic band around the toe and wait 5 minutes.
3. An incision is made at the base of the nail, about 3–4 mm from the edge, and then continued towards the side of the nail in an elliptical sweep to end up under the tip of the nail about 3–4 mm from the edge.
4. The ingrown skin (about 10 × 20 mm) is thus removed along with subcutaneous tissue (it is important that none of the skin remains around the edge of the nail) (Fig. 6.14).
5. Cauterise any bleeding points, e.g. with a silver nitrate stick.
6. A 3 mm thick Sofra-tulle square is then placed directly over the wound, followed by a single gauze square (to wrap the toe), then a simple 25 mm Elastoplast pressure dressing.

Note: Bleeding can be a problem when the patient walks, so place a small plastic bag over the foot before pulling on the shoe. The patient should elevate the foot at home for an hour or so.

Follow-up

• Next day, the patient should soak the foot in lukewarm water for 15–20 minutes, gradually peel off the old dressing and then apply several layers of fine mesh gauze and tape them into place.
• Repeat the soaking procedure *religiously* 3 times daily for 20 minutes.
• Follow up the patient weekly for 4 weeks—cauterise any granulation tissue (a sign of poor compliance) with silver nitrate and dress.

The 'plastic gutter' method

This simple method separates the ingrowing nail from the skin to allow healing.

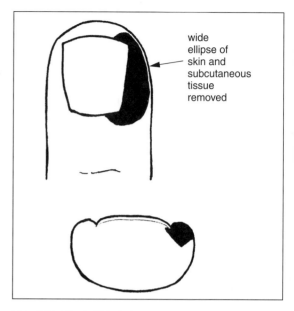

Fig. 6.14 Elliptical block dissection open method

Method

1. Cut a length (to match the nail) of tubing from a scalp vein plastic cannula and cut it down the middle to form a hemi-cylinder.
2. Under suitable local anaesthetic lift the skin around the ingrowing toenail with forceps and insert the tubing (Fig. 6.15). Leave it in place for one week covered with a dressing. It can be stitched to the skin.
3. Repeat if necessary.

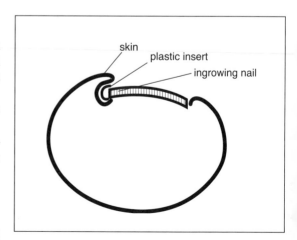

Fig. 6.15 Illustration of the 'plastic gutter' method

Tip for post-operative pain relief

Procedures on the toe, especially for ingrown toenails, can be very painful, especially during the night after the surgery.

Plan these procedures as the final appointment for the day and use the long-acting local anaesthetic bupivacaine 0.5% (Marcaine).

Paronychia

The extent of the procedure depends on the extent of the infection (Fig. 6.16). For all methods anaesthetise the finger or toe with a digital block.

Method 1: Lateral focus of pus

1. With a size 11 or 15 scalpel blade incise over the focus of pus (Fig. 6.17a).
2. Probe deeply until all pus is released.
3. Insert a small wick into the wound and allow to heal.

Method 2: Central focus of pus

Elevate the eponychial fold with a pair of fine artery forceps (Fig. 6.17b). This will release the pus.

Method 3: Infection adjacent to nail

Gently pack a fine wisp of cotton wool or gauze into the space between the paronychia and the nail and apply povidone-iodine. Dry and repeat as necessary. It should be relatively painless.

Method 4: Extensive infection under nail

1. If the infection extends under the nail, this fold should be pushed back proximally with a small retractor to expose the nail base.
2. Elevate the nail base bluntly and excise the proximal end of the nail with sharp scissors (Fig. 6.17c). (Alternatively, the nail can be removed.)

3. Apply petroleum jelly gauze dressing and use a light splint for 3 days.
4. The patient should be encouraged to wear gloves to keep the area dry.

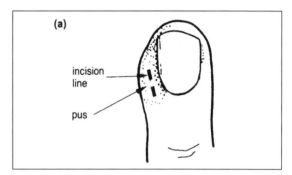

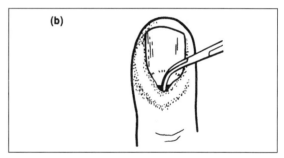

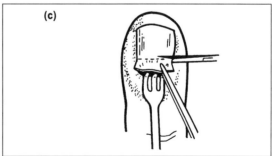

Fig. 6.17 Treatment of paronychia: **(a)** incision for lateral focus of pus; **(b)** elevation of eponychial fold; **(c)** excision of proximal end of nail   REPRODUCED FROM A. FORREST ET AL., *PRINCIPLES AND PRACTICE OF SURGERY*, CHURCHILL LIVINGSTONE, EDINBURGH, 1985, WITH PERMISSION

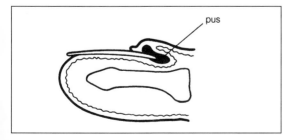

Fig. 6.16 Paronychia

Excision of nail bed

Method

1. Apply a tourniquet after digital or ring block.
2. Make skin incisions (Fig. 6.18a).
3. Avulse the nail using strong artery forceps.

4. Elevate the skin flaps (Fig. 6.18b).
5. Excise the nail bed carefully, including the undersurface of the overhanging skin (Fig. 6.18c).
6. Scrape the bone with a Volkman's spoon to ensure that no parts of the nail root remain.
7. Apply the phenolisation method also at this stage.
8. Suture the skin flaps (Fig. 6.18d).

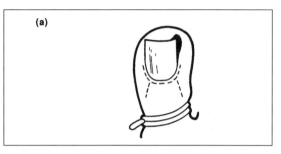

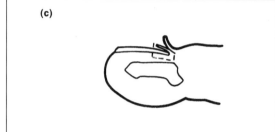

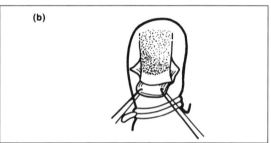

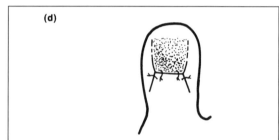

Fig. 6.18 Excision of nail bed: **(a)** skin incisions; **(b)** elevation of skin flap; **(c)** excision of nail bed; **(d)** suturing of skin flaps
REPRODUCED FROM A. FORREST ET AL., *PRINCIPLES AND PRACTICE OF SURGERY*, CHURCHILL LIVINGSTONE, EDINBURGH, 1985, WITH PERMISSION

Nail avulsion by chemolysis

Indication

Dystrophic toenails (e.g. from chronic fungal infection) in patients with peripheral vascular disease or other conditions where surgery is inadvisable.

Equipment

You will need:

- 40% salicylic acid ointment,
- plastic 'skin'.

Method

1. Apply plastic 'skin' spray to the skin around the nail to prevent possible skin maceration.
2. Apply 40% salicylic acid ointment to the nail. Use a liberal application, but confine it to the nail.
3. Cover with plastic wrap.

Post-procedure

- Reapply the ointment every 2 days.
- Maintain for about 4 weeks.

  This treatment will soften and destroy the nail.

7 Common trauma

General

Essential tips for dealing with trauma

Stab wounds

Always assume (and look for) the presence of nerve, tendon or artery injury.

Foreign bodies

Buried wooden splinters and slivers of glass are old traps—if suspected and not found on simple exploration, order high-resolution ultrasound which is good at detecting wood and glass.

Jumping or falling from a substantial height onto feet

Always consider a fractured calcaneum, talus, spine (especially lumbar) or pelvis and central dislocation of hip.

Cut finger or toe

Always look for a peripheral nerve injury.

Finger tourniquet

If using a small tourniquet such as a rubber band for haemostasis, clip on a small artery forcep so it is not forgotten when you finish.

Other cautionary tips

- You can get concussion from a heavy fall onto the coccyx/sacrum.
- Think of a sewing needle in the knees of women and in the feet of children for unexplained pain.
- Treat (evacuate) haematomas of the nasal septum and ear because they can collapse cartilage.

- Beware of pressure gun injuries into soft tissue, especially those involving oil and paint.
- Beware of a painful immobile elbow in a child—look for a fracture which can cause trouble later.
- Beware of the scaphoid fracture after a fall onto an outstretched hand.

Finger trauma

Finger injuries can be treated by simple means, providing there is neither tendon nor nerve injuries complicating the lacerations or compound fractures involved.

Finger tip loss

Not all finger tip loss demands an immediate graft or tidy-up amputation. If there is no exposed phalanx tip and the area of exposed subdermal tissue is small, conservative management is best. Remember that a grafted finger tip is insensate. If the amputated skin tip is available it should be replaced (use Steri-strips or a couple of small sutures), as it may take as a graft or merely act as a good biological dressing.

Large skin loss

Apply a split skin graft, preferably using a Goulian knife with three spacing devices.

Amputated finger

In this emergency situation, instruct the patient to place the severed finger directly into a fluid-tight sterile container, such as a plastic bag or sterile specimen jar. Then place this 'unit' in a bag containing iced water with crushed ice.

Note: Never place the amputated finger directly in ice or in fluid such as saline. Fluid makes the tissue soggy, rendering microsurgical repair difficult.

Care of the finger stump

Apply a simple, sterile, loose, non-sticky dressing and keep the hand elevated.

Finger tip dressing

A method of applying a dressing (using an adhesive dressing strip) for an injured finger tip is described.

Method

1. Cut a suitable length of the dressing strip almost as long as the finger.
2. Cut through the adhesive margins to the central non-adhesive dressing about 1–1.5 cm from the top (Fig. 7.1).
3. Remove the backing from the lower larger segment and apply to the injured side of the finger. Wrap the adhesive part around the circumference of the finger.
4. Now remove the backing from the upper segment and fold it backwards over the tip, with the adhesive margins wrapped around the finger to provide the most effective dressing.

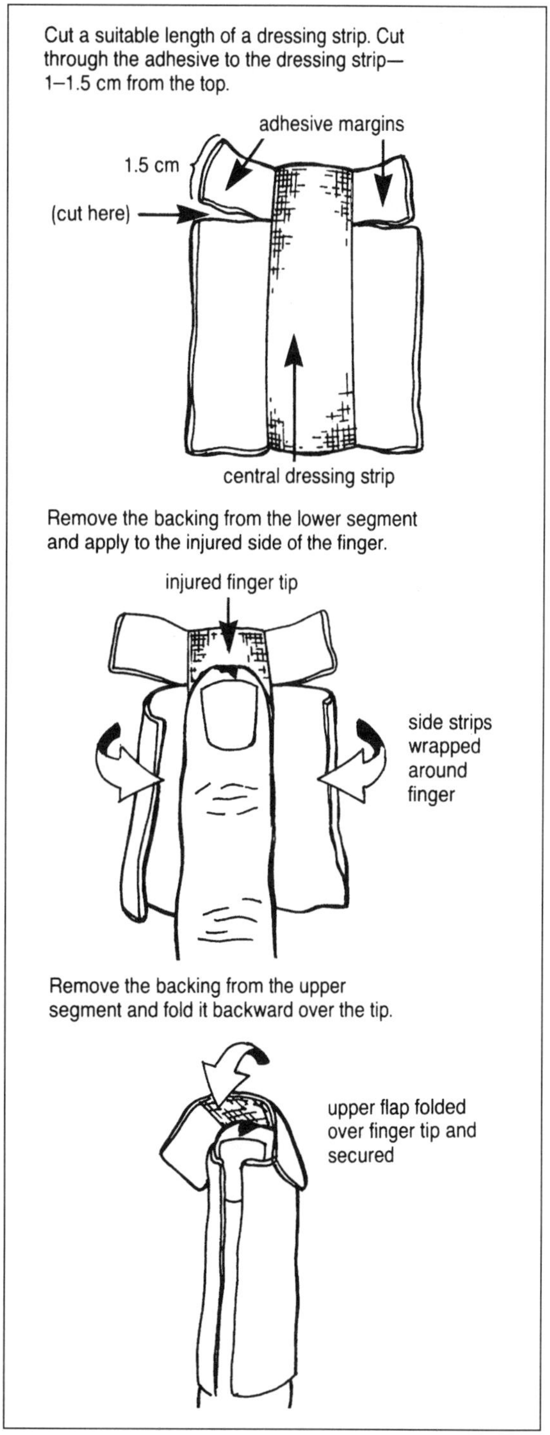

Cut a suitable length of a dressing strip. Cut through the adhesive to the dressing strip—1–1.5 cm from the top.

adhesive margins

1.5 cm

(cut here)

central dressing strip

Remove the backing from the lower segment and apply to the injured side of the finger.

injured finger tip

side strips wrapped around finger

Remove the backing from the upper segment and fold it backward over the tip.

upper flap folded over finger tip and secured

Fig. 7.1 Applying a finger tip dressing

Abrasions

Abrasions or 'gravel rash' vary considerably in degree and potential contamination. They are common with bicycle or motorcycle accidents and skateboard accidents. Special care is needed over joints such as the knee or elbow.

Management

- Clean meticulously, remove all ground-in dirt, metal, clothing and other material.
- Scrub out dirt with sterile normal saline under anaesthesia (local infiltration or general anaesthesia for deep wounds). Adequate local anaesthesia may also be achieved by coating the wound liberally with Xylocaine jelly 2% and leaving for 10 minutes.
- Treat the injury as a burn.
- When clean apply a protective dressing (some wounds may be left open).
- Use paraffin gauze and non-adhesive absorbent pads such as Melolin.
- Ensure adequate follow-up.
- Immobilise a joint that may be affected by a deep wound.

Haematomas

Haematoma of the pinna ('cauliflower ear')

When trauma to the pinna causes a haematoma between the epidermis and the cartilage, a permanent deformity known as 'cauliflower ear' may result. The haematoma, if left, becomes organised and the normal contour of the ear is lost.

The aim is to evacuate the haematoma as soon as practicable and then to prevent it re-forming. One can achieve a fair degree of success even on haematomas that have been present for several days.

Method

1. After cleansing the pinna with a suitable solution (e.g. cetrimide), insert a 25-gauge needle into the haematoma and aspirate the extravasated blood.
2. Position the needle at the lowest point while pressing the upper border of the haematoma gently between finger and thumb (Fig. 7.2a).
3. Apply a padded test tube clamp to the haematoma site and leave on for 30–40 minutes. The test tube clamp has large jaws that allow it to be placed over the haematoma site (Fig. 7.2b).

Generally, daily aspirations and clamping are sufficient to eradicate the haematoma completely.

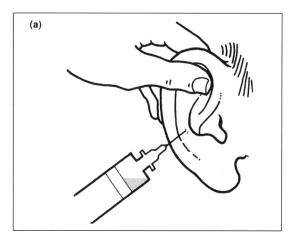

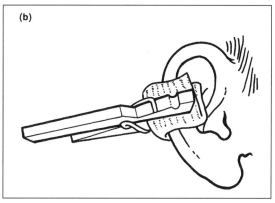

Fig. 7.2 Treatment of cauliflower ear

Haematoma of the nasal septum

Septal haematoma following injury to the nose can cause total nasal obstruction. It is easily diagnosed as a marked swelling on both sides of the septum when inspected through the nose (Fig. 7.3). It results from haemorrhage between the two sheets of muco-periosteum covering the septum. It may be associated with a fracture of the nasal septum.

Note: This is a most serious problem as it can develop into a septal abscess. The infection can pass readily to the orbit or the cavernous sinus through thrombosing veins and may prove fatal, especially in children. Otherwise it may lead to necrosis of the nasal septal cartilage followed by collapse and nasal deformity.

Treatment

- Remove the blood clot on both sides through an incision, under local anaesthetic. This must be done within 2 hours of injury.
- Prescribe systemic (oral) antibiotics, e.g. penicillin or erythromycin.
- Treat as a compound fracture if an X-ray reveals a fracture.

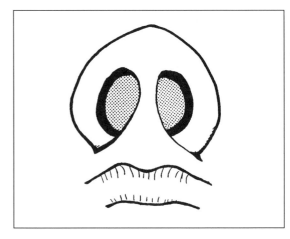

Fig. 7.3 Inferior view of nasal cavity showing bilateral swelling of septal haematoma

Pretibial haematoma

A haematoma over the tibia (shin bone) can be persistently painful and slow to resolve. An efficient method is, under very strict asepsis, to inject 1 mL of 1% of lignocaine and 1 mL of hyaluronidase and follow with immediate ultrasound. This may disperse or require drainage.

Roller injuries to limbs

A patient who has been injured by a wheel or by rollers passing over a limb can present a difficult problem. An arm caught in the wringers of an old-fashioned washing machine used to be a common example, but a more likely problem now is the wheel of a vehicle passing over a limb, especially a leg.

A freely spinning wheel is not so dangerous, but serious injuries occur when a non-spinning (braked) wheel passes over a limb, and then perhaps reverses over it. This leads to a 'degloving' injury due to shearing stress. The limb may look satisfactory initially, but skin necrosis will follow.

To manage a 'wheel over the limb' injury, treat it as a serious problem and admit the patient to hospital for observation. Surgical intervention with removal of necrotic fat may be essential. Fasciotomy with open drainage may also be an option.

Fractures

Testing for fractures

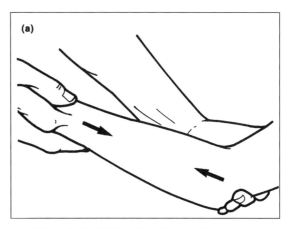

This method describes the simple principle of applying axial compression for the clinical diagnosis of fractures of bones. It applies especially to suspected fractures of bones of the forearm and hand, but also applies to all bones of the limbs.

Many fractures are obvious when applying the classic methods of diagnosis: pain, tenderness, loss of function, deformity, swelling and sometimes crepitus. It is sometimes more difficult if there is associated soft-tissue injury from a blow or if there is only a minor fracture such as a greenstick fracture of the distal radius.

If the bone is compressed gently from end to end, a fracture will reveal itself and the patient will feel pain. A soft-tissue injury of the forearm will show pain, tenderness, swelling and possibly loss of function. It will, however, not be painful if the bone is compressed axially—that is, in its long axis.

Walking is another method of applying axial compression, and this is very difficult (because of pain) in the presence of a fracture in the weight-bearing axis or pelvis. Hence, every patient with a suspected fracture of the lower limb should be tested by walking.

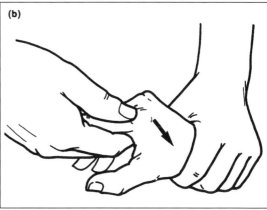

Fig. 7.4 Testing for fractures: **(a)** axial compression to detect a fracture of the radius or ulnar bones; **(b)** axial compression to detect a fracture of the metacarpal

Method

1. Grasp the affected area both distally and proximally with your hands.
2. Compress along the long axis of the bones by pushing in both directions, so that the forces focus on the affected area (fracture site; Fig. 7.4a). Alternatively, compression can be applied from the distal end with stabilising counterpressure applied proximally (Fig. 7.4b).
3. The patient will accurately localise the pain at the fracture site.

Spatula test for fracture of mandible

A simple office test for a suspected fractured mandible is to get the patient to bite on a wooden tongue depressor (or similar firm object).

Ask them to maintain this bite as you twist the spatula (Fig. 7.5). If they have a fracture, they cannot hang on to the spatula because of pain.

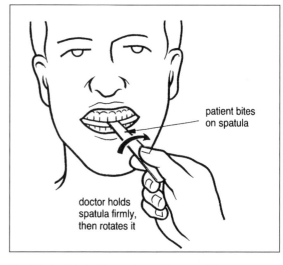

patient bites on spatula

doctor holds spatula firmly, then rotates it

Fig 7.5 Spatula test for fracture of the mandible

First aid management of fractured mandible

- Check the patient's bite and airway.
- Remove any free-floating tooth fragments and retain them.
- Replace any avulsed or subluxed teeth in their sockets.

Note: Never discard teeth.

- First aid immobilisation with a four-tailed bandage (Fig. 7.6).

Treatment

Refer for possible internal fixation.

A fracture of the body of the mandible will usually heal in 6–12 weeks (depending on the nature of the fracture and the fitness of the patient).

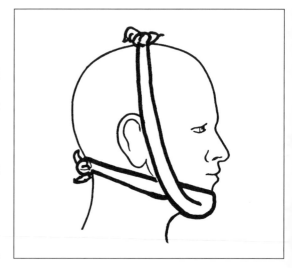

Fig. 7.6. Immobilisation of a fractured mandible in a four-tailed bandage

Fractured clavicle

There is a history of a fall onto the outstretched hand or elbow. The patient has pain aggravated by shoulder movement and usually supports the arm at the elbow and clasped to the chest. The most common fracture site is at the junction of the outer and middle thirds, or in the middle third.

Treatment

- St John elevated sling to support the arm—for 3 weeks.
- Figure-of-eight bandage (used mainly for severe discomfort).

- Early active exercises to elbow, wrist and fingers.
- Active shoulder movements as early as possible.

Special problem

Fracture at the lateral end of the bone. Consider referral for open reduction.

Healing time

4–8 weeks.
  The healing times for uncomplicated fractures are presented in Table 7.1, page 109.

Bandage for fractured clavicle

A figure-of-eight bandage can be made simply by inserting pads of cotton wool into pantyhose or stockings.

Fractured rib

A simple rib fracture can be extremely painful. The first treatment strategy is to prescribe analgesics such as paracetamol, and encourage breathing within the limits of pain.

  If pain persists in cases of single or double rib fracture with no complication, application of a rib support is most helpful.

The universal rib belt

A special elastic rib belt can provide thoracic support and mild compression for fractured ribs (Fig. 7.7). Despite its flexibility it gives excellent support and symptom relief while permitting adequate lung expansion.

  The elastic belt is 15 cm wide and has Velcro grip fastening, so it can be applied to a variety of chest sizes.

Healing time

3–6 weeks.

Towel method

The patient can wrap a standard-sized towel (folded lengthwise to a third of its width) around the chest

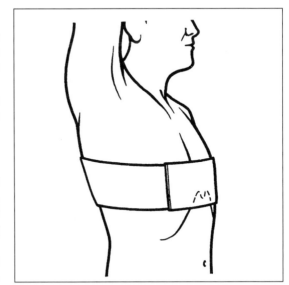

Fig 7.7 Method of application of rib belt

and secure it with a large safety pin. When the patient is about to cough, the towel can be pulled tight by the patient.

Phalangeal fractures

These fractures require as near perfect reduction as possible, careful splintage and, above all, early mobilisation once the fracture is stable—usually in 2 or 3 weeks.

Early operative intervention should be considered if the fracture is unstable.

Angulation is usually obvious, but it is most important to check for rotational malalignment, especially with torsional fracture. A simple method is to get the patient to make a fist of the hand and check the direction in which the nails are facing. Furthermore, each finger can be flexed in turn and checked to see if the fingertips point towards the tubercule of the scaphoid (palpable halfway along the base of the thenar eminence and 1.5 cm distal to the distal wrist crease).

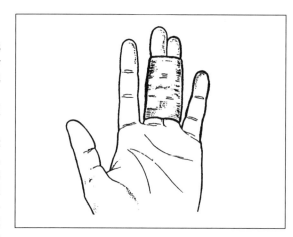

Fig. 7.8 Treatment of non-displaced phalanges by 'buddy strapping': the fractured finger is strapped to an adjacent healthy finger.

The phalanges

- Distal phalanges: usually crush fractures; generally heal simply unless intra-articular.
- Middle phalanges: tend to be displaced and unstable—beware of rotation.
- Proximal phalanges: are the greatest concern, especially of the little finger; intra-articular fractures usually need internal fixation.

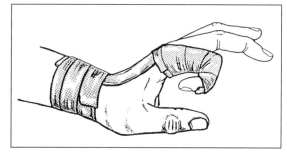

Fig. 7.9 Method of splinting a phalangeal fracture of the index finger by a posterior plaster slab

Treatment of uncomplicated fractures

For non-displaced phalanges with no rotational malalignment, strap the injured finger to the adjacent normal finger with an elastic garter or adhesive tape for 2–3 weeks, i.e. 'buddy strapping' (Fig. 7.8). Start the patient on active exercises.

If pain and swelling is a problem, splint the finger with a narrow dorsal or anterior slab (a felt-lined strip of malleable aluminium can be used) (Fig. 7.9). An alternative is to bandage the hand while the patient holds a tennis ball or appropriate roll of bandage in order to maintain appropriate flexion of all interphalangeal joints.

Slings for fractures

There are three slings in common use in first aid:

Sling	Main indications
Collar and cuff	Fractured humerus
Broad arm	Fractured forearm
St John	Fractured clavicle
	Dislocated acromioclavicular joint
	Subluxed acromioclavicular joint
	Infected or fractured hand

Collar and cuff sling

This is useful for the patient with a fractured humerus, because it allows gravity to realign the distal and proximal parts of the fractured bones.

Method

1. Using a narrow bandage, make a clove hitch (Fig. 7.10a). The cove hitch is made by fashioning two loops—one towards your body and the other away, leaving one end of the bandage longer than the other. Now place your fingers under the loops and bring them together.
2. Slide the loops over the wrist of the injured arm with the knot of the clove hitch on the thumb side of the wrist.
3. Gently flex the elbow and elevate the injured arm so that the fingers point towards the opposite shoulder (Fig. 7.10b).

4. Place the long end of the bandage around the neck and tie the bandage, using a reef knot (Fig. 7.10c).

The broad arm sling

This has multiple uses but is used mainly for injuries to the forearm and wrist.

Method

1. Place an open triangular bandage over the patient's chest, with the point of the triangle stretching beyond the elbow of the injured side. Place the flexed forearm over the bandage as shown (see Fig. 7.11a overleaf).
2. Carry the upper end of the bandage over the shoulder on the uninjured side, around the back of the neck. Ensure that the injured arm lies slightly above the horizontal position.
3. Tie the long ends of the bandage in the hollow above the collar bone of the injured side (see Fig. 7.11b overleaf).
4. Fold the corner adjacent to the injured elbow and secure it with a safety pin.

The St John sling

This sling, used for a fractured clavicle, dislocated acromioclavicular joint, or fractured or infected hand, supports the elbow and keeps the hand in elevation resting comfortably on the shoulder of the uninjured side. (*continues*)

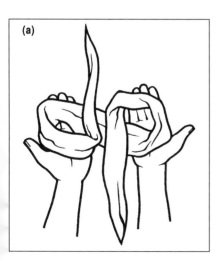

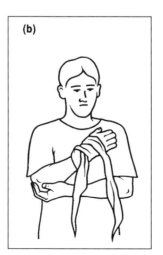

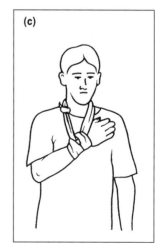

Fig. 7.10 **(a)** Preparing a clove hitch; **(b)** flex the elbow and elevate the injured arm; **(c)** applying a collar and cuff sling

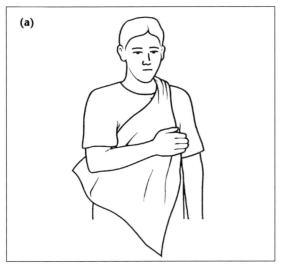
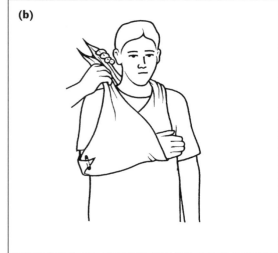

Fig. 7.11 **(a)** The broad arm sling: first step; **(b)** the broad arm sling

Method

1. Place an open triangular bandage over the patient's forearm and hand with the point of the triangle to the elbow and the upper end over the far shoulder.
2. Tuck the long edge of the bandage under the whole forearm to make a supporting trough (Fig. 7.12a).

3. Convey the lower dependent end around the patient's back to the front of the far shoulder.
4. Tie the ends as close to the fingers as possible (Fig. 7.12b).
5. Tuck the triangular point firmly in between the forearm and the bandage.
6. Secure the fold with a safety pin when the sling is firm, comfortable and at the correct elevation.

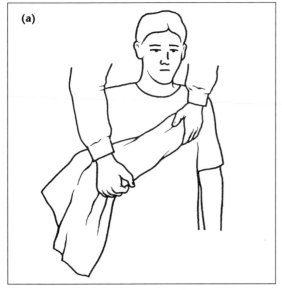
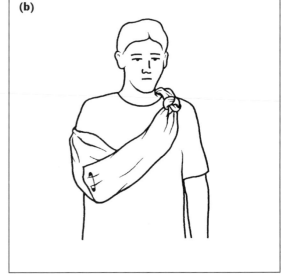

Fig. 7.12 **(a)** The St John sling: first step; **(b)** the St John sling

The makeshift sling

An effective sling can be made with a large jumper or windcheater.

Method

1. Place the sleeves of the jumper around the neck and knot the ends.
2. Guide the affected arm into the sleeve until a suitable recess is found.

Important principles for fractures

- Children under 8 years usually take half the time to heal.
- Have a check X-ray in 1 week (for most fractures).
- Radiological union lags behind clinical union.

Table 7.1 Healing of uncomplicated fractures (adults)

Fracture	(Approximate) average immobilisation time (weeks)
Rib	3–6 (healing time)
Clavicle	4–8 (2 weeks in sling)
Scapula	weeks to months
Humerus	
• neck	3–6
• shaft	8
• condyles	3–4
Radius	
• head of radius	3
• shaft	6
• Colles' fracture	4–6
Radius and ulna (shafts)	6–12
Ulna—shaft	8
Scaphoid	8–12
Metacarpals	
• Bennett's #	6–8
• other	3–4
Phalanges (hand)	
• proximal	3
• middle	2–3
• distal	2–3
Pelvis	Rest in bed 2–6
Femur	
• femoral neck	according to surgery
• shaft	12–16
• distal	8–12
Patella	3–4
Tibia	12–16
Fibula	6
Both tibia and fibula	12–16
Potts fracture	6–8
Lateral malleolus avulsion	3
Calcaneus	
• minor	4–6
• compression	14–16
Talus	12
Tarsal bones (stress #)	8
Metatarsals	4
Phalanges (toes)	0–3
Spine	
• spinous process	3
• transverse process	3
• stable vertebra	3
• unstable vertebra	9–14
• sacrum/coccyx	3

Other trauma

Primary repair of severed tendon

Immediate repair of cut tendons by primary suture is important, preferably by an experienced surgeon. Partial ruptures usually require no active surgery, although primary repair is recommended if greater than 40% of the tendon is severed.

Method for totally cut tendon

1. Debride the wound.
2. Pass a loop suture of 3/0 monofilament nylon on a straight needle into the tendon through the cut surface close to the edge to emerge 5 mm beyond and then construct a figure-of-eight suture as shown in Figure 7.13a–c.

3. Pull the two ends of the suture to take up the slack without bunching the tendon (Fig. 7.13d).
4. Repeat this with the other end of the tendon (Fig. 7.13e).
5. Tie the corresponding suture ends together in order to closely approximate the cut ends of the tendon (Fig. 7.13f).
6. Bury the knots deep between the tendon and cut the sutures short (Fig. 7.13g).

Post-operation

Hold the repaired tendons in a relaxed position with suitable splintage for 3–4 weeks.

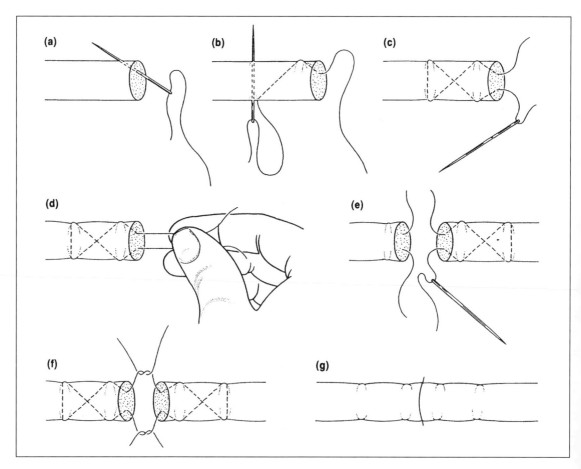

Fig. 7.13 Primary suture of a cut tendon: **(a–c)** Inserting figure-of-eight suture; **(d)** pulling the two ends of the suture; **(e)** inserting a similar suture in the other end of the tendon; **(f)** tying the sutures and burying the knots; **(g)** suture is completed

Burns

First aid

The immediate treatment of burns, especially for smaller areas, is immersion in cold running water such as tap water, for a minimum of 10–15 minutes (ideally 20 minutes). Do not disturb charred adherent clothing but remove wet clothing.

Chemical burns should be liberally irrigated with water. Apply 1 in 10 diluted vinegar to alkali burns and sodium bicarbonate solution for acid burns.

Refer the following burns to hospital:

- >9% surface area, especially in a child
- >5% in an infant
- all deep burns
- burns of difficult or vital areas (e.g. face, hands perineum/genitalia, feet)
- burns with potential problems (e.g. electrical, chemical, circumferential)
- suspicion of inhalational injury

Always give adequate pain relief. During transport, continue cooling by using a fine mist water spray.

Treatment

1. *Very superficial—intact skin.* Can be left with application of a mild antiseptic only. Review if blistering.
2. *Superficial—blistered skin.* Apply a dressing to promote epithelialisation (e.g. hydrocolloid sheets, hydrogel sheets) covered by an absorbent dressing

or (best option)

a retention stretch adhesive material (e.g. Fixomull, Mefix, Hypafix) with daily or twice daily cleaning of the serous ooze and reapplication of outer bandage. Leave 7 days. Fixomull can be left in place for up to 2 weeks.

Guidelines to patient for retention dressings

- First 24 hours: keep dry. If there is any ooze coming through the dressing, pat dry with a clean tissue.
- From day 2: wash over dressing twice daily. Use gentle soap and water, rinse then pat dry. Do not

soak. Rinse only. Do not remove the dressing as it may cause pain and damage to the wound. If the wound becomes red, hot or swollen or if pain increases, return to the clinic.
- From day 7: return to the clinic for removal of the dressing. Two hours prior to coming into the clinic, soak the dressing with olive oil then cover with Glad Wrap.

Note: Dressing must be soaked off with oil (e.g. olive, baby, citrus or peanut). Debride 'popped blisters'. Only pop blisters that interfere with dermal circulation.

3. *Deep burns.* If considerable ooze, apply the following in order:

- Solosite gel
- non-adherent neutral dressing (e.g. Melolin)
- layer of absorbent gauze or cotton wool (larger burns)

Change every 2–4 days with analgesic cover. Surgical treatment, including skin grafting, may be necessary.

Exposure (open method)

- Keep open without dressings (good for face, perineum or single surface burns).
- Renew coating of antiseptic cream every 24 hours.

Dressings (closed method)

- Suitable for circumferential wounds.
- Cover creamed area with non-adherent tulle (e.g. paraffin gauze).
- Dress with an absorbent bulky layer of gauze and wool.
- Use a plaster splint if necessary.

Burns to the hand

For superficial blistered burns to the hand or similar 'complex' shaped parts of the body apply strips of the retention stretch adhesive dressings as described above. They conform well to digits. Apply an outer bandage. At 7 days soak the dressings in oil for two hours prior to coming into the clinic.

Rapid testing of the hand for nerve injury

Following an injury to the arm or hand that has the potential for a nerve injury, it is important when one examines a hand to have a knowledge of simple tests that detect injuries to the three main nerves—the median, the ulnar and the radial.

The 'quick' hand test for nerve injury

Get the patient to make the following configurations:

- '4-fingered cone' (Fig. 7.14a)—if the patient can do this, the ulnar nerve is intact,

- '5-fingered cone' and ability to approximate the thumb (Fig. 7.14b)—success means the median nerve is intact,
- 'trigger test' for the thumb—that is, extension—if normal, the radial nerve is intact (Fig. 7.14c).

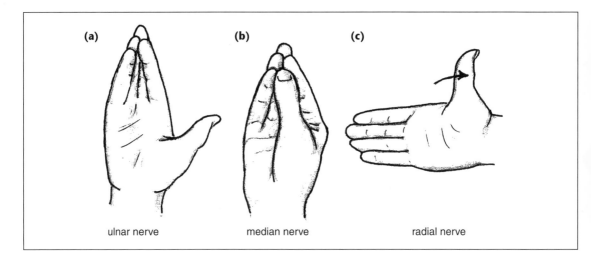

Fig. 7.14 Rapid testing of the hand for nerve injury

Froment's sign

Ask the patient to grip a sheet of paper forcefully between the thumbs and index fingers while the examiner tries to pull the paper away. A positive Froment's sign is strong flexion of the interphalangeal joint of the thumb. This occurs because of loss of action of adductor pollicis caused by injury to the deep branch of the ulnar nerve. Flexor pollicis longus overcompensates.

8 Removal of foreign bodies

General

Cautionary note

Failure to diagnose the presence of a foreign body has emerged as a common cause of malpractice actions against general practitioners. It is particularly important to locate and remove foreign bodies, especially splinters in children, glass slivers after motor vehicle accidents and pub brawls and metal objects such as needles in the feet of children.

Removal of maggots

The larvae of the common blowfly can find their way into the most unexpected corners of the body, and can be extremely difficult to remove.

This unusual problem is more likely to occur in unkempt people, such as alcoholics and itinerants, and in those with exposed wounds. Examples of sites that can become infested are the eye, the ear, traumatic wounds in comatose victims, and rodent ulcers.

The eye

The presence of maggots should be suspected when an unkempt person presents with a red eye and with marked swelling (Fig. 8.1). When disturbed, the maggots crawl for cover and are difficult to see and remove.

Method

1. Instil LA (e.g. amethocaine).
2. Instil two drops of eserine or pilocarpine to 'paralyse' the maggots.
3. Remove the maggots with fine forceps.

Wounds

A writhing mass of maggots can be a difficult problem, and has to be rendered inactive. The old 'trick' was to use chloroform, but ether is just as effective.

Method

1. Irrigate the infested wound with the anaesthetic until the activity ceases.
2. Carefully remove all the intruders.

Using dextrose

Apply 10% dextrose to the maggots. If unsuccessful apply 50% dextrose.

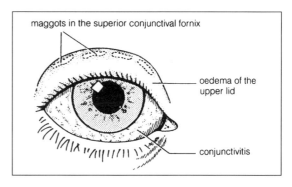

Fig. 8.1 Maggots in the eye

Removal of leeches

There are several varieties of leeches in this country, but the most troublesome are the small, black leeches that inhabit the damp forests of New South Wales, Victoria and Tasmania. The major problem is the difficulty of removing a parasite adhering firmly to such awkward anatomical sites as the eye, or the urethral meatus in men.

No attempt should be made to extract the leech manually. There are several methods of inducing leeches to 'jump off' rapidly:

- application of hot objects,
- application of salt,
- application of a detergent,
- application of toothpaste,
- slicing the leech in half with a knife.

Method

1. Carefully apply a hot object near the end of the leech. The object could be the hot tip of a snuffed out match (Fig. 8.2) or the heated end of a paper clip.
2. The leech soon lets go!

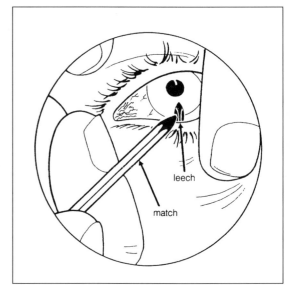

Fig. 8.2 Removal of leech from the eye

Removal of ring from finger

From time to time one is faced with the need to remove a ring from a swollen finger. Destruction of a possibly valuable piece of jewellery can often be avoided by the following.

Method

1. Using a needle, bent paper clip or bobby pin, pass a length of dental tape (the best), cord or string (or Mersilk) under the ring (Fig. 8.3a). The ring should be over the narrowest part of the phalanx for this.
2. Liberally apply petroleum jelly or moistened soap paste to the finger, distal to the ring. Wind about six turns of the string around the finger close to and immediately distal to the ring (Fig. 8.3b).
3. While holding the end (B) of the cord firmly, pull the proximal end (A) over the ring, roughly parallel to the long axis of the finger, unwinding it steadily in the same direction in which the distal coils were wound originally (Fig. 8.3c). The pressure of the cord is thus applied successively around the periphery of the ring, forcing it distally. The distal cords, by applying pressure, also help to reduce the oedema of the finger.

In many cases the ring slides off with little or no discomfort and without damage to ring or finger.
Sometimes a digital block may be necessary.

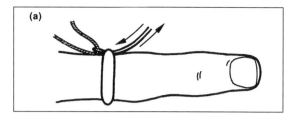

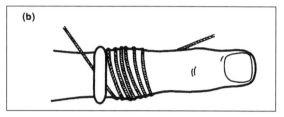

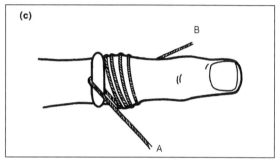

Fig. 8.3 Removal of ring from finger: **(a)** thread string through bobby pin or needle passed under ring; **(b)** wind string firmly round finger after liberally applying Vaseline; **(c)** hold firm at B and pull and unwind at A

Skin

Splinters under the skin

The splinter under the skin is a common and difficult procedural problem. Instead of using forceps or making a wider excision, one method is to use a disposable hypodermic needle to 'spear' the splinter (Fig. 8.4) and then use it as a lever to ease the splinter out through the skin.

Reactive objects such as thorns, spines and wood should be removed as soon as possible.

Superficial horizontal splinters

These use usually readily palpated under the skin. Apply antiseptic and infiltrate with local anaesthetic.

Incise the skin over the length of the splinter using a no. 15 scalpel blade, to completely expose the splinter. Lift it out with the scalpel blade or with forceps.

Alternatively, the overlying skin can be deroofed with a sterile 19-gauge needle in a feathering motion and then speared out with the aid of fine forceps.

The vertical splinter

This is more difficult but can be removed by making a superficial circular excision over the splinter followed by a deeper encircling incision to undermine the sides of the wound. The free central block of tissue containing the object can be picked out with fine forceps (Fig. 8.5).

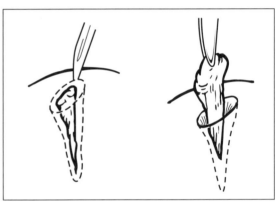

Fig. 8.5 Method of removal of the vertical splinter

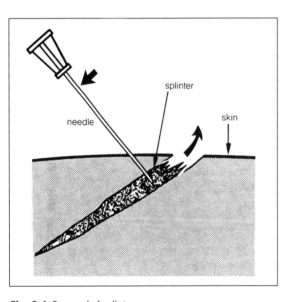

Fig. 8.4 Removal of splinters

Detecting fine skin splinters— the soft soap method

Problem

Finding fine foreign bodies in the skin that are difficult to see, such as cactus spurs and glass slivers.

Method

1. Spread soft soap very lightly over the skin. The soap permits easier identification of the foreign bodies.
2. Remove the foreign bodies with splinter (or other types) forceps.

Alternatively they can be removed with hair removal wax applied to the skin.

Detecting skin splinters

High-resolution ultrasound imaging by experienced operators can assist in both the diagnosis and removal of these foreign bodies. Table 8.1 shows the comparative efficacy of X-rays and ultrasound.

CT scans are also very effective.

Table 8.1 Efficacy of X-ray and ultrasound

Material	Plain X-ray	Ultrasound
Wood	Poor	Good
Glass	Good	Good
Metal	Good	Good
Plastic	Moderate	Good
Plant (e.g. thorns)	Poor	Good

Detecting metal fragments

A simple tip for detecting subcutaneous metal pieces is to use a magnet and run it over the skin. If the metal 'tents' the skin, this is the site to make the incision.

Embedded ticks

Some species of ticks can be very dangerous to human beings, especially to children. If they attach themselves to the head and neck, a serious problem is posed. As it is impossible to distinguish between dangerous and non-dangerous ticks, early removal is mandatory. The tick should be totally removed, and the mouthparts of the tick must not be left behind. Do not attempt to grab the tick by the body and tug. This is rarely successful in dislodging the tick, and more toxin is thereby injected into the host.

As an office procedure, many practitioners grasp the tick's head as close to the skin as possible with fine forceps or tweezers, and pull the tick out sideways with a sharp rotatory action. This is acceptable, but not as effective as the methods described here.

First aid bush removal method

1. Saturate the tick with petrol, kerosene or insect repellant such as Rid, and leave for 3 minutes.
2. Loop a strong thread around the tick's head as close to the skin as possible, and pull sharply.

Alternative methods

- Apply tea-tree oil 12-hourly—leave 24 hours and remove.

- Apply 5% acetic acid firmly onto the tick with a cotton bud. Wait 30 seconds, then slowly turn the end of the bud until the tick is dislodged.

Shock freezing

Freeze the tick with liquid nitrogen Kryospray and remove it in toto.

Lignocaine anaesthetic method

Infiltrate 1% lignocaine under and around the head of the tick. It should then be easily extracted because of immobilisation and eversion of the mouth parts. If not, move on to the office procedure.

Loop of suture material method

1. Select a long length of 3/0 nylon or silk.
2. Loop it over the tick and tie a single knot.
3. Holding the nylon flush with the skin, slowly tighten the knot over the neck of the tick.
4. Pull off the tick with a sharp rotatory action.

Office procedure

1. Infiltrate a small amount of LA in the skin around the site of embedment.
2. With a no. 11 or 15 scalpel blade make the necessary very small excision, including the

(continues)

mouth parts of the tick to ensure total removal (Fig. 8.6).

3. The small defect can usually be closed with a Bandaid (or Steri-strips).

Punch biopsy method

A very practical method is to inject local anaesthetic and then use a punch biopsy to remove the entire tick. If the punch will not fit over the tick cut it behind its head and then punch out the head parts. Use a cross pulley stitch (Fig. 2.5, page 34) to close the wound.

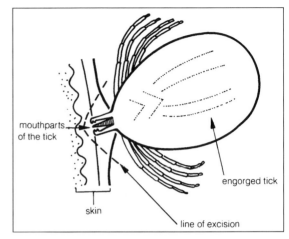

Fig. 8.6 Removing the embedded tick

Embedded fish hooks

Five methods of removing fish hooks are presented here, some relying on removal in a direction continuous with their direction of entry to conform with the nature of the barb, others requiring removal in the reverse direction, against the barb. Method 4 or 5 is recommended as first-line management.

Method 1

1. Inject 1–2 mL of LA in front of and then below the hook.
2. Cut the shank with wire cutters or pliers below the eye (Fig. 8.7a). Alternatively, repeated bending at this point will cause the shank to snap.
3. With a needle holder grasp the shank, press the point of the barb through the skin and remove.

Method 2

1. A sharp pull in the direction shown (Fig. 8.7b) will in most cases make the barb continue on its natural path and come out through the skin.
2. It can then be cut off easily and the rest of the hook extracted.

No surgical instruments are required, simply a pair of pliers or wire cutters, but all personnel present should close their eyes when the barb is cut off.

Method 3

1. Inject 1–2 mL of LA around the fish hook.
2. Grasp the shank of the hook with strong artery forceps.
3. Slide a D11 scalpel blade in along the hook, sharp edge away from the hook, to cut the tissue and free the barb (Fig. 8.7c).
4. Withdraw the hook with the forceps.

Method 4

This method, used by some fishermen, relies on a loop of cord or fishing line to forcibly disengage and extract the hook intact. It requires no anaesthesia and no instruments—only nerves of steel, especially for the first attempt.

1. Take a piece of string about 10–12 cm long and make a loop. One end slips around the hook as a double loop, the other hooking around one finger of the operator.
2. Depress the shank with the other hand in the direction that tends to disengage the barb.
3. At this point give a very swift, sharp tug along the cord. (Some find that using a ruler in the loop to flick out the hook is ideal.)
4. The hook flies out painlessly in the direction of the tug (Fig. 8.7d).

Note: You must be bold, decisive, confident and quick, as half-hearted attempts do not work.

For difficult cases, some local anaesthetic infiltration may be appropriate. Instead of a short loop of cord, a long piece of fishing line double-looped around the hook and tugged by the hand will work.

Method 5

This method, regarded by some as the best, involves 'flicking' the hook out by traversing its path of entry into the skin.

1. Loop a length of fishing tackle around the eye of the hook.
2. Loop a length of string around the front curve of the hook.
3. Keep the fishing tackle taut by holding it firmly in a straight line with the non-dominant hand.
4. Now pull sharply outwards with the dominant hand so that it flicks the hook out (Fig. 8.7e).

Caution: Take care not to let the hook fly off uncontrollably.

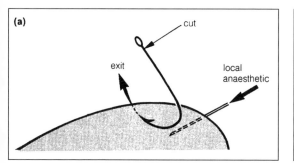

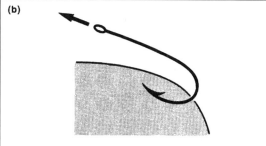

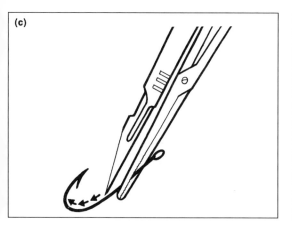

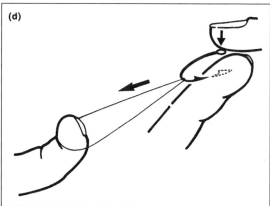

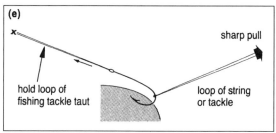

Fig. 8.7 Five methods of removing fish hooks: **(a)** cutting the shank; **(b)** cutting the barb; **(c)** cutting a skin path; **(d)** intact removal; **(e)** using double string method

Penetrating gun injuries

Injuries to the body from various types of guns present decision dilemmas for the treating doctor. The tips below represent guidelines including special sources of danger to tissues from various foreign materials discharged by guns.

Gunshot wounds

Airgun

The rule is to remove subcutaneous slugs but to leave deeper slugs unless they lie within and around vital structures (e.g. the wrist). A special, common problem is that of slugs in the orbit. These often do little damage and can be left alone, but referral to an ophthalmologist would be appropriate.

0.22 rifle (pea rifle)

The same principles of management apply but the bullet must be localised precisely by X-ray. Of particular interest are abdominal wounds, which should be observed carefully, as visceral perforations can occur with minimal initial symptoms and signs.

0.410 shotgun

The pellets from this shotgun are usually dangerous only when penetrating from a close range. Again, the rule is not to remove deep-lying pellets—perhaps only those superficial pellets that can be palpated.

Pressure gun injuries

Injection of grease, oil, paint and similar substances from pressure guns (Fig. 8.8) cause very serious injuries, requiring decompression and removal of the substances.

Grease gun and paint gun

High-pressure injection of paint or grease into the hand requires urgent surgery if amputation is to be avoided. There is a deceptively minor wound to show for this injury, and after a while the hand feels comfortable. However, ischaemia, chemical irritation and infection can follow, with gangrene of the digits, resulting in, at best, a claw hand due to sclerosis. Treatment is by immediate decompression and meticulous removal of all foreign material and necrotic tissue.

Oil injection

Accidental injection of an inoculum in an oily vehicle into the hand also creates a serious problem with local tissue necrosis. If injected into the digital pulp, this may necessitate amputation. Such injections are common on poultry farms, where many fowl-pest injections are administered.

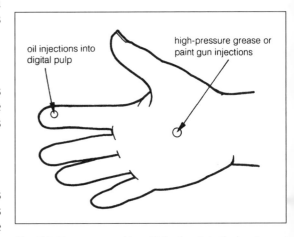

Fig. 8.8 Dangerous accidental injections into the hand

Ear, nose and throat

Removal of various foreign bodies

Removal of foreign bodies (FBs) from the nose in children is a relatively urgent procedure because of the risks of aspiration. The same mechanical principles of removal apply to the ear.

The nose should be examined using a nasal speculum under good illumination. The tip of the nose should be raised and pressed with the tip of a thumb. Do not attempt to remove foreign bodies from the nose by grasping with 'ordinary' forceps.

Summary of methods of removal

1. It is best to pass an instrument behind the FB and pull it forward. Examples of instruments are:

   - a eustachian catheter (Fig. 8.9a),
   - a probe to roll out FB,
   - a bent hair pin,
   - a bent paper clip.

2. Snaring the FB is the method most suitable for soft foreign bodies (e.g. paper, foam rubber, cotton wool). It is more applicable to the nose. Examples of instruments are:

   - a foreign-body remover (Fig. 8.9b),
   - crocodile forceps (Fig. 8.9c).

3. Application of suction which uses instruments such as:

   - a rubber catheter,
   - a fine sucker.

4. Irritation of FBs in nose (e.g. white pepper sprinkled in nose to induce sneezing).

Probe technique

The method shown in Figure 8.10 simply requires good vision, using a head mirror or head light and a thin probe.

Method

1. Insert the probe under and just beyond the FB (Fig. 8.10a).
2. Lever it in such a way that the tip of the probe 'rolls' the FB out of the obstructed passage (Fig. 8.10b,c).

   This technique seems to be successful with both hard and soft foreign bodies. (*continues*)

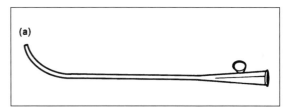

(a)

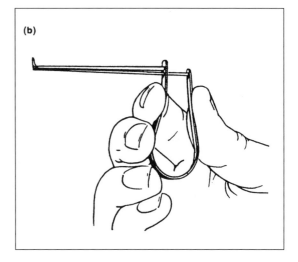

(b)

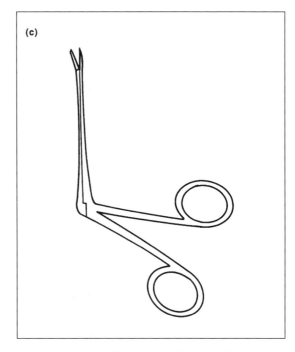

(c)

Fig. 8.9 Instruments for removal of foreign bodies: **(a)** eustachian catheter; **(b)** foreign-body remover; **(c)** crocodile forceps

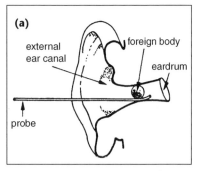 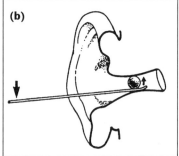 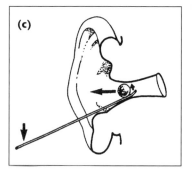

Fig. 8.10 Removal of foreign body from ear: **(a)** probe inserted under foreign body; **(b)** tip of probe is lifted by depressing outer end of probe; **(c)** continued levering 'rolls' the foreign body out

Bent hairpin technique

This method requires an old-fashioned hairpin (the type with crinkly edges) bent to an angle of about 30°.

Method

1. Push the pin back beyond the FB.
2. Depress the pin to ensnare the object.
3. Gently withdraw the FB (Fig. 8.11).

This method is relatively painless and highly effective; other methods of removing FBs may push them deeper into the nares.

Bent paper clip technique

A simple, effective and disposable instrument can be made with a paper clip.

Method

1. As demonstrated in Figure 8.12, open the paper clip with the hairpin bends at both ends intact.

2. Angulate the smaller end of the clip. The sharp ends of the hairpin bends should be bent towards the straight stems of the clip so that they do not cause trauma. The degree of angulation can be increased by the use of small-artery forceps if desired. The larger loop acts as a handle to get an effective grip.
3. The angulated end, passed gently over the foreign body in the nose or ear canal, acts as a scoop to remove the foreign body.

Note: It is important to remember that only foreign bodies that can easily be seen in the ear or nose could be removed by this method. The paper clip instrument is not suitable for the removal of deeper foreign bodies. Patient co-operation is also very important.

Rubber catheter suction technique

The following is a relatively simple and painless way of removing foreign bodies from the ears and noses of children.

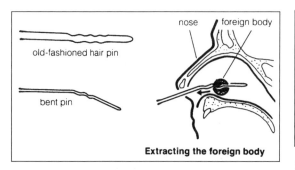

Fig. 8.11 Extracting the foreign body using a hairpin

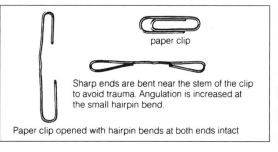

Fig. 8.12 Extracting the foreign body using a bent paper clip

The only equipment required is a straight rubber catheter (large type) and perhaps a suction pump. The procedure causes minimal distress to a frightened child, avoids the need for a general anaesthetic, and is less traumatic than mechanical extraction for objects such as a round bead.

Method

1. Cut the end of the catheter at right angles (Fig. 8.13a).
2. Smear the rim of the cut end with petroleum jelly.
3. Apply this end to the FB and then apply suction.

Oral suction may be used for a recently placed or 'clean' object, but gentle pump suction, if available, is preferred (Fig. 8.13b).

It is advisable to pinch close the suction catheter until close to the foreign body, as the hissing noise may frighten the child.

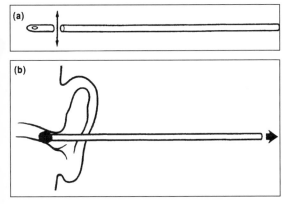

Fig. 8.13 Extracting the foreign body using a rubber catheter: **(a)** catheter cut straight across near its extremity; **(b)** application of suction (orally or by pump)

Pneumatic otoscopic attachment vacuum technique

The following method is ideal for the removal of a foreign body from the nose or ear of a child where it can be very difficult to extract without the use of a general anaesthetic. The method is similar to using a rubber catheter with the end cut off, and applying it to the foreign body using oral suction.

Method

- Use the pneumatic otoscope attachment by removing the end fitting.
- Squeeze the bulb to create a vacuum effect.
- Place the end of the rubber tubing against the foreign body (Fig. 8.14).
- Release the hand-squeeze on the bulb in order to create suction.
- Extract the object.

This method works very well for smooth, round foreign bodies such as beads.

Tissue glue and plastic swab technique

Method

This technique employs the simple method of applying a rapidly setting adhesive to bond the FB to the extracting probe. It works best in dry conditions and for a smooth non-impacted foreign body.

1. Apply a thin coat of cyanoacrylate or tissue glue to the end of a hollow plastic swab stick or orange stick.
2. Insert the stick into the ear canal (or nostril) to allow the glue to bond with the FB (if clearly accessible and suitable) for about 1 minute.

(continues)

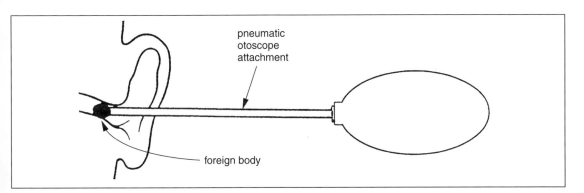

pneumatic otoscope attachment

foreign body

Fig. 8.14 The rubber tubing is placed against the foreign body

3. Remove the FB using gentle traction, perhaps assisted by external pressure from the fingers.

Caution: Avoid touching the skin or mucous membrane.

If glue is accidentally applied to the skin, dissolve the glue with acetone.

The 'kiss and blow' technique

This method is used for a co-operative child with a firm, round foreign body impacted in the anterior nares.

Method

1. Place your mouth over the child's mouth, blowing into the mouth until you feel a slight resistance. (This indicates that the glottis is closed.)

2. Then blow much harder to cause the foreign body to 'pop out'.

To encourage co-operation with the technique the child can be asked to give the doctor a 'kiss' (or any ruse to allow placement of the lips over the child's open mouth).

On all occasions that this technique has been used (adapted from an article in *The New England Medical Journal*), the foreign bodies 'popped out' after two attempts, thus avoiding general anaesthetic with intubation.

Insects in ears

Live insects should be killed by first instilling olive oil or Waxsol drops, then syringing the ear with warm water. Dead flies that have originally been attracted to pus are best removed by suction. Maggots are best killed by eserine drops, although other fluids should work. Syringing the ear is then appropriate.

Note: 2mL of 1% lignocaine introduced by the blunt end of a syringe or via a cut-off 'butterfly' needle (or other piece of plastic tubing) is also effective.

A moth in the ear

This is a very distressing sensation for the patient, who invariably telephones urgently at night with the problem.

First aid method

Instruct the patient to insert drops of olive oil or a similar preparation into the ear to kill the moth (Fig. 8.15a).

Note: Ideally olive oil should be gently warmed by, e.g., placing the bottle under running hot water from a tap for a short while.

Office procedure

Simply syringe the moth out of the ear with tepid water (Fig. 8.15b).

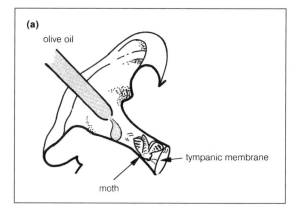

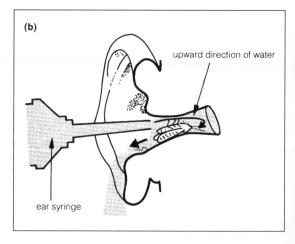

Fig. 8.15 Insect in ear: **(a)** first aid; **(b)** office procedure

General principles about a foreign body in the ear

The main danger of a foreign body in the ear lies in its careless removal.

Syringing is very effective and safe for small foreign bodies.

Vegetable foreign bodies, e.g. peas, swell with water and are better not syringed.

Insects commonly become wedged in the meatus, especially in the tropics. They can be syringed or removed with forceps under vision.

Maggots cause a painful ear and their removal is difficult—insufflation of pulv. calomel is usually effective treatment.

Cotton wool in the ear

A common problem is the finding of the cotton wool tip of a 'cotton bud' which has become dislodged from injudicious self ear toilet. It can be seen deep in the ear canal.

Method

Obtain a dental broach and fashion a very small hook on the end. When inserted in the ear canal under vision, this hook can easily engage some threads of cotton and then extraction of the foreign body is simple (Fig. 8.16).

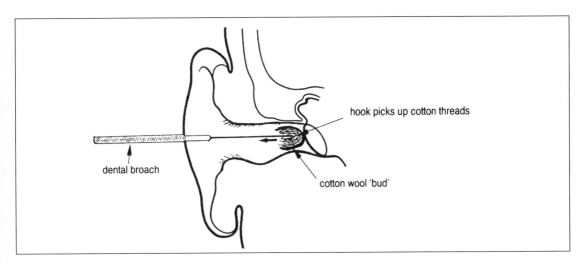

hook picks up cotton threads

dental broach

cotton wool 'bud'

Fig. 8.16 Removal of cotton wool bud from ear

Fish bones in the throat

After spraying the throat with local anaesthetic, use a frontal mirror and dental mirror to find the bone.

To overcome the difficulty of not having a spare hand to remove the bone, use a laryngoscope having localised the bone and remove with packing forceps or intubation forceps.

Anogenital

Extricating the penis from a zipper

The patient has accidentally entrapped the foreskin of his penis in his 'fly' zipper. He will already have tried to extricate himself, and further manoeuvring will not only be painful but will continue to impact the skin.

The following are simple and effective techniques, which free the skin but ruin the zipper.

Method

1. Cut the zipper from the trousers for access.

2. Infiltrate LA beneath the entrapped foreskin, or infiltrate the skin at the base of the penis (ring block).
3. Grasp the zip fastener with pliers or any similar 'crushing clamp'. Apply pressure until the zip breaks and the skin is freed (Fig. 8.17a).

Alternatively, cut across the closed section of the zipper, keeping as close as possible to the fastener (Fig. 8.17b), with a suitable instrument such as a sharp scalpel, and the zipper will fall apart.

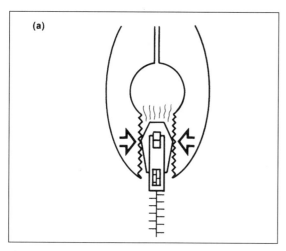
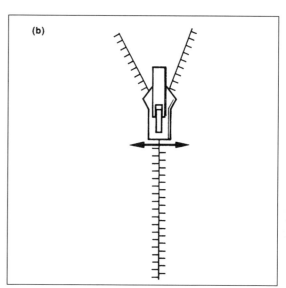

Fig. 8.17 Extracting penis from zipper

Removal of impacted vaginal tampon

The problem associated with this procedure is the unpleasant odour that envelops the surgery, causing considerable embarrassment to both patient and doctor.

Management

Under good vision, the tampon is seized with a pair of sponge-holding forceps and quickly immersed under water. A bowl of water (an old ice cream container is suitable) is kept as close to the introitus as possible. This results in minimal malodour.

Method

1. *Inspection:* usually in the Sims position with a Sims speculum (other positions can be used).
2. *Removal:* the tampon is grasped with a sponge-holding forceps (dorsal position; Fig. 8.18a).
3. *Disposal:* the tampon is quickly plunged under water without releasing the forceps (Fig. 8.18b). The tampon and water can be immediately flushed down the toilet (except in septic tank systems or where drainage problems exist).

It may be preferable to use another disposal method, such as taking the forceps and tampon outside and inserting the tampon into a self-sealing plastic bag.

Note: The Master Plumbers Association warns against flushing tampons down toilets because of their tendency to block systems.

Gloved and extraction method

The tampon can be grasped with the gloved hand and then invaginated into the glove which acts as a receptacle for disposal.

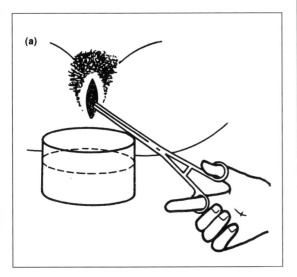

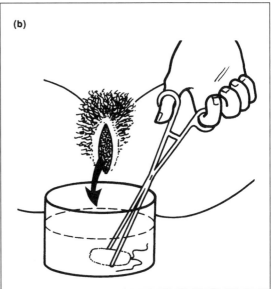

Fig. 8.18 Removal of tampon

Faecal impaction

Faecal impaction, manifested as an aggregation of hard faeces in the rectum on rectal examination and associated with constipation or spurious diarrhoea, can be a difficult problem. It often presents in children and the elderly. A good method of doing a rectal examination on a home visit (in the absence of gloves in the doctor's bag) is to apply moist soap around the finger and caked under the nail (in case of breakage), then plastic wrap and finally petroleum jelly (e.g. Vaseline).

Before resorting to a good, old-fashioned '3H' enema (hot water, high, and a hell of a lot) use a Microlax 5 mL enema. This can be carried in the doctor's bag, is very easy to insert and most effective.

Manual disimpaction

Rarely, one has to resort to manual disimpaction, which is a most offensive procedure for all concerned. However, the procedure can be rendered virtually odourless if the products are milked or scooped directly into a pan or container of water. A large plastic cover helps to restrict permeation of the smell.

Discomfort and embarrassment are reduced by this and adequate premedication (e.g. intravenous diazepam, or even IV morphine if hard faecoliths are present).

Removal of vibrator from vagina or rectum

Manual removal of a vibrator or similar object from the vagina usually presents no problem, but removal from the rectum (if high) can be difficult without general anaesthesia.

9 Musculoskeletal medicine

Temporomandibular joint

Temporomandibular dysfunction

A tender and perhaps clicking temporomandibular joint (TMJ) is a relatively common problem presenting to the general practitioner. In the absence of obvious malocclusion and organic disease, such as rheumatoid arthritis, simple exercises can alleviate the annoying problem in about 2 weeks. Three methods are described as alternatives to splint therapy.

Method 1

1. Obtain a cylindrical (or similar-shaped) rod of soft wooden or plastic material, approximately 15 cm long and 1.5 cm wide. An ideal object is a large carpenter's pencil or piece of soft wood.
2. Instruct the patient to position this at the back of the mouth so that the molars grasp the object with the mandible thrust forward.
3. The patient then rhythmically bites on the object with a grinding movement (Fig. 9.1) for 2–3 minutes at least three times a day.

Method 2

1. Instruct the patient to rhythmically thrust the lower jaw forward and backward in an anterior–posterior direction with the mouth slightly open, rather like a cheeky schoolchild exposing the bottom lip (Fig. 9.2).
2. This exercise hurts initially but should soon lead to relief of the uncomplicated TMJ syndrome.

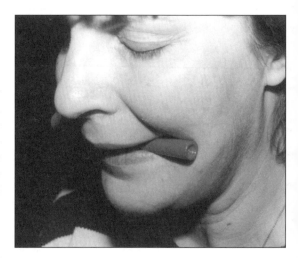

Fig. 9.1 Chewing the 'pencil' exercise

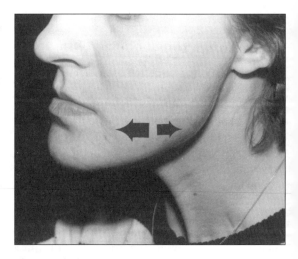

Fig. 9.2 The lower jaw-thrust exercise

Method 3: The 'six-by-six' program

This is a specific program (separate from the exercises above) recommended by some dental surgeons. The six exercises should be done six times each time, six times a day. It takes 1 minute to do them. Instruct the patient as follows:

1. Hold the front one-third of your tongue to the roof of your mouth and take six deep breaths.
2. Hold the tongue to the roof of your mouth and open your mouth six times. Your jaw should not click.
3. Hold your chin with both hands, keeping the chin still. Without letting your chin move, push up, down and to each side. Remember not to let your chin move.
4. Hold both hands behind your neck and pull the chin in.

5. Push on the upper lip so as to push the head straight back.
6. Pull your shoulders back as if to touch the shoulder blades together.

Repeat each exercise six times, six times a day.
Note: Patients should use a visual cue to remind them to do the exercises.

These exercises should be pain-free. If they hurt, do not push patients to the limit until the pain eases.

Method 4: Resisted 'jaw' opening

For this isometric contraction method the patient grasps the jaw mainly on the jaw angle and strongly resists opening of the jaw. This simple exercise is repeated many times a day.

The TMJ 'rest' program

This program is reserved for an acutely painful TMJ condition.

- When eating, avoid opening your mouth wider than the thickness of your thumb and cut all food into small pieces.
- Do not bite any food with your front teeth—use small bite-size pieces.
- Avoid eating food requiring prolonged chewing, e.g. hard crusts of bread, tough meat, raw vegetables.

- Avoid chewing gum.
- Always try to open your jaw in a hinge or arc motion. Do not protrude your jaw.
- Avoid protruding your jaw, e.g. talking, applying lipstick.
- Avoid clenching your teeth together—keep your lips together and your teeth apart.
- Try to breathe through your nose at all times.
- Do not sleep on your jaw: try to sleep on your back.
- Practise a relaxed lifestyle so that your jaws and face muscles feel relaxed.

Dislocated jaw

The patient may present with a unilateral or bilateral dislocation. The jaw will be 'locked' and the patient unable to articulate.

Method

1. Get the patient to sit upright with the head against the wall.
2. Wrap a handkerchief around both thumbs and place the thumbs over the lower molar teeth, with the fingers firmly grasping the mandible on the outside.
3. Firmly thrusting with the thumbs, push downward towards the floor and at the same time press upwards on the chin with the fingers (Fig. 9.3).

This action invariably reduces the dislocation, with the reduction being reinforced by the fingers rotating the mandible upward as the thumbs thrust downward.

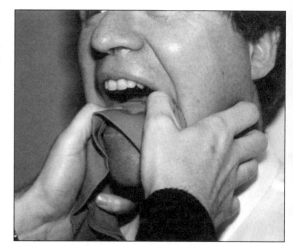

Fig. 9.3 Method of reduction of dislocated jaw

The spine

Recording spinal movements

Method 1

Simple diagrams obviate the need for copious notes when recording the range of movement of the cervical spine. They are of particular value to the 'whiplash' accident patient, who requires repeated assessment and accurate recording. Done serially, the diagrams are an excellent guide to progress, and assist in the compilation of medicolegal reports.

The neck movement grid (Fig. 9.4a) provides a two-dimensional field on which to record movements of the neck as viewed when standing behind and above the patient (looking down on the patient's head). Not only is the range of movement written on the grid, but pain can be recorded also.

Table 9.1 shows the movements recorded for the patient in Figure 9.4b.

Table 9.1 'Whiplash' accident patient: Neck movement record

Flexion	full and pain-free
Extension	50% (of normal), painful through range
Left rotation	40%, painful at end of range
Right rotation	60%
Left lateral flexion	40%
Right lateral flexion	70%

Method 2

One can use a special direction of movement (DOM) diagram to record movements for all spinal levels. Figure 9.4c illustrates restricted and painful movements (blocked, indicated by II) in flexion, left lateral flexion and left rotation but pain-free extension, right lateral flexion and right rotation (free movements).

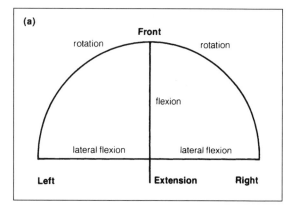

(a)

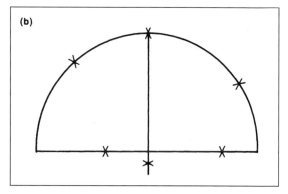

(b)

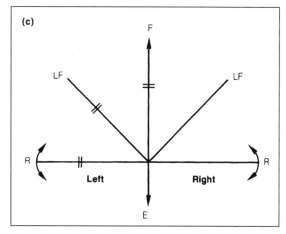

(c)

Fig. 9.4 The neck movement grid (viewed from above the patient) PART 9.4(c) REPRODUCED FROM C. KENNA & J. MURTAGH, *BACK PAIN AND SPINAL MANIPULATION*, BUTTERWORTHS, SYDNEY, 1989, WITH PERMISSION

Spinal mobilisation and manipulation

Spinal mobilisation and manipulation are examples of physical therapy that can be very beneficial in many spinal conditions where hypomobility that causes pain and stiffness is present.

These therapies improve the range of joint movement, decrease stiffness and reduce pain. Mobilisation of the spine is a safe procedure but manipulation can have serious sequelae, especially if given inappropriately to the cervical spine. For the cervical spine, mobilisation is a relatively simple and most effective technique, while manipulation should be left to the experts.

Key concepts

- Mobilisation is a gentle, coaxing, repetitive, rhythmic movement within the range of movement of the joint (Fig. 9.5).
- Manipulation is a high-velocity thrust at the end range (Fig. 9.5).
- If in doubt, use mobilisation in preference to manipulation.
- Always mobilise or manipulate in the direction of no pain.
- Manipulation is generally more effective and produces a faster response, but requires accurate diagnosis and greater skill, and can aggravate some spinal problems.

Important contraindications to spinal manipulation

- Disease of the spine (e.g. osteoporosis, neoplasm, rheumatoid arthritis).
- Neurological changes.
- Evidence of nerve root compression (e.g. pain in the leg).
- Instability of spine following trauma.
- Cerebrovascular disease (for neck).
- Anticoagulation therapy.
- The elderly patient.

A golden rule: Opposite movement, no pain. This generally means that manipulation achieves a gapping or opening up of the painful side.

Anterior directed gliding—an example of spinal mobilisation

The technique of anterior directed gliding, also termed posterior-anterior mobilisation, can be applied directly to the spinous process centrally (Fig. 9.6) or over tender points unilaterally. It is a very simple technique, directed either with the thumbs (placed side by side) or the pisiform process of the leading hand (for central mobilisation only). This

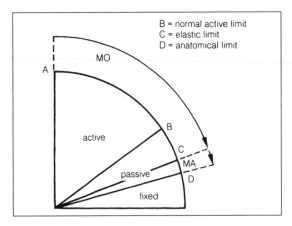

Fig. 9.5 Schematic representation of movement (by rotation) of a joint: mobilisation (MO), A–C; manipulation (MA), C–D

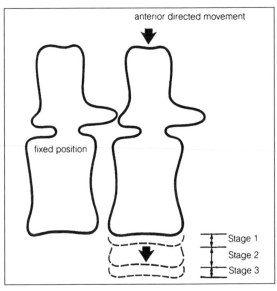

Fig. 9.6 Anterior directed central gliding mobilisation, illustrating the three stages of mobilisation   REPRODUCED FROM C. KENNA & J. MURTAGH, *BACK PAIN AND SPINAL MANIPULATION*, BUTTERWORTHS, SYDNEY, 1989, WITH PERMISSION

method is suitable for anywhere along the spine, but particularly for the cervical spine and more so at lateral tender points.

Method (using thumbs)

1. The patient lies prone, with head turned to one side and arms by the side.
2. For the thoracic and lumbar spines, stand at the patient's side and place your thumbs over the tender area. For the cervical spine, stand behind the patient's head.
3. Lean over the patient with your arms perfectly straight and head and shoulders over the treatment area.
4. Obtain an oscillatory movement by gently rocking the upper trunk up and down, with pressure being transmitted to your thumbs by the shoulders and arms.
5. Go as deeply as possible without causing pain.
6. Provide a small-amplitude, controlled oscillation at the rate of 2 per minute. Maintain this for about 30–60 seconds, with two or three repeats in one treatment session.

Cervical spine

Clinical problems of cervical origin

Pain originating in the cervical spine is commonly, although not always, experienced in the neck. The patient may complain of headache, or pain around the ear, face, shoulder, arm, scapulae or upper anterior chest.

If the cervical spine is overlooked as a source of pain, the cause of symptoms will remain masked and mismanagement will follow.

Possible symptoms

- Neck pain.
- Neck stiffness.
- Headache.
- Migraine-like headache.
- Arm pain (referred or radicular).
- Facial pain.
- Ear pain (periauricular).
- Scapular pain.
- Anterior chest pain.
- Torticollis.
- Dizziness/vertigo.
- Visual dysfunction.

Figure 9.7 indicates the typical directions of referred pain. Surprisingly, headache, which is commonly caused by cervical problems, is often not considered by clinicians.

Pain in the arm (brachialgia) is common, and tends to cover the shoulder and upper arm area indicated in Figure 9.7. This is the zone of referred pain that is not caused by nerve root compression. It can be a difficult diagnostic dilemma, because pain reference from the fifth cervical nerve segment (C_5) involves musculoskeletal, neurological and visceral

structures. Virtually all shoulder structures are innervated by C_5.

The practitioner must first determine whether the pain originates in the cervical spine or the shoulder joints, or in both simultaneously, or some other structure. The often missed diagnosis of polymyalgia rheumatica should be considered in the elderly patient presenting with pain in the zone indicated, especially if bilateral.

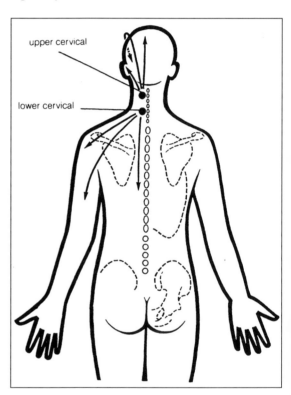

Fig. 9.7 Possible common directions of referred pain from the cervical spine   REPRODUCED FROM C. KENNA & J. MURTAGH, *BACK PAIN AND SPINAL MANIPULATION*, BUTTERWORTHS, SYDNEY, 1989, WITH PERMISSION

Locating tenderness in the neck

Palpation of the neck to determine the precise level of pain or tenderness can be difficult; however, if the surface anatomy of the neck is clearly defined, the affected level can easily be determined.

Method

1. The patient lies prone on the examination couch with hands (palms up) resting on the forehead. The shoulders should be relaxed.
2. Systematically palpate the spinous processes of the cervical vertebrae:

   - C_2 (axis) is the first spinous process palpable beneath the occiput.
   - C_7 is the largest 'fixed' and most prominent process at the base of the neck.
   - C_6 is also prominent and easily palpable, but usually 'disappears' under the palpating finger with extension of the neck.
   - the spinous process of C_1 (atlas) is not palpable, but the tip of the transverse process is: it lies between the angle of the jaw and the mastoid process.
   - the spinous processes of C_3, C_4 and C_5 are difficult to palpate because of cervical lordosis, but their level can be estimated (see Fig. 9.8).

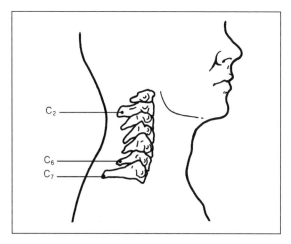

Fig. 9.8 Relative sizes of spinous processes of cervical spine

Acute torticollis

An amazingly effective treatment for an acute wry neck is muscle energy therapy, which relies on the basic physiological principle that the contracting and stretching of muscles leads to the automatic relaxation of agonist and antagonist muscles.

Note: Lateral flexion or rotation or a combination of movements can be used, but treatment in rotation is preferred. The direction of contraction can be away from the painful side (preferred) or towards the painful side, whichever is most comfortable for the patient.

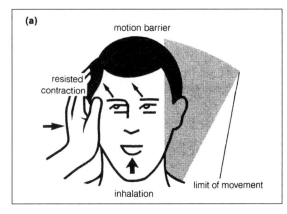

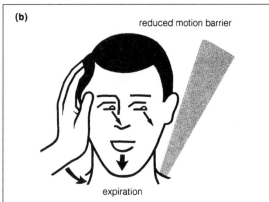

Fig. 9.9 Acute torticollis: **(a)** isometric contraction phase for problem on left side; **(b)** relaxation phase towards the affected (left) side   REPRODUCED FROM C. KENNA & J. MURTAGH, *BACK PAIN AND SPINAL MANIPULATION*, BUTTERWORTHS, SYDNEY, 1989, WITH PERMISSION

Method

1. Explain the method to the patient, with reassurance that it is not painful.
2. Rotate the patient's head passively and gently towards the painful side to the limit of pain (the motion barrier).
3. Place your hand against the head on the side opposite the painful one. The other (free) hand can be used to steady the painful level—usually C_3–C_4.
4. Ask the patient to push the head (in rotation) as firmly as possible against the resistance of your hand. The patient should therefore be producing a strong isometric contraction of the neck in rotation away from the painful side. Your counterforce (towards the painful side) should be firm and moderate (never forceful), and should not 'break' through the patient's resistance. To reinforce the effect of this contraction (although not essential), you can ask the patient to inhale and hold the breath and also to look upward in the direction of the contracting muscles (Fig. 9.9a).
5. After 5–10 seconds (average 7 seconds) ask the patient to relax; then passively stretch the neck gently towards the patient's painful side. During this phase the patient is asked to exhale slowly and to look downward to that side (Fig. 9.9b).

6. The patient will now be able to turn the head a little further towards the painful side.
7. This sequence is repeated at the new and improved motion barrier. Repeat three to five times until the full range of movement returns.
8. Ask the patient to return the following day for another treatment, although the neck may now be almost normal.

The patient can be taught self-treatment at home using this method.

Traction to the neck

Traction to the neck can be given by machine but can also be applied manually, with or without the use of a belt. It is ideal for treating nerve root irritation with arm pain, and acute neck pain with headache.

Method

1. The patient lies supine, relaxed, with arms by the side and head at the end of the couch.
2. Stand at the head of the couch, with one hand clasping the occipital area and the other holding the chin (Fig. 9.10).
3. Traction is achieved by using body weight, not the arms alone. Hence, you should lean back during traction.

Special notes

- Avoid traction on an extended neck: use a neutral position for upper cervical problems and flexion (20°–40°) for middle to lower problems.
- Always take up traction slowly and release gently.

The belt method

It is best to use a belt (a modified car seat belt or camping gear belt) for neck traction. The belt is applied around the waist and is then looped over the wrist and hands, which fit comfortably under the occiput. Traction is applied by leaning back and allowing the body weight to exert the force.

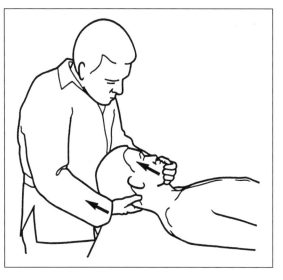

Fig. 9.10 Longitudinal traction to the neck for a mid-cervical problem REPRODUCED FROM C. KENNA & J. MURTAGH, *BACK PAIN AND SPINAL MANIPULATION*, BUTTERWORTHS, SYDNEY, 1989, WITH PERMISSION

A simple traction technique for the cervical spine

This technique demonstrates the use of longitudinal traction of the neck, especially for the upper cervical spine, as a muscular energy therapy. Co-ordination of breathing is considered to be a most effective facilitator of this method. It is very safe and gentle, and particularly helpful in the elderly with painful dysfunctional necks.

Method

1. The patient sits on the chair (sitting is preferable to lying supine), with the head in a 'neutral' position.
2. Stand behind the patient and place the palms of your hands on the sides of the patient's face (to spread the pressure evenly around the face and not in one or two sites).
3. Ask the patient to simultaneously breathe in and look upwards (without extending the neck).
4. Hold the patient's neck in a fixed position with very slight traction during this inspiration phase (Fig. 9.11a). The neck muscles will contract during this phase.
5. Ask the patient to then exhale while looking down. Apply a gentle but firm upward stretch (Fig. 9.11b). Maintain this traction for about 7 seconds.
6. Repeat this procedure about 4 times, applying traction during each expiration phase.

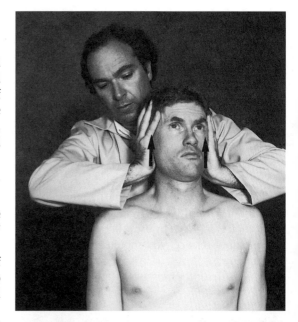

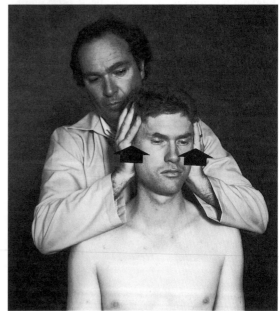

Fig. 9.11 Simple traction technique: **(a)** the therapist applies slight traction during inspiration and upward gaze; **(b)** the therapist applies firm traction during expiration and downward gaze

Neck rolls and stretches

Indications

Dysfunction of neck, including tenderness and stiffness, usually following injury.

Method

The objective is to produce a smooth, circular motion to the end range in all directions so that stretching occurs at the end range.

1. Patients are instructed to 'draw circles in the air' (Fig. 9.12a) or 'roll their head around their halo'. A wide arc of movement is not necessary, provided that stretch is obtained.
2. The roll is performed at a slow to medium pace, so that tender or painful areas can be avoided by moving just short of this level. As stretch is obtained, these areas become less painful, allowing further stretching.
3. Patients can be taught to stretch the neck themselves (Fig. 9.12b), including the use of a muscle energy technique. No matter how stiff the neck initially, it is surprising how much immediate improvement can be obtained from simple, gentle, lateral stretching.

Patients should be instructed to train themselves into a permanent daily habit of rolling the neck to assess flexibility.

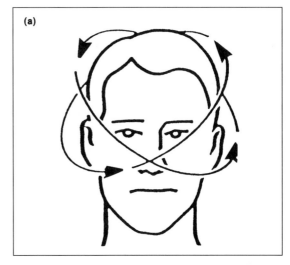

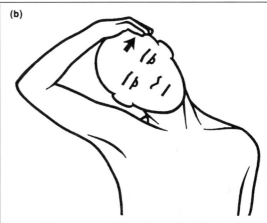

Fig. 9.12 Exercises for dysfunctional neck: **(a)** the slow neck roll; **(b)** stretching neck into lateral flexion   REPRODUCED FROM C. KENNA & J. MURTAGH, *BACK PAIN AND SPINAL MANIPULATION*, BUTTERWORTHS, SYDNEY, 1989, WITH PERMISSION

Thoracic spine

Anterior directed costovertebral gliding

This unilateral mobilisation method is directed at the tender costotransverse joint of the thoracic spine. The joint, which is about 4–5 cm from the midline, is arguably the commonest source of musculoskeletal pain in the thoracic spine. The tender area determined by palpation is the target for mobilisation.

Method

1. With the pad of the thumbs applied over the rib (Fig. 9.13), apply a rhythmic oscillating movement (about 2 per second) at right angles.
2. Maintain this for 30–60 seconds with as much pressure as possible without causing discomfort.

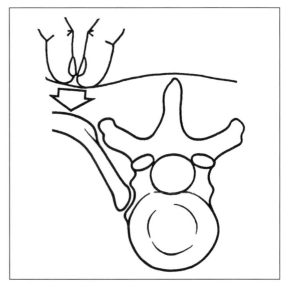

Fig. 9.13 Costovertebral gliding mobilisation   REPRODUCED FROM C. KENNA & J. MURTAGH, *BACK PAIN AND SPINAL MANIPULATION*, BUTTERWORTHS, SYDNEY, 1989, WITH PERMISSION

Thoracic spinal manipulation

Thigh extension thrust technique

This is very effective in the treatment of painful spinal dysfunction of the upper thoracic spine (T_1–T_7). The technique involves extension of the upper thoracic spine over the therapist's thigh. A low couch is necessary, or the therapist can stand on a stool or chair at the head of a high couch.

Method

1. Stand at the head of the couch and flex your thigh and knee on the couch.
2. The patient lies supine on the couch and positions the spine on your thigh so that the tender area lies just above your knee.
3. The patient clasps hands firmly behind the neck.
4. Insert your arms through the patient's arms (as far as possible) to grasp the patient around the sides of the thorax.
5. Take up the slack by gently stretching the patient over your thigh.
6. Extend the patient's thoracic spine firmly and suddenly over your thigh by simultaneously lifting and rotating the patient's trunk towards you, dropping your body back and down towards the floor and thrusting with your forearms down across the patient's outer clavicular region (Fig. 9.14). It is a carefully controlled, decisive, but relatively gentle movement.

The sternal thrust ('Nelson hold') method

This is a time-honoured method for patients with upper to mid-thoracic dysfunction. It is similar to the thigh extension method (and is used as an alternative), but involves a sternal (chest) thrust from the therapist.

Method

1. Although the patient can be standing for this method, it is best to have them sitting across the couch with their back to you (buttocks to the edge of the couch), ideally with the head at the same level as yours.
2. Stand behind the patient and place a soft object such as a rolled-up towel on the back, with the upper edge just below the painful level.
3. Slide the hands in front of the patient's axillae and grasp the wrists.
4. Gently but firmly extend the patient's back against your chest in a lifting movement as you also extend your back.
5. Ask the patient to breathe in and breathe out, and to relax.
6. When the patient is relaxed, take up the slack, increase the stretching lift and backward extension, and apply a sharp forward thrust with your chest (Fig. 9.15).

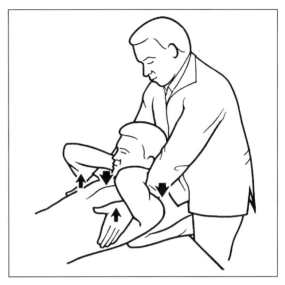

Fig. 9.14 Upper thoracic spinal manipulation: the thigh extension technique, illustrating the direction of the applied forces   REPRODUCED FROM C. KENNA & J. MURTAGH, *BACK PAIN AND SPINAL MANIPULATION*, BUTTERWORTHS, SYDNEY, 1989, WITH PERMISSION

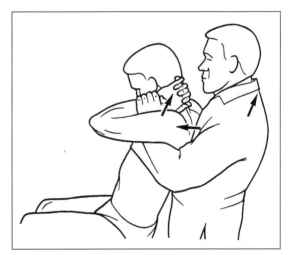

Fig. 9.15 The sternal thrust method   REPRODUCED FROM C. KENNA & J. MURTAGH, *BACK PAIN AND SPINAL MANIPULATION*, BUTTERWORTHS, SYDNEY, 1989, WITH PERMISSION

Manipulation for the mid-thoracic spine

Of the dozens of manipulative thrusts for dysfunction of the thoracic spine (T_3–T_8), the most effective is the postero-anterior indirect thrust, using the underlying hand as a block over the affected area.

Method

1. The patient lies supine on a low couch, with a pillow supporting the head.
2. The patient folds the arms across the body with hands resting on opposite shoulders, the uppermost forearm being the one furthest from you.
3. Roll the relaxed patient towards you.
4. Place your cupped hand (Fig. 9.16a) on the spine at the painful level, with this level in the palm.
5. Roll the patient back onto the hand, which should feel comfortable (if not, readjust).
6. Lean well over the patient, placing your forearm directly on theirs, and grasp the patient's far elbow with your hand.
7. Rest your chest on your uppermost arm.
8. Ask the patient to inhale and exhale fully.
9. As the patient commences to exhale, lean down to take up the slack on your bottom hand.
10. Towards the end of exhalation, apply a sharp downward thrust with your chest and upper arm directly through the patient's chest onto your hand (Fig. 9.16b).

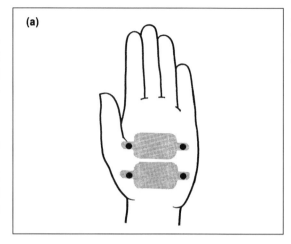

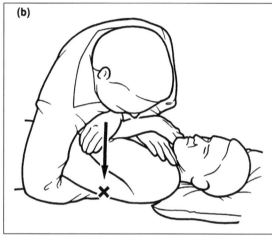

Fig. 9.16 Mid-thoracic manipulation: **(a)** cupped hand position, showing position of the vertebrae on the hand—note how the spinous processes run along the long axis and occupy the hollow of the hand; **(b)** manipulation to mid-thoracic spine—note the direction of the applied force (X indicates blockage with the hand) REPRODUCED FROM C. KENNA & J. MURTAGH, *BACK PAIN AND SPINAL MANIPULATION*, BUTTERWORTHS, SYDNEY, 1989, WITH PERMISSION

Thoracolumbar stretching and manipulation

Rotation in the sitting position

In this very effective technique, the patient fixes the pelvis by straddling a low couch or a chair; the couch provides the better position, because it allows greater flexibility of the trunk.

The main indications are unilateral pain at the thoracolumbar junction. The method can be used also for pain (unilateral and bilateral) of the lumbar spine and the lower thoracic spine. The usual rules and contraindications apply. The technique must be co-ordinated with deep breathing.

Method

1. The patient straddles the end of the couch and sits firm and erect. Alternatively the patient can straddle a chair, facing the back of the chair with a pillow used against the chair to protect the thighs.

It must be a standard, open chair, with a carpeted floor.
2. The patient crosses the arms over the chest so that the hands rest on the opposite shoulders. The patient should be comfortable throughout the procedure, and proper padding should rest against the inner thighs.
3. Stand directly behind the patient. Adopt a firm, wide-based stance.
4. Grasp the patient's shoulders with your hands.
5. Ask the patient to take a deep breath in, exhale fully and relax.
6. When you feel the patient relax, grasp the shoulders and rotate the patient's trunk steadily and firmly, away from the painful side, to the limit of rotation. Before rotation is attempted the patient must be at the absolute limit of stretch. Gently oscillate the trunk at this position of full stretch.
7. If any sharp pain is reproduced at this end range abandon the treatment. *(continues)*

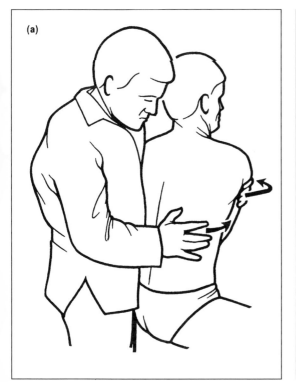
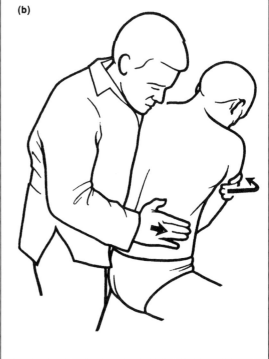

Fig. 9.17 Thoracolumbar manipulation: **(a)** rotation in sitting technique for thoracolumbar region (right-sided problem); **(b)** rotation in sitting technique for lumbar spine (right-sided problem)   REPRODUCED FROM C. KENNA & J. MURTAGH, *BACK PAIN AND SPINAL MANIPULATION*, BUTTERWORTHS, SYDNEY, 1989, WITH PERMISSION

Mobilisation: consists of performing a gentle, repetitive, oscillatory rotation of the trunk at this end range for up to 30 seconds.

Manipulation: consists of a sharp, well-controlled rotation.

Variations of this technique

An alternative and better strategy is to 'hug' the patient's trunk, using the arm that embraces the trunk to grasp the arm near the elbow on the side to be rotated. The thrusting hand can be applied to a specific area of the back corresponding to the level of pain. Thus, a type of 'push-pull' manoeuvre can be achieved, with the embracing arm pulling into rotation and the other hand pushing to achieve a complementary smooth rotation of the trunk. Co-ordinate this with breathing so the rotation only occurs during the relaxed exhaled stage.

Figure 9.17a demonstrates the technique for a right-sided problem at the thoracolumbar junction, while Figure 9.17b demonstrates the technique for low lumbar pain. Both rotations are to the left, since rotation to the right reproduces pain.

Lumbar spine
Drawing and scale-marking for back pain

A very useful procedure to assess the nature of patients' back pain is to ask them to draw the location of their pain on a sheet with blank outlines of the body. They can indicate also their perception of the intensity of the pain on a scale on the same page. The basic sheet is illustrated in Figure 9.18a, while examples of this application are provided in Figures 9.18b and c overleaf. *(continues)*

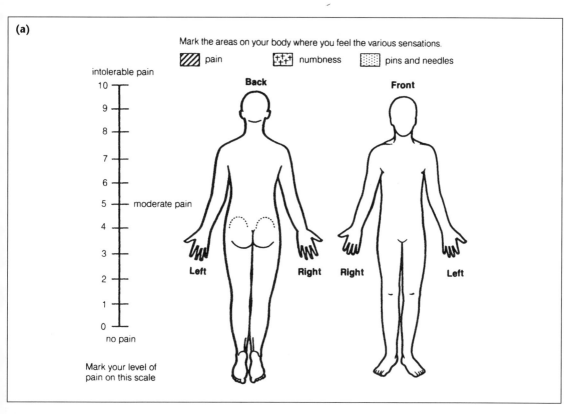

Fig. 9.18 Drawing and scale-marking for back pain: **(a)** basic sheet

(b)

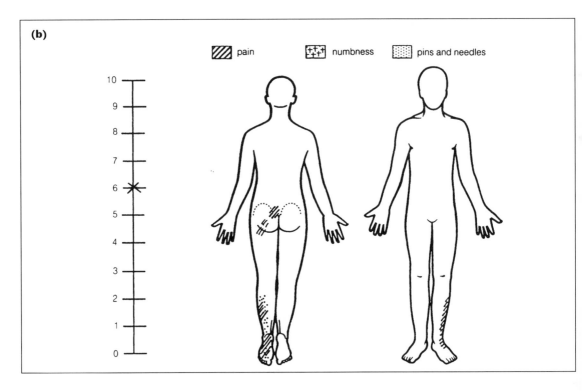

(c)

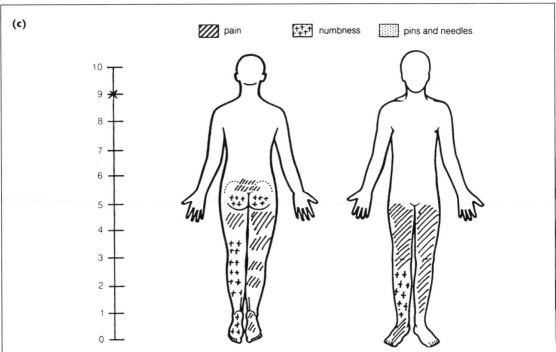

Fig. 9.18 Drawing and scale-marking for back pain: **(b)** drawing by a patient with L_5–S_1 disc prolapse causing S_1 nerve root compression (left side); **(c)** drawing by a patient with psychologically based problem (conversion reaction)

Reference points in the lumbar spine

A working knowledge of the bony landmarks of the lumbar spine is vitally important for determining the level of the spinal pain and for procedures such as epidural injections and lumbar punctures.

This anatomical knowledge is readily determined by using the iliac crests as the main reference point.

Method

1. For the examination the patient should be relaxed, lying prone, with the arms by the sides.
2. Standing behind and below the patient, place your fingers on the top of the iliac crests and your thumbs at the same level on the midline of the back. This level will correspond with the fourth and fifth lumbar interspace (Fig. 9.19), or slightly higher at the fourth lumbar spinous process.
3. Consequently, the thumbs will either feel the L_4–L_5 gap or the L_4 spinous process.

(When inspecting X-rays of the lumbar spine, it becomes apparent that the upper limits of the iliac crest usually lie opposite the L_4–L_5 interspace.)

The reference points should be marked and the level of each lumbar spinous process can then be identified.

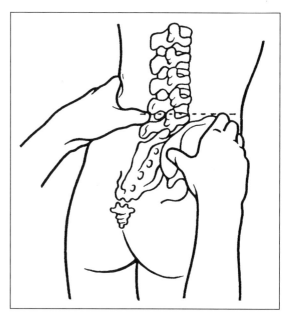

Fig. 9.19 Illustration of bony landmarks of the lumbosacral spine   REPRODUCED FROM C. KENNA & J. MURTAGH, *BACK PAIN AND SPINAL MANIPULATION*, BUTTERWORTHS, SYDNEY, 1989, WITH PERMISSION

Tests for non-organic back pain

Several tests are useful in differentiating between organic and non-organic back pain (e.g. that caused by depression or complained of by a known malingerer).

Magnuson's method (the 'migratory pointing' test)

1. Request the patient to point to the painful sites.
2. Palpate these areas of tenderness on two occasions separated by an interval of several minutes, and compare the sites.

Between the two tests divert the patient's attention from his or her back by another examination.

Burn's 'kneeling on a stool' test

1. Ask the patient to kneel on a low stool, lean over and try to touch the floor.
2. The person with non-organic back pain will usually refuse on the grounds that it would cause great pain or that he or she might overbalance in the attempt.

Patients with even a severely herniated disc usually manage the task to some degree (Fig. 9.20a,b).

The 'axial loading' test

1. Place your hands over the patient's head and press firmly downward (Fig. 9.21).
2. This will cause no discomfort to (most) patients with organic back pain.

(*continues*)

The 'hip and shoulder rotation' test

1. Examine for pain by rotating the patient's hips and shoulders while the feet are kept in place on the floor (Fig. 9.22).

2. The manoeuvre is usually painless in those with an organically based back disorder.

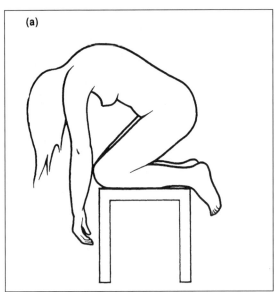 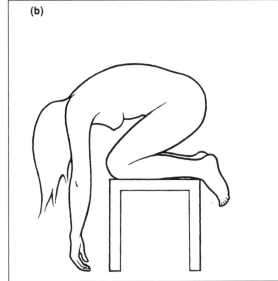

Fig. 9.20 Back pain tests: **(a)** abnormal attempt to kneel on a stool; **(b)** normal attempt to kneel on a stool

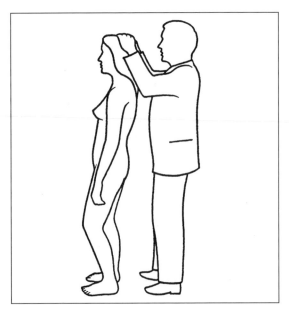 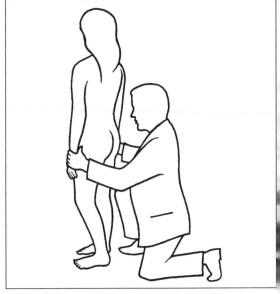

Fig. 9.21 The 'axial loading' test

Fig. 9.22 The 'hip and shoulder rotation' test

Movements of the lumbar spine

There are three main movements of the lumbar spine. As there is minimal rotation, which mainly occurs at the thoracic spine, rotation is not so important. The movements that should be tested, and their normal ranges, are as follows:

- extension (20°–30°) (Fig. 9.23a),
- lateral flexion, left and right (30°) (Fig. 9.23b),
- flexion (75°–90°: average 80°) (Fig. 9.23a).

Measurement of the angle of movement can be made by using a line drawn between the sacrum and large prominence of the C_7 spinous process.

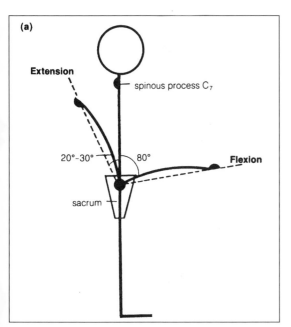
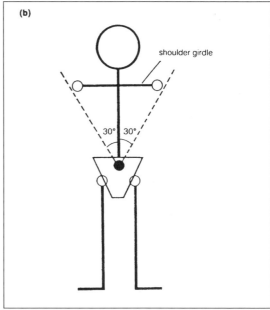

Fig. 9.23 **(a)** illustration of degrees of movement of the lumbar spine in flexion and extension; **(b)** illustration of the degree of lateral flexion of the lumbar spine   REPRODUCED FROM C. KENNA & J. MURTAGH, *BACK PAIN AND SPINAL MANIPULATION*, BUTTERWORTHS, SYDNEY, 1989, WITH PERMISSION

Nerve roots of leg and level of prolapsed disc

Pain in the leg from discogenic lesions in the lumbosacral spine is commonly due to pressure on the L_5 or S_1 nerve roots. Unlike discogenic lesions in the cervical spine, more than one nerve root can be involved with prolapses of the L_4–L_5 or L_5–S_1 discs, but this is uncommon.

Working guidelines are given in Table 9.2 and Figure 9.24.

Table 9.2 Typical lumbosacral disc causes of various clinical problems

Problem	Usual causative disc prolapse
L_3 nerve root lesion	L_2–L_3
L_4 nerve root lesion	L_3–L_4
L_5 nerve root lesion	L_4–L_5
S_1 nerve root lesion	L_5–S_1
Severe low back pain, no leg pain	L_4–L_5
Severe sciatica, minimal low back pain	L_5–S_1
Low back pain with lateral deviation of spine	L_4–L_5

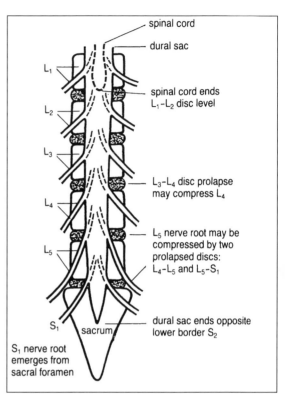

Fig. 9.24 Posterior 'window' view of lumbosacral spine, illustrating the relationships of the nerve root to the intervertebral discs   REPRODUCED FROM C. KENNA & J. MURTAGH, *BACK PAIN AND SPINAL MANIPULATION*, BUTTERWORTHS, SYDNEY, 1989, WITH PERMISSION

The slump test

The slump test is an excellent provocation test for lumbosacral pain and more sensitive than the straight leg raising test. It is a screening test for a disc lesion and dural tethering. It should be performed on patients who have low back pain with pain extending into the leg, and especially for posterior thigh pain.

A positive result is reproduction of the patient's pain, and may appear at an early stage of the test (when it is ceased).

Method

1. The patient sits on the couch in a relaxed manner.
2. The patient then slumps forward (without excessive trunk flexion), then places the chin on the chest.
3. The unaffected leg is straightened.
4. The affected leg only is then straightened (Fig. 9.25).
5. Both legs are straightened together.
6. The foot of the affected straightened leg is dorsiflexed.

Note: Take care to distinguish from hamstring pain. Deflexing the neck relieves the pain of spinal origin, not hamstring pain.

Significance of the slump test

- It is positive if the back or leg pain is reproduced.
- If positive, it suggests disc disruption.
- If negative, it may indicate lack of serious disc pathology.
- If positive, one should approach manual therapy with caution.

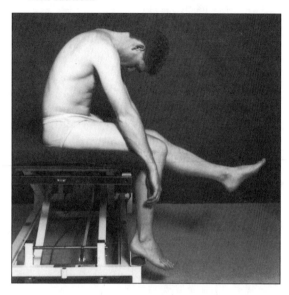

Fig. 9.25 The slump test: illustrating one of the stages

Schober's test (modified)

Schober's test is a useful objective means of measuring the mobility of the lumbar spine. The test described here is a modified version.

A measurement of less than 5 cm of movement is indicative of hypomobility, and was used initially to detect the seronegative spondyloarthropathy—ankylosing spondylitis. Related spondyloarthropathies include Reiter's disease, psoriasis and inflammatory bowel disorders. Other hypomobile spines are found with lumbar spondylosis (degenerative disease) and intervertebral disc disorders.

Method

1. Stand the patient erect and mark the spine in line with the 'dimples of Venus' (the posterior superior iliac spines). This corresponds to the spinous process of S_2.
2. Place another mark 10 cm above the first and a third mark 5 cm below the first mark.
3. Ask the patient to bend forward (flexion), as if to touch the toes, to the point of maximal flexion.
4. Now measure the distance between the upper and lower marks.

Interpretation

- Normal is greater than 5 cm increase in length.
- Less than 5 cm represents hypomobility.

Manual traction for sciatica

Although traction is usually administered by machines, it can also be performed manually, often with great benefit.

Indication

• Low back pain (central or unilateral), with or without sciatica, where the pain is acute and spinal manipulation is contraindicated. Particularly useful for sciatica radiating to the foot.

Rules

• Traction can be used on both legs simultaneously or just one leg (usually opposite the side of pain).
• Commence traction to both legs simultaneously; if this double method proves ineffective, traction can be applied to a single leg (Fig. 9.26), preferably the leg opposite to the painful side at first and then to the painful leg.

Method

1. The patient lies prone or supine (the author prefers the prone position), and can grasp the end of the table for support. This provides suitable counterpressure.
2. Stand at the feet of the patient and grasp the foot or feet firmly around the ankle. (It is advisable to use a belt around your waist, as this allows the body weight to supply the force, making possible a smooth, gentle and well-controlled traction. Although your hands can be used, the arms tire quickly and cannot sustain the traction.)
3. Apply the belt (such as a car seat belt or packing belt from a camping store) to the legs by looping it over your hands and apply body weight by leaning backwards on the belt. This action provides the traction force.

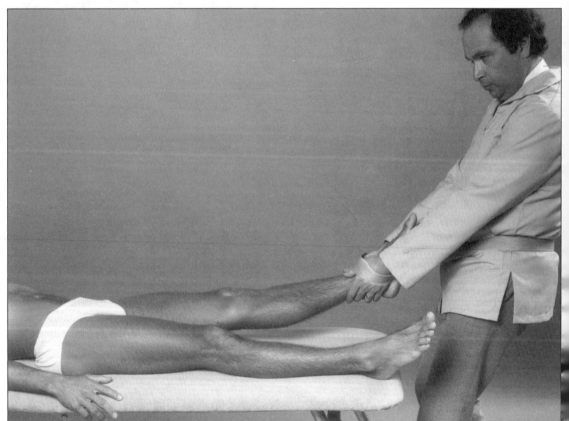

Fig. 9.26 Longitudinal traction applied to one leg with patient lying supine

4. Apply the traction gently until the symptoms begin to ease, and then maintain at this level for about 2 minutes. A gentle oscillatory force can be applied if this proves to be effective.
5. A key point is to keep talking to the patient, to determine what is happening as the traction is applied.

- If the pain increases, stop (ease off gently).
- If the pain decreases, maintain or increase traction.
- If the pain is unchanged, apply stronger traction.

Rotation mobilisation for lumbar spine

This technique is very useful for acute low back pain of the spine, especially where manipulation is contraindicated or of doubtful value. Patients tend to prefer gentler mobilisation to spinal manipulation. There are several grades of this technique.

Method

1. The patient lies on the pain-free side, with the head supported by a pillow.
2. The lower shoulder is pulled forwards by grasping the arm at the elbow and gently rotating the spine. The uppermost arm rests on the lateral wall of the chest.
3. The uppermost leg is flexed at the hip (30°–90°) and the knee flexed to a right angle. The patient places the palm of the lowermost hand under the head.
4. You stand behind the patient, opposite the pelvis.
5. Place both hands over the pelvis and apply a gentle, small-amplitude oscillatory movement (Fig. 9.27).
6. This is a gentle 'push and pull' method, with emphasis on the push.
7. The rocking movement occupies 30–60 seconds. It can be repeated two or three times on any one treatment visit.

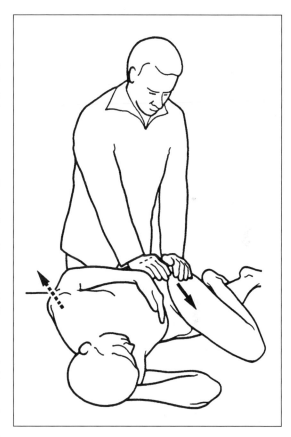

Fig. 9.27 Lumbar mobilisation in rotation (for left-sided pain)   REPRODUCED FROM C. KENNA & J. MURTAGH, *BACK PAIN AND SPINAL MANIPULATION*, BUTTERWORTHS, SYDNEY, 1989, WITH PERMISSION

Lumbar stretching and manipulation technique 1

This is a traditional method used for a thrusting manipulative movement but steady stretching is simpler and safer.

Method

1. The patient lies on the pain-free side, reasonably squarely on the lower shoulder. The body should be in a straight line with the lower leg extended. The upper leg (on the painful side) can be either falling freely over the side of the couch or flexed with the foot tucked into the popliteal fossa of the lower leg. The lower arm should lie comfortably in front of the trunk. Alternatively, the hand of the lower arm can be placed under the head.
2. Stand behind the patient at the level of the patient's waist.
3. Ask the patient to take a deep breath and breathe out.
4. When the patient has exhaled and relaxed, use one hand to push the trochanteric area of the hip forwards, and the other to gently force the front of the shoulder downwards (Fig. 9.28). It is best to keep hands in contact with the skin (avoid grasping clothing).
5. Apply steady rotational movement until a full stretch is applied to both shoulder and hip. Do not force the shoulder down too hard—take care to keep it firm and steady during the stretch.
6. Maintain sustained pressure for about 7 seconds at the end range.
7. Repeat this stretch twice.

Manipulation: If desired, this position can be used to apply a sharp rotational thrust to the hip with the force along the axis of the femur.

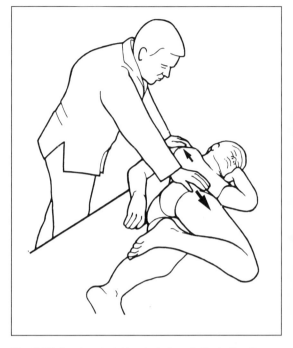

Fig. 9.28 Lumbar stretching technique 1: illustrating the direction of the applied stretching forces
REPRODUCED FROM C. KENNA & J. MURTAGH, *BACK PAIN AND SPINAL MANIPULATION*, BUTTERWORTHS, SYDNEY, 1989, WITH PERMISSION

Lumbar stretching and manipulation technique 2

This is the ideal stretching or manipulative technique for the lumbar spine and is the procedure of first choice for lumbar problems. It is designed to mobilise the lower lumbosacral segments which are responsible for most of the problems in the lower back.

The stretch

Method

1. The patient lies on the pain-free side in a relaxed position with the head on a pillow facing the therapist. The uppermost leg is flexed at the hip and the knee, both to about 45 degrees, with the foot tucked into the popliteal fossa of the lower leg.
2. Position yourself at the level of the patient's waist.
3. Ask the patient to turn his or her head and look up at the ceiling.
4. Carefully rotate the trunk by grasping the patient's lowermost arm just above or around the elbow and gently pulling the arm outwards.
5. Maintain smooth slow rotation of the trunk until you sense it is taut down to the upper lumbar spine.

6. Fix the trunk by asking the patient to place the hand of this arm under the head.
7. Rest the fleshy part of your upper forearm against the patient's shoulder and upper chest via the axilla, and your other forearm over the ischium, just below the iliac crest.
8. Ensure that you are properly balanced.
9. Apply a distracting force for several seconds, gently rocking back and forth with the forearms as you move towards maximal rotating stretch. This stretching is usually sufficient to achieve the desired therapeutic effect (Fig. 9.29a and b).

The manipulation

If desired, especially for a 'locked' lumbosacral level, this position can be used to perform a sharp manipulative thrust—but only from the position of full stretch.

Method

1. When all the slack is taken up by your forearms, ask the patient to take a deep breath and exhale.

(continues)

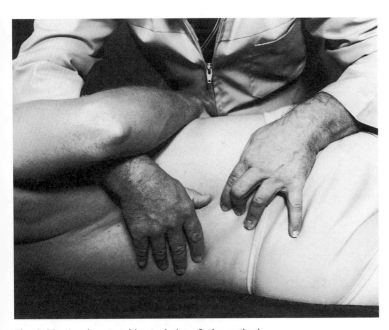

Fig. 9.29a Lumbar stretching technique 2: the method

2. At the end of the exhalation execute a sharp increase of rotatory pressure through both forearms, especially through the short lever to the pelvis.

Note: It is important not to dig the elbow of the proximal arm into the patient's body, since this can be painful. Likewise it is important to find a position for the distal forearm which is comfortable for the patient, and to avoid using the point of the elbow for thrusting, as the buttock area is very sensitive to sharp pressure.

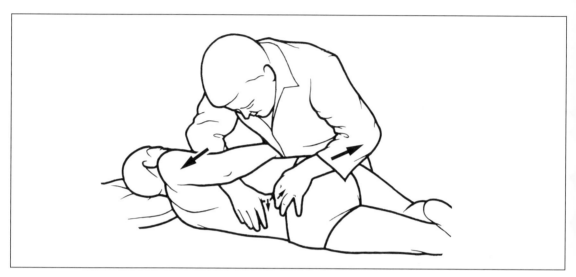

Fig. 9.29b Lumbar stretching technique 2: illustrating the direction of the applied stretching forces
REPRODUCED FROM C. KENNA & J. MURTAGH, *BACK PAIN AND SPINAL MANIPULATION*, BUTTERWORTHS, SYDNEY, 1989, WITH PERMISSION

Exercise for the lower back

The following yoga-like exercise is highly recommended for patients with pain in the lumbosacral
spine, usually after any muscle spasm has resolved.

Guidelines

It is preferable to perform the exercise on a couch
or very firm bed, but it can be done on the floor.
It can be performed repeatedly throughout the day
but should be repeated at least twice a day for about
3–5 minutes at a time.

Method

1. Lie on your back.
2. Bend the leg on the painful side and stretch it
   across the body while turning the head to the
   opposite side.

3. If possible, hang onto the side of the bed or couch
   with your free hand (the hand that is on the same
   side as the leg which is crossed over).
4. Use the other hand to grasp the bent leg at the
   level of the knee and increase the stretch as far as
   possible (Fig. 9.30).
5. Relax and return to the resting position.
6. Repeat on the opposite side, especially if that side
   also hurts.
7. Repeat several times, concentrating on stretching
   the painful joints.

Note: If someone pins your shoulders to the floor
or bed while you are performing this exercise, the
stretch is better.

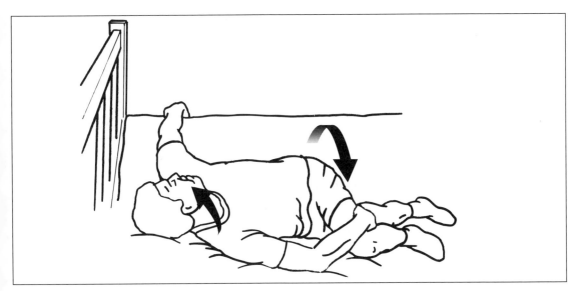

Fig. 9.30 An ideal exercise for the lower back (right side illustrated)

Shoulder

Dislocated shoulder

Types of dislocation:

- anterior (forward and downward)—95% of dislocations,
- posterior (backward)—difficult to diagnose,
- recurrent anterior dislocation.

Anterior dislocation of the shoulder

Management

An X-ray should be undertaken to check the position and exclude an associated fracture. Reduction can be achieved under general anaesthesia (easier and more comfortable) or with intravenous pethidine ± diazepam. The following methods can be used for anterior dislocation.

Kocher method

1. The patient's elbow should be flexed to 90° and held close to the body.
2. Slowly rotate the arm laterally (externally).
3. Adduct the humerus across the body by carrying the point of the elbow.
4. Rotate the arm medially (internally).

Hippocratic method

Apply traction to the outstretched arm by a hold on the hand with countertraction from a stockinged foot in the medial wall of the axilla. This levers the head of the humerus back. It is a good method if there is an associated avulsion fracture of the greater tuberosity.

Milch method (does not require anaesthesia or sedation)

1. The patient reclines at 30° and with guidance slowly bends the elbow to 90° (Fig. 9.31a).
2. The patient is asked to lift the arm up slowly with the elbow bent so that they can pat the back of their head (requires considerable reassurance and encouragement).
3. At this position, traction along the line of the humerus (with countertraction) achieves reduction (Fig. 9.31b).

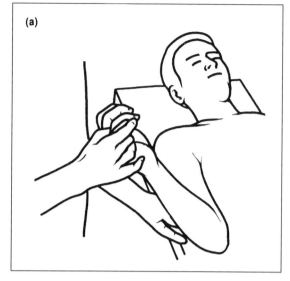

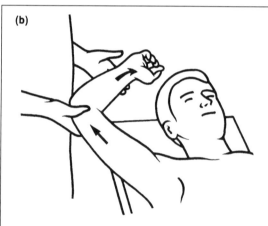

Fig 9.31 Milch method for reduction of dislocated shoulder: **(a)** starting position with elbow bent to 90°; **(b)** patient bringing hand up to touch back of head

Scapula pressure method

1. The patient lies prone with the dislocated arm hanging freely over the table.
2. Steady traction is applied to the arm by an assistant.
3. Firm pressure is then applied by the 'butt' of the hand to the inferolateral border of the scapula. The pressure is directed towards the glenohumeral joint.

Free-hanging method

The free-hanging method is relatively painless, yet simple. It is gentler than traditional methods, without rotational forces or direct pressure to the glenohumeral joint. It can be used with or without an intravenous analgesic or relaxant, which is not usually required for recurrent dislocation or in the elderly patient.

Preparation

1. Insert a 'butterfly' needle into a vein on the dorsum of the non-involved hand.
2. Prepare two solutions: (a) 10 mg of diazepam diluted to 5 mL with isotonic saline; (b) 50 mg of pethidine diluted to 5 mL with isotonic saline.
3. The patient sits at right angles to the chair with only half the buttock on the seat. The affected arm hangs freely over a pillow placed on the back of the chair and tucked into the axilla. The hand with the intravenous needle rests on the opposite knee (for easy access to the practitioner).
4. You sit on a very low stool, facing the back of the chair.

Method

1. With both hands working simultaneously on the dislocated limb, grasp the patient's wrist with one hand and exert a steady, downward pressure.
2. Place the other hand in the axilla, with the palm exerting a direct outward pressure against the upper part of the shaft of the humerus (Fig. 9.32).
3. When appropriate muscle relaxation is achieved, the head of the humerus slips up and over the glenoid rim.

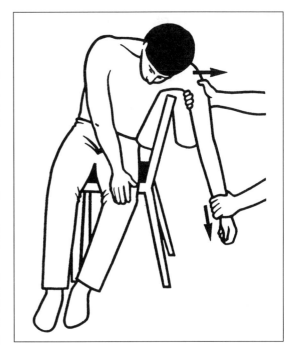

Fig. 9.32 Reduction of the dislocated shoulder

Analgesia and relaxation (if necessary)

Steady traction should be maintained during administration of analgesic; 2.5 mL pethidine (25 mg) is given intravenously over 60 seconds (and may be repeated), then 1 mL diazepam (2 mg) a minute, until reduction is achieved.

Note: Carefully monitor the patient's vital signs.

The Mt Beauty analgesia-free method

This technique, described by Zagorski, aims to reduce anterior shoulder dislocation without the need for any sedating or narcotic analgesics. It is very helpful in more remote situations and is ideal for recurrent dislocation. Fractures must be excluded.

Method (e.g. left-sided dislocation)

- Explain the procedure to the patient, emphasising its gentleness.
- The patient sits upright in a straight-backed chair (no arm rests).
- An assistant stands behind the patient with a hand on each shoulder to prevent tilting of the shoulder girdle.
- The doctor kneels facing the patient with the left knee beside the patient's knees.
- The patient rests his or her left hand on the doctor's left shoulder.

- The doctor places his or her left hand on the patient's forearm just distal to the elbow (Fig. 9.33).
- Very gentle downward traction is applied as the patient, distracted somewhat by conversation, is encouraged to relax (there should be no pain).
- The doctor's right hand feels for relaxation of the shoulder and the position of the humeral head as downward traction is maintained (it usually reduces after 1–2 minutes).
- If not reduced by now, very gentle external rotation is applied by leaning around the outside of the patient away from the affected side. Reduction is heralded by a gentle click.

Rules

- Patient must be relaxed and distracted.
- Patient must not tilt to one side.
- Gentle steady traction to avoid spasm and pain.

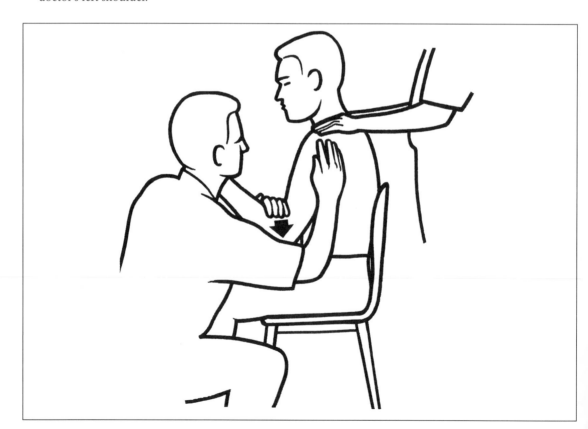

Fig. 9.33 Reduction of dislocated shoulder by gentle steady traction (as shown) in seated position

Recurrent dislocation of shoulder

For this condition, there is a way of effecting reduction without the use of force.

Method

1. The patient sits comfortably on a chair with legs crossed.

2. The patient then interlocks hands and elevates the upper knee so that the hands grip the knee (Fig. 9.34).

3. The knee is allowed to lower gradually so that its full weight is taken by the hands. At the same time the patient has to concentrate on relaxing the muscles of the shoulder girdle.

Recurrent dislocation requires definitive surgery.

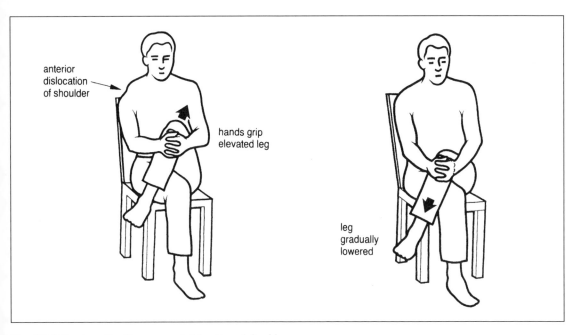

Fig. 9.34 Simple method for recurrent dislocation of shoulder

Impingement test for supraspinatus lesions

This is probably the most effective test for the rotator cuff, as it forces impingement of the greater tuberosity under the acromion. Supraspinatus tendinous lesions are the most common cause of pain in the shoulder.

Method 1

1. The patient places the arms in the position of semiflexion (90° of forward flexion) and internal rotation with the forearms in full pronation.
2. You then test resisted flexion by pushing down as the patient pushes up against this movement (Fig. 9.35).
3. If pain is reproduced, this is called a positive 'impingement sign', and is a very sensitive test for the upper components of the rotator cuff, especially supraspinatus.

Method 2

The 'emptying the can' method is an even better test for supraspinatus tendinitis. It is almost identical to Method 1 except that the affected arm is moved 30° laterally (i.e. horizontal flexion) in the horizontal plane as though to empty a can of drink. Resisted elevation is tested in this position.

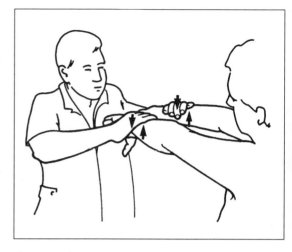

Fig. 9.35 The impingement test: resisted flexion in semiflexion, internal rotation and pronation

Elbow

Pulled elbow

This typically occurs in children under 8 years of age, usually at 2–3 years, when an adult applies sudden traction to the child's extended and pronated arm: the head of the radius can be pulled distally through the annular radioulnar ligament (Fig. 9.36a).

Symptoms and signs

- The crying child refuses to use the arm.
- The arm is limp by the side or supported in the child's lap.
- The elbow is flexed slightly.
- The forearm is pronated or held in mid-position (Fig. 9.36b).

Treatment method

1. Gain the child's confidence. Ask the parent to hold the unaffected arm.
2. Hold the child's hand (on the affected side) as if to shake it.
3. Place one hand around the child's elbow to give support, pressing the thumb over the head of the radius.
4. With the other hand, firmly twist the forearm into full supination (Fig. 9.36c).
5. Fully flex the forearm. A popping sound indicates relocation of the radial head.

An alternative method is to very gently alternate pronation and supination through a small arc as you flex the elbow.

If you cannot get the child's co-operation apply a 'high' sling and send them home. It may reduce spontaneously within a few days.

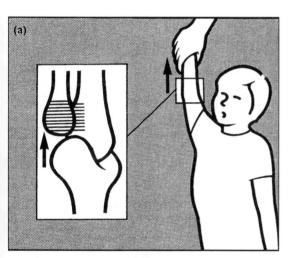

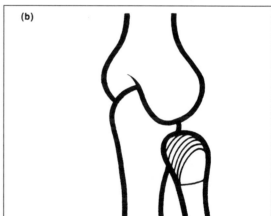

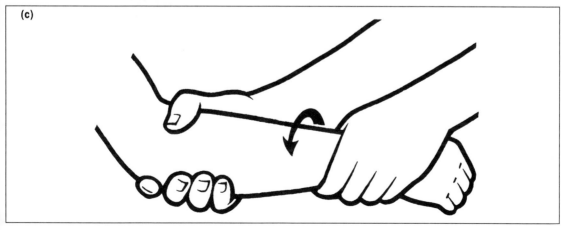

Fig. 9.36 Pulled elbow: **(a)** mechanism of injury; **(b)** annular ligament displaced over head of radius; **(c)** reduction

Dislocated elbow

A dislocated elbow is caused by a fall on the out-stretched hand, forcing the forearm backwards to result in posterior and lateral displacement (Fig. 9.37). The peripheral pulses and sensation in the hand must be assessed carefully. Check the function of the ulnar nerve before and after reduction.

Usual treatment

Attempt reduction with the patient fully relaxed under anaesthesia. It is important to apply traction to the flexed elbow but allowing it to extend approximately 20–30° to enable correction of the lateral displacement with the hand pushing from the side and then the posterior displacement by pushing the olecranon forward with the thumbs.

A simple method of reduction

This method reduces an uncomplicated posterior dislocation of the elbow without the need for anaesthesia or an assistant. The manipulation must be gentle and without sudden movement.

Method

1. The patient lies prone on a stretcher or couch, with the forearm dangling towards the floor.
2. Grasp the wrist and *slowly* apply traction in the direction of the long axis of the forearm (Fig. 9.38).
3. When the muscles feel relaxed (this might take several minutes), use the thumb and index finger of the other hand to grasp the olecranon and guide it to a reduced position, correcting for any lateral shift.
4. After reduction the arm is held in a collar-and-cuff sling, with the elbow flexed above 90°, for 1–3 weeks.

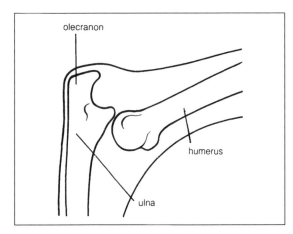

Fig. 9.37 Dislocated elbow: uncomplicated posterior dislocation

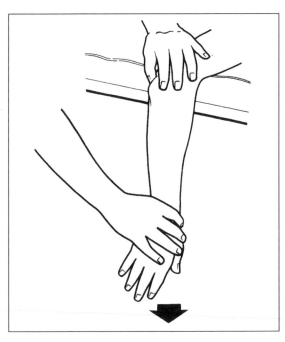

Fig. 9.38 Method of reduction by traction on the dependent arm

Tennis elbow

A simple cure—the wringing exercise

Chronic tennis elbow can be cured by a simple wringing exercise using a small hand towel.

Method

1. Roll up the hand towel.
2. With the arms extended, grasp the towel with the wrist of the affected side placed in slight flexion.
3. Then exert maximum wring pressure (Fig. 9.39):

   - first fully flexing the wrist for 10 seconds,
   - then fully extending the wrist for 10 seconds,
   - alternate flexion and extension between hands.

This is an isometric 'hold' contraction.

Frequency

This exercise should be performed only twice a day, initially for 10 seconds in each direction. After each week, increase the time by 5 seconds in each twisting direction until 60 seconds is reached (week 11). This level is maintained indefinitely. Apply ice for 10 minutes after completion, especially last thing at night.

Note: Despite severe initial pain, the patient must persist, using as much force as possible.

Review at 6 weeks (there is usually some relief by 4–6 weeks), to ensure that the patient is doing the exercise exactly as instructed.

(continues)

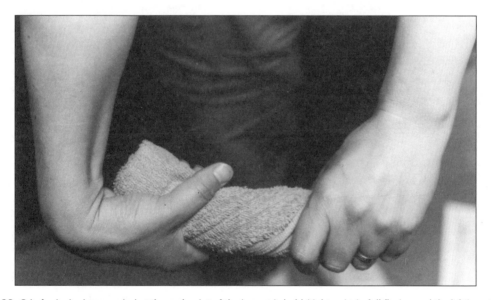

Fig. 9.39 Grip for 'wringing exercise' at the end point of the isometric hold (right wrist in full flexion and the left in extension)

Exercises

Stretching and strengthening exercises for the forearm muscles represent the best management for tennis elbow. The muscles are strengthened by the use of hand-held weights or dumbbells. A suitable starting weight is 0.5 kg, building up gradually (increasing by 0.5 kg) to 5 kg, depending on the patient.

Method

1. To perform this exercise the patient sits in a chair beside a table.
2. The arm is rested on the table so that the wrist extends over the edge.
3. The weight is grasped with the palm facing downwards (Fig. 9.40a).
4. The weight is slowly raised and lowered by flexing and extending the wrist.
5. The flexion/extension wrist movement is repeated 10 times, with a rest for 1 minute and the program repeated twice.

This exercise should be performed every day until the patient can play tennis, work or use the arm without pain.

For medial epicondylitis (forearm tennis elbow, golfer's elbow), perform the same exercises but with the palm of the hand facing upward (Fig. 9.40b).

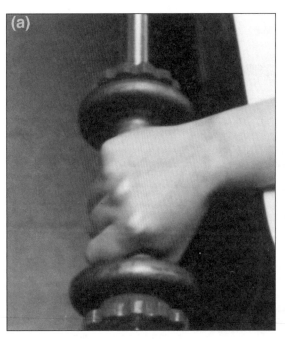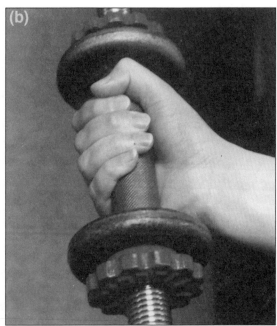

Fig. 9.40 Tennis elbow: **(a)** dumbbell exercise for classical case (palm facing down); **(b)** dumbbell exercise for medial epicondylitis—forearm tennis elbow, golfer's elbow (palm facing up)

Wrist and hand

De Quervain's tenosynovitis and Finkelstein's test

De Quervain's disease is a stenosing tenosynovitis of the abductor pollicus longus or extensor pollicus brevis tendons over the radial styloid of the wrist, or both. It results from repetitive activity, such as that engaged in by staple gun operators on assembly lines, or from direct trauma.

Symptoms

The major symptoms are:

- pain during pinch grasping,
- pain on thumb and wrist movement.

Tetrad of diagnostic signs

Four key diagnostic signs are:

1. tenderness to palpation over and just proximal to the radial styloid;
2. localised swelling in the area of the radial styloid;
3. positive Finkelstein's sign;
4. pain on active extension of thumb against resistance.

Finkelstein's test

Method

1. The patient folds the thumb into the palm with the fingers of the involved hand folded over the thumb.
2. Rotate the wrist in an ulnar direction (medially) to gently stretch the involved tendons (Fig. 9.41).
3. A positive test is indicated by reproduction of or increased pain.

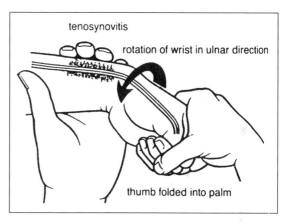

Fig. 9.41 Finkelstein's test

Simple tests for carpal tunnel syndrome

The carpal tunnel syndrome, caused by compression of the median nerve, is a common disorder that is usually easily diagnosed from the history. The most common and easily recognised symptoms are early-morning numbness and tingling or burning in the distribution of the median nerve in the hand. In the physical examination for the suspected carpal tunnel syndrome, a couple of simple tests can assist with confirming the diagnosis. These are Tinel's test and Phalen's test.

The Tinel test

1. Hold the wrist in a neutral or flexed position, and tap over the median nerve at the flexor surface of the wrist. This should be over the retinaculum just lateral to the palmaris longus tendon (if present) and the tendons of flexor digitorum superficialis (Fig. 9.42a).
2. A positive Tinel's sign produces a tingling sensation (usually without pain) in the distribution of the median nerve.

The Phalen test

1. The patient approximates the dorsum of both hands, one to the other, with wrists maximally flexed and fingers pointed downward (Fig. 9.42b).
2. This position is held for 60 seconds.
3. A positive test reproduces tingling and numbness along the distribution of the median nerve.

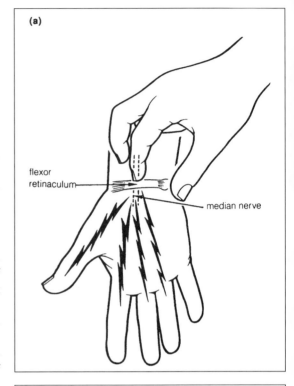

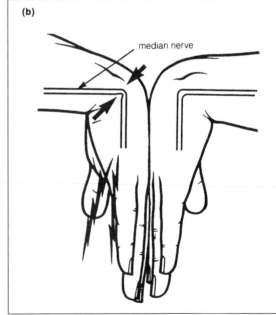

Fig. 9.42 Carpal tunnel syndrome: **(a)** Tinel sign for diagnosis; **(b)** Phalen's test to reproduce symptoms

Simple reduction of dislocated finger

This method employs the principle of using the patient's body weight as the distracting force to achieve reduction of the dislocation. It is relatively painless and very effective. Getting a good grip is very important, so wrap a small strip of zinc oxide adhesive plaster around the finger.

Method

1. Face the patient, both in standing positions.
2. Firmly grasp the distal part of the dislocated finger.
3. Request the patient to lean backwards, while maintaining the finger in a fixed position (Fig. 9.43).
4. As the patient leans back, sudden, painless reduction should spontaneously occur.

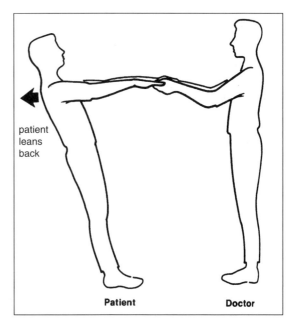

Fig. 9.43 Reduction of dislocated finger

Strapping a finger

Method

1. Instead of strapping an injured finger circumferentially, it is more comfortable and more effective to place a single strip of adhesive tape 2.5 cm or less in width on the dorsum of the finger from the tip of the nail to the carpometacarpal line (Fig. 9.44a).
2. The direction of the tape should follow the line of the extensor tendon (Fig. 9.44b). The effect is the use of the skin traction as a suspensory sling for the finger. The flexor and extensor tendons are allowed to relax with a decrease in position maintenance strain and pain. At the same time the finger is free to flex with recovery, and frozen finger is unlikely.
3. The degree of mobility of the finger is adjusted by altering the tension along the line of the tape.

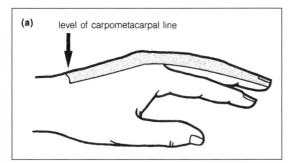
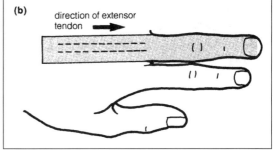

Fig. 9.44 Strapping a finger

Mallet finger

A forced hyperflexion injury to the distal phalanx can rupture or avulse the extensor insertion into its dorsal base. The characteristic swan neck deformity is due to retraction of the lateral bands and hyper-extension of the proximal interphalangeal joint.

The 45° guideline

Without treatment, the eventual disability will be minimal if the extensor lag at the distal joint is less than 45°; a greater lag will result in functional difficulty and cosmetic deformity.

Treatment

Maintain hyperextension of the distal inter-phalangeal joint for 6 weeks, leaving the proximal interphalangeal joint free to flex. Even with treatment the failure rate is high—only about 50–60% recover.

Equipment

- Friar's balsam (will permit greater adhesion of tape).
- Non-stretch adhesive tape, 1 cm wide: two strips approximately 10 cm in length.

Method

1. Paint the finger with friar's balsam (compound benzoin tincture).
2. Apply the first strip of tape in a figure-of-eight conformation. The centre of the tape must engage and support the pulp of the finger. The tapes must cross dorsally at the level of the distal inter-phalangeal joint and extend to the volar aspect of the proximal interphalangeal joint without inhibiting its movement (Fig. 9.45a).
3. Apply the second piece of tape as a 'stay' around the midshaft of the middle phalanx (Fig. 9.45b).

Reapply the tape whenever extension of the distal interphalangeal joint drops below the neutral position (usually daily, depending on the patient's occupation). Maintain extension for 6 weeks.

Other splints

There are a variety of splints. A popular one is a simple plastic mallet finger splint.

Surgery

Open reduction and internal fixation are reserved for those cases where the avulsed bony fragment is large enough to cause instability leading to volar subluxation of the distal interphalangeal joint.

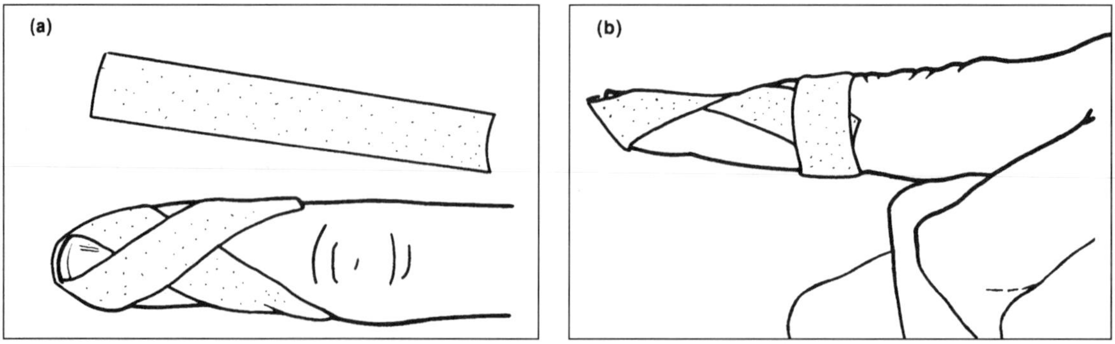

Fig. 9.45 'Mallet finger': **(a)** application of first tape; **(b)** application of 'stay' tape

Boutonnière deformity

The 'button hole' deformity is a closed rupture of the extensor tendon apparatus over the PIP joint (Fig. 9.46).

Treatment of uncomplicated deformity

1. Splint the PIP joint in full extension for 8–10 weeks.
2. Leave the DIP joint free for movement (Fig. 9.47).

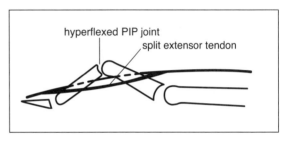

Fig. 9.46 Illustration of the mechanism of a boutonnière deformity

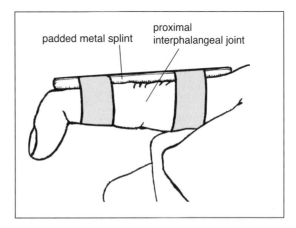

Fig. 9.47 Method of splinting for a boutonnière deformity

Tenpin bowler's thumb

Tenpin bowler's thumb is a common stress syndrome in players. It usually presents as a soft-tissue swelling at the base of the thumb web (Fig. 9.48), with associated pain and stiffness of the digits used for bowling.

Management

The patient will need:

- rest,
- massage,
- to bevel the bowling ball holes to reduce friction,
- an intralesional injection of 0.25 mL of long-acting corticosteroid mixed with local anaesthetic (resistant cases).

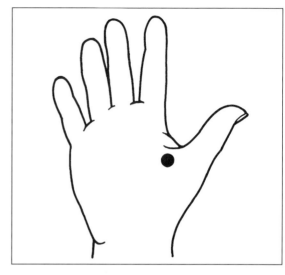

Fig. 9.48 Site of tender 'mass' at base of thumb web

Skier's thumb (gamekeeper's thumb)

A special injury is skier's thumb (also known as gamekeeper's thumb) in which there is ligamentous disruption of the metacarpophalangeal joint with or without an avulsion fracture of the base of the proximal phalanx at the point of ligamentous attachment (Fig. 9.49). This injury is caused by the thumb being forced into abduction and hyper-extension by the ski pole as the skier pitches into the snow.

Diagnosis is made by X-ray with stress views of the thumb. Incomplete tears are immobilised in a scaphoid type of plaster for 3 weeks, while complete tears and avulsion fractures should be referred for surgical repair.

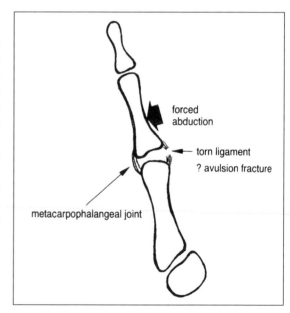

Fig 9.49 Skier's thumb

Colles' fracture

Features

- A supination fracture of distal 3 cm of radius.
- Caused by a fall onto an outstretched hand.
- The fracture features (Fig. 9.50):
  —impaction,
  —posterior displacement and angulation,
  —lateral (radial) displacement and angulation,
  —supination.

Method of reduction

Under appropriate anaesthesia:

- Traction on hand (to disimpact).
- An assistant maintains countertraction.
- Pronate.
- Ulnar deviation for 10° (to correct radial displacement).
- Flexion (10–15°).

Immobilise the wrist and forearm in a well-padded, below-elbow plaster for 3 weeks—forearm in full pronation, wrist in corrected position described above.

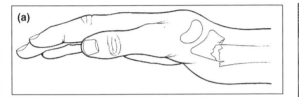

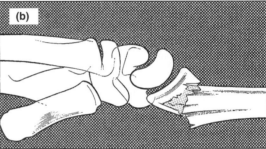

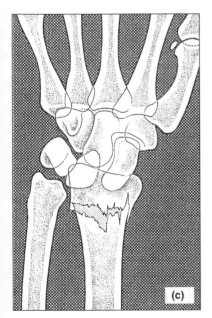

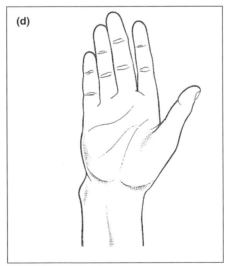

Fig. 9.50 Colles' fracture: **(a)** dinner-fork deformity; **(b)** lateral X-ray view; **(c)** anteroposterior X-ray view; **(d)** radial (lateral) tilt of distal segment

Hip

Age relationship of hip disorders

Hip disorders have a significant age relationship (Fig. 9.51).

- Children can suffer from a variety of serious disorders of the hip, e.g. developmental dysplasia (DDII), Perthes' disorder, tuberculosis, septic arthritis and slipped upper capital epiphysis

(SCFE) all of which demand early recognition and management.

- SCFE typically presents in the obese adolescent (10–15 years) with knee pain and a slight limp.
- Every newborn infant should be tested for DDH, which is diagnosed early by the Ortolani and Barlow tests (abnormal third or clunk on abduction). However, ultrasound examination is the investigation of choice and is more sensitive than the clinical examination, especially after 8 weeks.

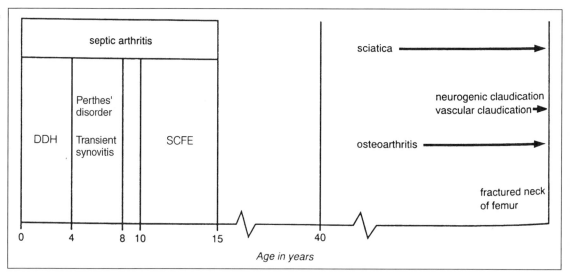

Fig. 9.51 Typical ages of presentation of hip disorders

Pain referred to the knee

Referred pain from the hip to the knee is one of the time-honoured traps in medicine. The hip joint is mainly innervated by L_3, hence pain is referred from the groin down the front and medial aspects of the thigh to the knee (Fig. 9.52). Sometimes the pain can be experienced on the anteromedial aspect of the knee only. It is not uncommon that children with a SCFE present with a limp and knee pain.

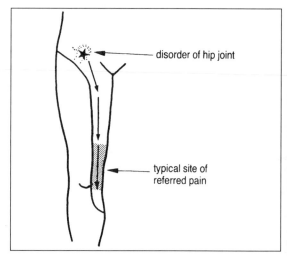

Fig. 9.52 Possible area of referred pain from disorders of the hip joint

Diagnosis of early osteoarthritis of hip joint

The four-step stress test

Degeneration of the hip joint is a common problem in general practice, and may present with pain around the hip or at the knee. Early diagnosis is very useful, and certain tests may detect the problem. It is worth remembering that, of the six main movements of the hip joint, the earliest to be affected are internal rotation, abduction and extension. A special stress test is described here that is sensitive to diagnosing disease in the hip.

Method

1. Lay the patient in the supine position.
2. Flex the hip to about 120°.
3. Adduct to about 20°–30° (Fig. 9.53).
4. Internally rotate.
5. Compress the joint through pressure down the axis of the femur.

Dysfunction of the joint may be evident when internal rotation is attempted. Any internal rotation may be virtually impossible because of stiffness or pain.

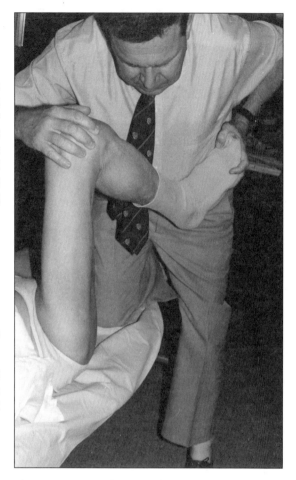

Fig. 9.53 Stress test for osteoarthritis of the hip

The 'hip pocket nerve' syndrome

If a man presents with 'sciatica', especially confined to the buttock and upper posterior thigh (without local back pain), consider the possibility of pressure on the sciatic nerve from a wallet in the hip pocket. This problem is occasionally encountered in people sitting for long periods in cars (e.g. taxi drivers). It appears to be related to the increased presence of plastic credit cards in wallets.

Surface anatomy

The sciatic nerve leaves the pelvis through the greater sciatic foramen and emerges from beneath the piriformis muscle at a position just medial to the midpoint of a line between the medial surface of the ischial tuberosity and the tip of the greater trochanter (Fig. 9.54). The lateral border of the nerve usually lies at this midpoint. It lies deep to the gluteus medius in the buttock.

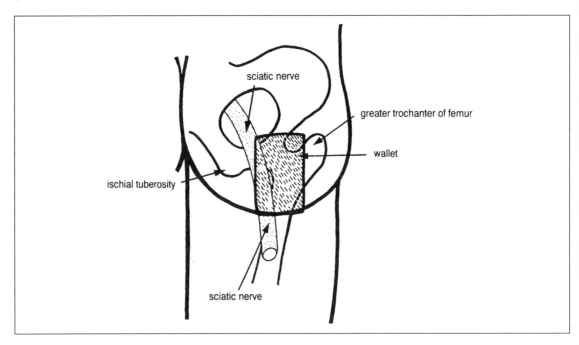

Fig. 9.54 'Hip pocket nerve' syndrome: location and relations of sciatic nerve in the buttock

Ischial bursitis

'Tailor's bottom' or 'weaver's bottom', which is occasionally seen is a bursa overlying the ischial tuberosity. Irritation of the sciatic nerve may coexist and the patient may appear to have sciatica.

Features

- severe pain when sitting, especially on a hard chair,
- tenderness at or just above the ischial tuberosity.

Treatment

- Infiltration into the tender spot of a mixture of 4 mL of 1% lignocaine and 1 mL of LA corticosteroid (avoid the sciatic nerve).
- Foam rubber cushion with two holes cut out for ischial prominences.

Patrick or Fabere test

To test hip and sacroiliac joint disorders.

Fabere is an acronym for Flexion, Abduction, External Rotation and Extension of the hip.

Method

1. The patient lies supine on the table and the foot of the involved side and extremity are placed on the opposite knee.
2. The hip joint is now flexed, externally rotated and abducted. (This position stresses the hip joint, so that inguinal pain on that side is a pointer to a defect in the hip joint or surrounding soft tissue.)
3. The range of motion for the hip joint in this position can be taken to the endpoint (thus fixing the femur in relation to the pelvis), by pressing the knee downward and simultaneously pressing on the region of the anterior superior iliac spine of the opposite side (Fig. 9.55). This stresses the hip joint as well as the sacroiliac joint on that side.

Thus, if low back pain is reproduced, the cause is likely to be a disorder of the sacroiliac joint. Such a lesion is uncommon, but is seen in nursing mothers and in those with inflammatory disorders of the joint (e.g. ankylosing spondylitis and Reiter's disease) and with infection (e.g. tuberculosis).

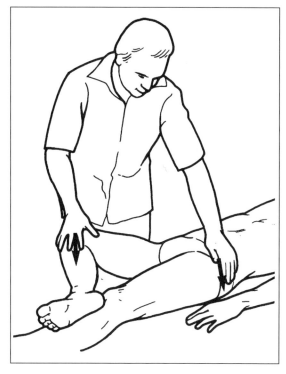

Fig. 9.55 The Patrick (Fabere) test for right-sided hip or sacroiliac joint regions, illustrating directions of pressure from the examiner

Snapping or clicking hip

Some patients complain of a clunking, clicking or snapping hip. This represents a painless, annoying problem.

Causes

One or more of the following:

- A taut iliotibial band (tendon of tensor fascia femoris) slipping backwards and forwards over the prominence of the greater trochanter.
- The iliopsoas tendon snapping across the ilio-pectineal eminence.
- The gluteus maximus sliding across the greater trochanter.
- Joint laxity.

Treatment method

There are two major components of the treatment:
(a) explanation and reassurance;
(b) exercises to stretch the iliotibial band.

1. The patient lies on the 'normal' side, and flexes the affected hip (with the leg straight and a weight around the ankle; Fig. 9.56) to a degree that produces a stretching sensation along the lateral aspect of the thigh.
2. This iliotibial stretch should be performed for 1–2 minutes, twice daily.

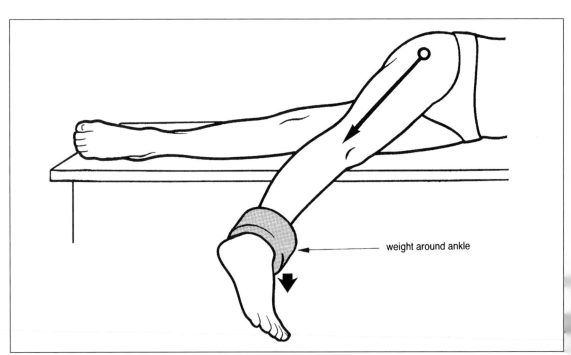

weight around ankle

Fig. 9.56 Clicking hip treatment

Dislocated hip

Posterior dislocation of the hip is usually caused by a direct blow to the knee of the flexed leg (knee and hip flexed).

The painful shortened leg is held in:

- internal rotation,
- adduction,
- slight flexion (9.57a).

Principles of management

- Adequate analgesia, e.g. IM morphine for pain.
- X-rays to confirm diagnosis and exclude associated fracture.
- Reduction of the dislocated hip under relaxant anaesthesia.
- Follow-up X-ray to confirm reduction and exclude any fractures not visible on the first X-ray.

Method of reduction A

Standard method

With the patient under relaxant anaesthesia and lying on the floor and with an assistant steadying or fixing the pelvis by downward pressure:

- Apply traction as the hip is flexed to 90°.
- Then apply gentle external rotation and abduction (maintaining traction) with hand pressure over the femoral head.

Method of reduction B

Dependent reduction method

This is especially useful if there is an associated fracture of the femur on the same side (Fig. 9.57b).

The anaesthetised patient lies prone on the table:

- Drop the leg and flex the dislocated hip over the edge of the table.
- Apply steady downward traction on the flexed hip.
- Gently rotate externally with hand pressure on femoral head (from gluteal region).

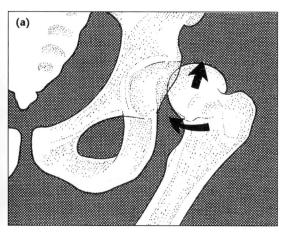 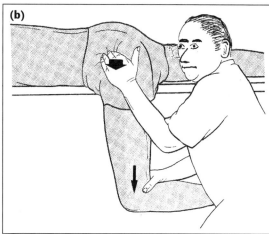

Fig. 9.57 **(a)** Posterior dislocation of hip with internal rotation; **(b)** dislocated hip: dependent reduction method

Knee

Inspection of the knees

Remembering the terminology

Sometimes it is difficult to recall whether 'knock knees' is known as genu valgum or genu varus. A useful method is to remember that the 'l' in valgum stands for 'l' in lateral. Valgum refers to deviation of the bone distal to the joint, namely the tibia in relation to the knee.

In the normal knee, the tibia has a slight valgus angulation in reference to the femur, the angulation being more pronounced in women.

The common types of knee deformity are:

- genu valgum, 'knock knees' (Fig. 9.58a),
- genu recurvatum, 'back knee' (Fig. 9.58b),
- genu varum, 'bowed legs' (Fig. 9.58c).

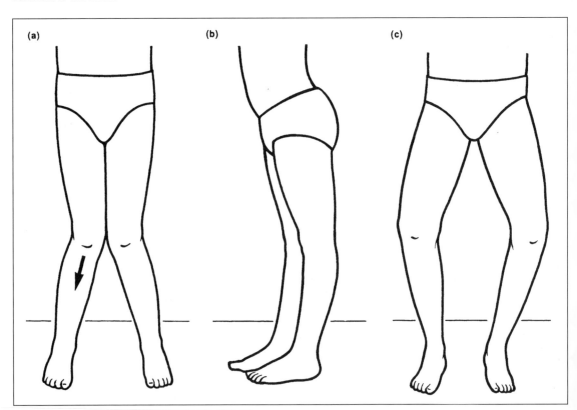

Fig. 9.58 Knee deformities: **(a)** genu valgum ('knock knees'): tibia deviates laterally from knee; **(b)** genu recurvatum ('back knee'); **(c)** genu varum ('bowed legs')

Common causes of knee pain

A UK study has highlighted the fact that the commonest cause of knee pain is simple ligamentous strains and bruises due to overstress of the knee or other minor trauma. Traumatic synovitis may accompany some of these injuries. Some of these so-called strains may include a variety of recently described syndromes such as the synovial plica syndrome, patellar tendinitis and infrapatellar fat-pad inflammation (Fig. 9.59).

Low-grade trauma of repeated overuse such as frequent kneeling may cause prepatellar bursitis known variously as 'housemaid's knee' or 'carpet layer's knee'. Infrapatellar bursitis is referred to as 'clergyman's knee'.

Osteoarthritis of the knee, especially in the elderly, is a very common problem. It may arise spontaneously or be secondary to previous trauma with associated internal derangement and instability.

The most common overuse problem of the knee is the patellofemoral joint pain syndrome (often previously referred to as chondromalacia patellae).

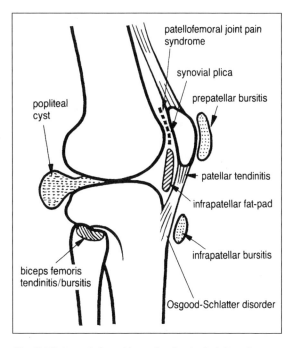

Fig. 9.59 Lateral view of knee showing typical sites of various causes of knee pain

Diagnosis of meniscal injuries of the knee

Injuries to the medial and lateral menisci of the knee are common in contact sports, and are often associated with ligamentous injuries.

Table 9.3 is a useful aid in the diagnosis of these injuries. There is a similarity in the clinical signs between the opposite menisci, but the localisation of pain in the medial or lateral joint lines helps to differentiate between the medial and lateral menisci (Fig. 9.60).

Note: The diagnosis of a meniscal injury is made if three or more of the five examination findings ('signs' in Table 9.3) are present.

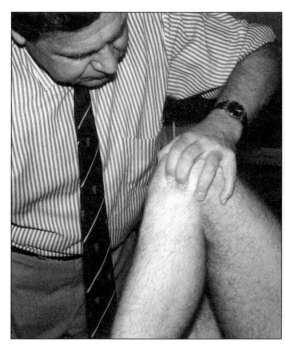

Fig. 9.60 Localised tenderness over the outer joint line with injury to the lateral meniscus

Table 9.3 Typical symptoms and signs of meniscal injuries

	Medial meniscus tear	**Lateral meniscus tear**
Mechanism	• Abduction (valgus) force • External rotation of lower leg on femur	• Adduction (varus) force • Internal rotation of leg on femur
Symptoms		
1. Knee pain during and after activity	Medial side of knee	Lateral side of knee
2. Locking	yes	yes
3. Effusion	+ or −	+ or −
Signs		
1. Localised tenderness over joint line (with bucket handle tear)	Medial joint line	Lateral joint line (may be cyst)
2. Pain on hyperextension of knee	Medial joint line	Lateral joint line
3. Pain on hyperflexion of knee joint	Medial joint line	Lateral joint line
4. Pain on rotation of lower leg (knee at 90°)	On external rotation	On internal rotation
5. Weakened or atrophied quadriceps	May be present	May be present

Lachman test

The Lachman test is a sensitive and reliable test for the integrity of the anterior cruciate ligament. It is an anterior draw test with the knee at 15° of flexion. At 90° of flexion, the draw may be negative but the anterior cruciate torn.

Test method

1. Position yourself on the same side of the examination couch as the knee to be tested.
2. The knee is held at 15° of flexion by placing a hand under the distal thigh and lifting the knee into 15° of flexion.
3. The patient is asked to relax, allowing the knee to 'fall back' into the steadying hand and roll slightly into external rotation.
4. The anterior draw is performed with the second hand grasping the proximal tibia from the medial side (Fig. 9.61) while the thigh is held steady by the other hand.
5. The feel of the endpoint of the draw is carefully noted. Normally there is an obvious jar felt as the anterior cruciate tightens. In an anterior cruciate-deficient knee there is excess movement and no firm endpoint. The amount of draw is compared with the opposite knee. Movement greater than 5 mm is usually considered abnormal.

Note: Functional instability due to anterior cruciate deficiency is best elicited with the pivot shift test. This is more difficult to perform than the Lachman test.

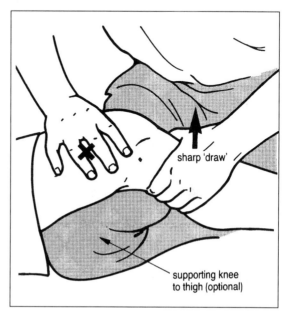

sharp 'draw'

supporting knee to thigh (optional)

Fig. 9.61 Lachman test

Overuse syndromes

The knee is very prone to overuse disorders. The pain develops gradually without swelling, is aggravated by activity and relieved with rest. It can usually be traced back to a change in the sportsperson's training schedule, footwear, technique or related factors. It may be related also to biomechanical abnormalities ranging from hip disorders to feet disorders.

Overuse injuries include:

- patellofemoral joint pain syndrome ('jogger's knee', 'runner's knee'),
- patellar tendinitis ('jumper's knee'),

- synovial plica syndrome,
- infrapatellar fat-pad inflammation,
- anserinus bursitis/tendinitis,
- biceps femoris tendinitis,
- semimembranous bursitis/tendinitis,
- quadriceps tendinitis/rupture,
- popliteus tendinitis,
- iliotibial band friction syndrome ('runner's knee'),
- the hamstrung knee.

It is amazing how often palpation identifies localised areas of inflammation (tendinitis or bursitis) around the knee, especially from overuse in athletes and in the obese elderly (Fig. 9.62a,b).

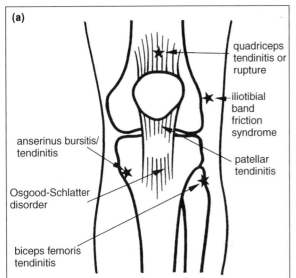
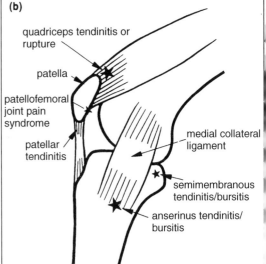

Fig. 9.62 Typical painful areas around the knee for overuse syndromes: **(a)** anterior aspect; **(b)** medial aspect

Patellar tendinitis ('jumper's knee')

'Jumper's knee' or patellar tendinitis (Fig. 9.63a) is a common disorder of athletes involved in repetitive jumping sports, such as high jumping, basketball, netball, volleyball and soccer. The diagnosis is often missed because of the difficulty of localising signs.

The condition is best diagnosed by eliciting localised tenderness at the inferior pole of the patella with the patella tilted.

Method

1. Lay the patient supine in a relaxed manner with head on a pillow, arms by the side and quadriceps relaxed (*a must*).
2. The knee should be fully extended.
3. Tilt the patella by exerting pressure over its superior pole. This lifts the inferior pole.
4. Now palpate the surface under the inferior pole. This allows palpation of the deeper fibres of the patellar tendon (Fig. 9.63b).
5. Compare with the normal side.

Very sharp pain is usually produced in the patient with patellar tendinitis.

Treatment

Explanation and conservative management including activity modification, stretching exercises and a strengthening program is the first-line treatment. However, the problem can be stubborn, and surgery has an important place in the management.

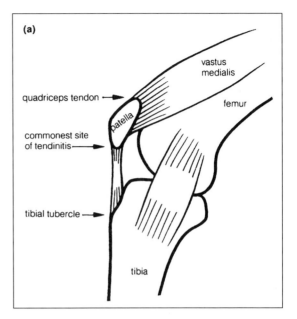

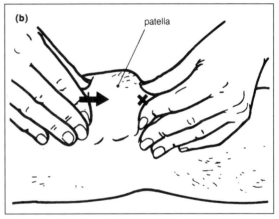

Fig. 9.63 Patellar tendinitis: **(a)** diagram of knee; **(b)** method of palpation

Anterior knee pain

Pain felt in the anterior part of the knee is very common and is most commonly caused by the patellofemoral joint pain syndrome. It needs to be distinguished from arthritis of the knee joint. It is common in sports medicine and is referred to sometimes as 'jogger's knee', 'runner's knee' or 'cyclist's knee'.

Diagnosis and treatment of patellofemoral joint pain syndrome

This syndrome, also known as chondromalacia patellae, is characterised by pain and crepitus around the patella during activities that require flexion of the knee under loading (e.g. climbing stairs).

Signs

Patellofemoral crepitation during knee flexion and extension is often palpable, and pain may be reproduced by compression of the patella onto the femur as it is pushed from side to side with the knee straight or flexed (Perkin's test).

Method for special sign (Fig. 9.64)

1. Have the patient supine with the knee extended.
2. Grasp the superior pole of the patella and displace it inferiorly.
3. Maintain this position and apply patellofemoral compression.
4. Ask the patient to contract the quadriceps (a good idea is to get the patient to practise quadriceps contraction before applying the test).
5. A positive sign is reproduction of pain under the patella and hesitancy in contracting the muscle.

Treatment

Figure 9.65 illustrates a simple quadriceps exercise. A series of isometric contractions are each held for about 4 seconds and alternated with relaxation of the leg. This exercise can be repeated many times in one period and throughout the day.

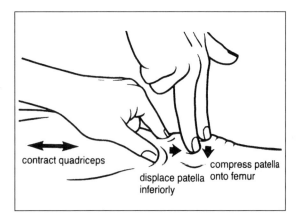

Fig. 9.64 Special sign of patellofemoral joint pain syndrome

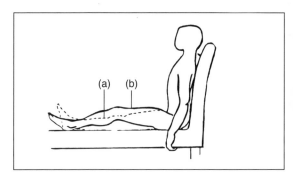

Fig. 9.65 Quadriceps exercise: tighten muscle by straightening the knee to position (a) from the relaxed position (b)

Dislocated patella

Typical features

- An injury of children and young adults (especially females).
- Caused by contraction of quadriceps with a flexed knee.
- There is always lateral displacement.
- Knee may be stuck in flexion.

Method of immediate reduction

The following can be attempted without anaesthesia (preferably immediately after the injury) or by using pethidine and IV diazepam as a relaxant:

- Place your thumb under the lateral edge of the patella.
- Push it medially as you extend the knee.

Important points

- Exclude an osteochondral fracture with X-rays.
- Post-reduction rest with knee splinted in extension and crutches for 4–6 weeks.
- Arthroscopic inspection and repair may be advisable.
- Recurrent dislocation in young females (14–18 years) requires surgery.

Leg

Overuse syndromes in athletes

Athletes, especially runners and joggers, are prone to painful problems in the lower legs (Fig. 9.66). Diagnosis of the various syndromes can be difficult, but Table 9.4 will be a useful guide. The precise anatomical site of the painful problem is the best pointer to a diagnosis.

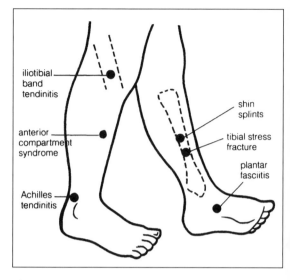

Fig. 9.66 Common sites of lower leg problems

Table 9.4 Clinical comparisons of overuse syndromes

Syndrome	Symptoms	Cause	Treatment
Anterior compartment syndrome	Pain in the anterolateral muscular compartment of the leg, increasing with activity. Difficult dorsiflexion of foot, which may feel floppy.	Persistent fast running (e.g. squash, football, middle-distance running).	Modify activities. Surgical fasciotomy is the only effective treatment.
Iliotibial band tendinitis	Deep aching along lateral aspect of knee or lateral thigh. Worse running downhill, eased by rest. Pain appears after 3–4 km running.	Running up hills by long-distance runners and increasing distance too quickly.	Rest from running for 6 weeks. Special stretching exercises. Correct training faults and footwear. Consider injection of LA and corticosteroids deep into tender areas.
Tibial stress syndrome or shin splints	Pain and localised tenderness over the distal posteromedial border of the tibia. Bone scan for diagnosis.	Running or jumping on hard surfaces.	Relative rest for 6 weeks. Ice massage. Calf (soleus stretching). NSAIDs. Correct training faults and footwear.
Tibial stress fracture	Pain, in a similar site to shin splints, noted after running. Usually relieved by rest. Bone scan for diagnosis.	Overtraining on hard (often bitumen) surfaces. Faulty footwear.	Rest for 6–10 weeks. Casting not recommended. Graduated training after healing.
Tibialis anterior tenosynovitis	Pain, over anterior distal third of leg and ankle. Pain at beginning and after exercise ± swelling, crepitus. Pain on active or resisted ankle dor-siflexion.	Overuse—excessive downhill running.	Rest, even from walking. Injection of LA and corticosteroid within tendon sheath.
Achilles tendinitis	Pain in the Achilles tendon aggravated by walking on the toes. Stiff and sore in the morning after rising but improving after activity.	Repeated toe running in sprinters or running uphill in distance runners.	Relative rest. Ice at first and then heat. 10 mm heel wedge. Correct training faults and footwear. NSAIDs. Consider steroid injection.
Plantar fasciitis	Pain in medial or control aspect of base of the heel, worse with weight bearing. Sharp pain upon getting up to walk after sitting.	Running on uneven surfaces with feet pronated.	Relative rest. Orthotics in shoes. Injection of LA and corticosteroid.

Torn 'monkey muscle'

The so-called torn 'monkey muscle', or 'tennis leg', is actually a rupture of the medial head of gastrocnemius at the musculoskeletal junction where the Achilles tendon merges with the muscle (Fig. 9.67). This painful injury is common in middle-aged tennis and squash players who play infrequently and are unfit.

Clinical features

- a sudden sharp pain in the calf (the person thinks he or she has been struck from behind, e.g. by a thrown stone),
- unable to put heel to ground,
- walks on tip toes,
- localised tenderness and hardness,
- dorsiflexion of ankle painful,
- bruising over site of rupture.

Management

- RICE treatment for 48 hours.
- Ice packs immediately for 20 minutes and then every 2 hours when awake (can be placed over the bandage).
- A firm elastic bandage from toes to below the knee.
- Crutches can be used if severe.
- A raised heel on the shoe (preferably both sides) aids mobility.
- Commence mobilisation after 48 hours rest, with active exercises.
- Physiotherapist supervision for gentle stretching massage and then restricted exercise.

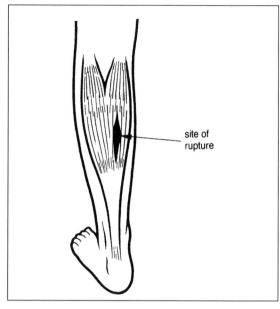

site of rupture

Fig. 9.67 'Tennis leg' or 'monkey muscle'—illustrating typical site of rupture of the medial head of gastrocnemius at the junction of muscle and tendon (left leg)

Complete rupture of Achilles tendon

A complete rupture of the Achilles tendon can be misdiagnosed because the patient is able to plantar flex the foot by virtue of the deep long flexors. Two tests should be performed to confirm the diagnosis.

Palpation of tendon

Palpate for a defect in the Achilles tendon. This defect could be masked by haematoma if the examination is performed more than a couple of hours after the injury.

The 'calf' squeeze test

With the patient prone and both feet over the edge of the couch, squeeze the gastrocnemius soleus complex of both legs. Plantar flexion of the foot indicates an intact Achilles tendon (Fig. 9.68a); failure of plantar flexion indicates total rupture (Fig. 9.68b).

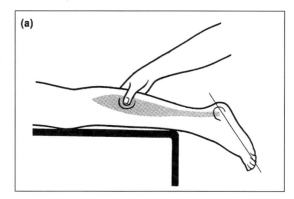

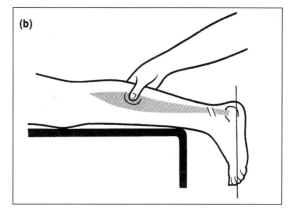

Fig. 9.68 Calf squeeze test for ruptured Achilles tendon: **(a)** intact tendon, normal plantar flexion; **(b)** ruptured tendon, foot remains stationary

Treatment of sprained ankle

Most of the ankle 'sprains' or tears involve the lateral ligaments (up to 90%), while the stronger tauter (deltoid) ligament is less prone to injury.

The treatment of ankle ligament sprains depends on the severity of the sprain. Most grade I (mild) and II (moderate) sprains respond well to standard conservative measures and regain full, pain-free movement in 1–6 weeks, but controversy surrounds the most appropriate management of grade III (complete tear) sprains.

Grades I & II sprains

R rest the injured part for 48 hours, depending on disability
I ice pack for 20 minutes every 3–4 hours when awake for the first 48 hours
C compression bandage, e.g. crepe bandage
E elevate to hip level to minimise swelling
A analgesics, e.g. paracetamol
R review in 48 hours, then 7 days
S special strapping

Use partial weight bearing with crutches for the first 48 hours or until standing is no longer painful, then encourage early full weight bearing and a full range of movement with isometric exercises. Use warm soaks, dispense with ice packs after 48 hours. Walking in sand, e.g. along the beach, is excellent rehabilitation. Aim towards full activity by 2 weeks.

Strapping of ankle

Method

1. Maintain the foot in a neutral position (right angles to leg) by getting the patient to hold the foot in that position by a long strap or sling.
2. Apply small protective pads over pressure points.
3. Apply one or two stirrups of adhesive low-stretch 6–8 cm strapping from halfway up the medial side, around the heel and then halfway up the lateral side to hold the foot in slight eversion (Figs. 9.69a,b).
4. Apply an adhesive bandage, e.g. Acrylastic (6–8 cm), which can be rerolled and reused.
5. Reapply in 3–4 days.
6. After 7 days, remove and use a non-adhesive tubular elasticised support until full pain-free movement is achieved.

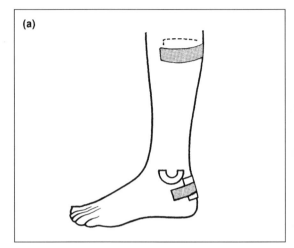

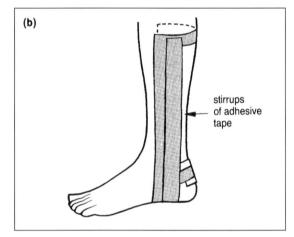

stirrups of adhesive tape

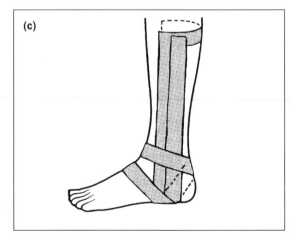

Fig. 9.69 Supportive strapping for a sprained ankle: **(a)** Step 1 apply protective pads and stay tape; **(b)** Step 2 apply stirrups to hold foot in slight eversion; **(c)** Step 3 apply an ankle lock tape

Mobilisation of the subtalar joint

The medial-lateral gliding mobilisation of the subtalar joint is indicated by a loss of function of the subtalar ankle joint, commonly with chronic post-traumatic ankle stiffness, with or without pain. The commonest cause is the classic 'sprained' ankle.

The objective of therapy is to increase the range of inversion and eversion.

Method

1. The patient lies on the side (preferably the problematic side), with the affected leg resting on the table. The foot hangs over the end of the table with the lower leg supported by a flexible support, such as a rolled-up towel, small pillow, sandbag or lumbar roll. The foot is maintained in dorsiflexion by support against the therapist's thigh.
2. Stand at the foot of the table facing the patient's leg.
3. Grasp the patient's leg with the stabilising hand just above the level of the malleolus.
4. The mobilising hand firmly grasps the calcaneum.
5. Apply a firm force to the foot at right angles to the long axis of the foot, so that an even up and down (medial-lateral) rocking movement is achieved. The movement should be smooth (not too forceful or jerky) and of consistent amplitude (Fig. 9.70).

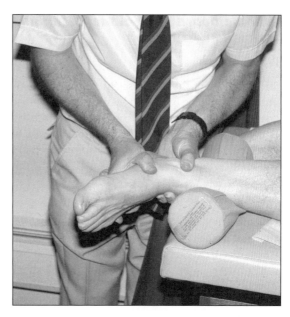

Fig. 9.70 Position of foot for mobilisation of the subtalar joint

Wobble board (aeroplane) technique for ankle dysfunction

Proprioception exercises

Strengthening of the leg muscles and the ligaments of the ankle can be improved by the use of a wobble board. The patient stands on the board and shifts his or her weight from side to side in neutral, forward or extended body positions to improve proprioception and balance.

An improvised wobble board

Patients can construct a simple wobble board by attaching a small piece of 2 or 4 inch (10 cm × 10 cm × 5 cm (deep)) wood to the centre of a 2 foot (30 cm) square piece of plywood or similar wood about 2 cm thick.

Alternative

Patients can simply place their slab of wood on a dome-shaped mound of earth.

The 'aeroplane' exercise

1. Instruct the patient to stand in a neutral position and shift his or her weight from side to side to improve balance and proprioception.
2. After 2 or 3 days, perform the balancing exercises by leaning forwards in addition to using the neutral position (Fig. 9.71).
3. After a further 2 or 3 days, practise the exercise by leaning backwards—thus adding to the difficulty of the exercise.

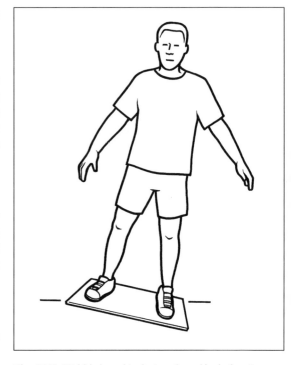

Fig. 9.71 Wobble board technique for ankle dysfunction

Tibialis posterior tendon rupture

Rupture of the tibialis posterior tendon after inflammation, degeneration or trauma is a relatively common and misdiagnosed disorder. It causes collapse of the longitudinal arch of the foot, leading to a flat foot. It is uncommon for patients to feel obvious discomfort at the moment of rupture. Most cases in middle age can be treated conservatively. Severe problems respond well to surgical repair, which is usually indicated in athletes.

Features

- Middle-aged females and athletes.
- Usually presents with 'abnormal' flat foot.
- Pain in region navicular to medial malleolus.
- Gross eversion of the foot.
- 'Too many toes' test (Fig. 9.72).
- Single heel raise test (unable to raise heel).
- On palpation, thickening or absence of tibialis posterior tendon.

'Too many toes' test

More toes are seen on the affected side when the feet are viewed from about 3 metres behind the patient (Fig. 9.72).

Useful investigations

- Ultrasound (the most economical).
- MRI and CT scan—gives the clearest image.

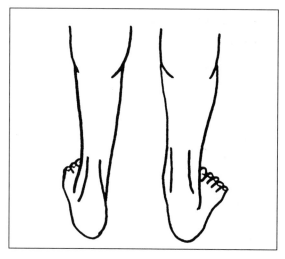

Fig. 9.72 Tibialis posterior rupture (right foot): the 'too many toes' posterior view

Plastering tips

Plaster of Paris

The bucket of water

- Line the bucket with a plastic bag for easy cleaning.
- The water should be deep enough to allow complete vertical immersion.
- Use cold water for slow setting.
- Use tepid water for faster setting.
- Do not use hot water: it produces rapid setting and a brittle plaster.

The plaster rolls

- Do not use plaster rolls if water has been splashed on them.
- Hold the roll loosely but with the free end firm and secure (Fig. 9.73).
- Immerse in water until bubbles have ceased coming from the plaster surface. Ensure that the centre of the plaster is fully wet.
- Drain surface water after removal from the bucket.
- Gently squeeze the roll in the middle: do not indent.
- Use about 2 × 10 cm and 1 × 8 cm rolls for below elbow and upper limb plasters.
- Use 4 × 15 cm rolls for below knee leg plaster.

Padding

- Use Velband or stockinet under the plaster.
- With Velband, moisten the end of the roll in water to allow it to adhere to the limb.
- For legs, make extra padding around pressure areas such as the ankle and heel.
- Use two layers of padding but avoid multiple layers.

Method

1. Use an assistant to support the limb where possible (e.g. hold the arm up with fingers of stockinet).
2. Lay the bandage on firmly but do not pull tight.
3. Lay it on quickly. Avoid dents.
4. Overlap the bandage by about 25% of its width.
5. Use only the flat of the hand so as to achieve a smooth cast.

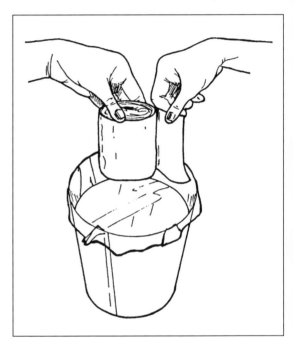

Fig. 9.73 Holding the plaster roll

Preparation of a volar arm plaster splint

A volar arm plaster splint can be prepared with minimal mess and maximal effectiveness by following this procedure.

Procedure

1. Measure the length of the required plaster splint.
2. Select Velband of the same width as the plaster and measure a length slightly more than twice the length of the splint.
3. On a flat bench top, lay out the length of the Velband on a piece of newspaper or undercloth.
4. Fold the plaster (10 cm roll for adults) according to the number of strips required and after immersing it in cool or lukewarm water and draining off excess water, place it on the Velband as shown in Figure 9.74.
5. Fold the Velband over the plaster to produce a 'sandwich' effect.
6. Using the fingers through the upper layer of Velband, mould two to three ridges along the length of the plaster on the outer surface of the slab. This provides reinforced strength for the splint.
7. Take a crepe bandage and apply the splint to the arm with appropriate moulding to hold the wrist in about 30° of extension.
8. This method can be adapted for plaster slabs for other areas.

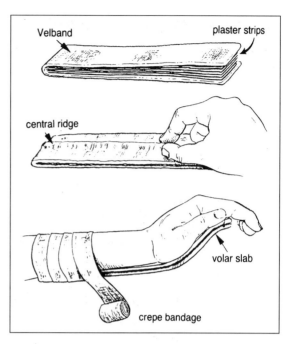

Fig. 9.74 Preparation of volar arm plaster splint

Leg support for plaster application

The awkward task of applying a leg plaster including a plaster cylinder can be aided by the use of a simple supportive device (Fig. 9.75).

The support, which should be at least 30 cm high, can be made by pinning a broad leather strap across a U-shaped frame.

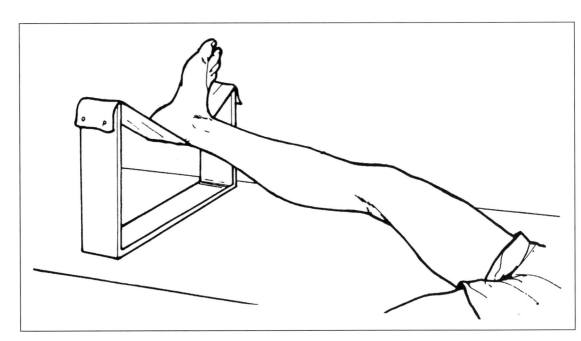

Fig. 9.75 Supportive device for application of leg plaster

Waterproofing your plaster cast

A suitable plastic protective cover for a plaster cast, especially for one on the arm, is a veterinary plastic glove which is ideally long and fits on the arm like a mega 'glove'. These are the gloves used in rural practice!

A long-lasting plaster walking heel

To avoid the plaster underlying the walking heel (incorporated into a leg plaster) becoming soft and therefore uncomfortable for walking (thus requiring repair), the following method can be used (Fig. 9.76).

It involves incorporating a small piece of masonite (or similar wooden material) into the plaster cast at the time of affixing the heel. This is performed 24 hours after application of the original base plaster cast.

Method

1. Apply a thin layer of plaster of Paris to the underside of the base of the cast.
2. Place the piece of masonite (or wood) against the plaster.
3. Place the heel over the wood.
4. Wrap adhesive plaster (such as Elastoplast) around the wood and heel to 'fix' the unit.
5. Apply the final coating of plaster of Paris to fix the heel.
6. Weight bearing can commence 24 hours later.

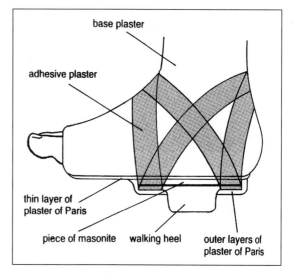

Fig. 9.76 Plaster walking heel

Supporting shoe for a walking plaster

Method A

An economical method is to get the patient to bring an old pair of rubber sneakers and cut out the front half (including the tongue) but leave the laces intact. On review (day 2), the plaster cast is filled into the sneaker and tied over with the laces.

Method B

A better alternative to the walking heel is the 'open-toe cast shoe', with its open heel and toe areas that can accommodate a wide variety of foot and cast types. The rocker sole, which is manufactured from EVA (a synthetic rubber), has three layers and minimises microtrauma to joints. The upper is made from reinforced canvas with Presto-flex adhesive straps.

The shoes come in at least three sizes and fit neatly onto the plaster. They can be washed and will last throughout the life of a normal walking plaster. The shoes are available from various surgical suppliers.

Use of silicone filler

An economical walking plaster can be improvised by obtaining silicone filler (preferably resin type) from your hardware store and layering it over the base of the plaster with extra thickness over pressure areas.

10 Orodental problems

Knocked-out tooth

If a permanent (second) tooth is knocked out (i.e. in an accident or fight) but is intact, it can be saved by the following, immediate procedure. The tooth should not be out of the mouth for longer than 15–20 minutes from the time of injury.

Method

1. Using a sterile glove hold the tooth by its crown and replace it in its original position, preferably immediately (Fig. 10.1); if dirty, put it in milk before replacement or, better still, place it under the tongue and 'wash' it in saliva. Alternatively, it can be placed in contact lens saline or the solution in the 'Dentist in A Box' kit (www.dentistinabox.com.au/~dentabox). *Note:* Do not use water, and do not rub (it removes dentine) or wipe it or touch the root.
2. Fix the tooth by moulding strong silver foil (e.g. a milk bottle top or cooking foil) over it and the adjacent teeth. Moulding foil can be difficult: an

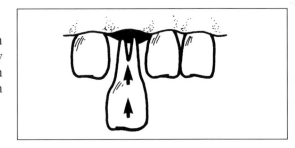

Fig. 10.1 Replacement of a knocked-out tooth

alternative is to suture with a figure-of-eight silk suture to encompass the tooth. It can also be secured to the two adjoining teeth with a strip of tape cut from a disc in the 'Dentist in A Box' kit.

3. Refer the patient to his or her dentist or dental hospital as soon as possible. Tell the patient to avoid exerting any direct biting force on the tooth.

Note: If a blood clot is present, remove it after a nerve block. Teeth replaced within 20–30 minutes have a 90% chance of successful reimplantation.

Loosening of a tooth

Loosening is excessive movement of a permanent tooth with no displacement.

Splint the mobile tooth to a neighbouring tooth with the splinting material from the kit (see above). Alternatively, use chewing gum or Blu-Tack. Refer the patient to a dentist.

Chipped tooth

Cover the exposed area, which is usually painful, with dental tape. Recover and store the tooth fragment for use by the dentist. If possible, secure the broken fragment with splinting material from the kit. Refer the patient to a dentist.

Bleeding tooth socket

First aid treatment method

Instruct the patient to bite very firmly on a rolled-up handkerchief over the bleeding socket. This simple measure is sufficient to achieve haemostasis in most instances. Biting on a recently used tea bag is another suggestion.

Surgical treatment for persistent bleeding

1. Remove excess blood clot, using a piece of sterile gauze.
2. Bite on a firm gauze pack.
3. If still bleeding, insert a suture. (Chromic or plain catgut is suitable.)
4. Using a reverse suture, approximate the anterior and posterior mucosal remnants (Fig. 10.2). The idea is not to close the socket but to tense the mucoperiosteum against the bone.

Avoid aspirin, rinsing and alcohol.

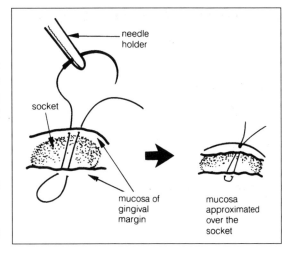

Fig. 10.2 Treatment for persistent bleeding of tooth socket

Dry tooth socket

Clinical features

- Tooth extraction 1–3 days earlier.
- Very severe pain, unrelieved by analgesics.
- Continuous pain on the side of the face.
- Foetid odour.
- Mainly in the lower molars, especially the third (wisdom teeth).

Examination shows a socket with few or no blood clots, and sensitive bone surfaces covered by a greyish-yellow layer of necrotic tissue.

Treatment method

1. Self-limiting healing 10–14 days.
2. Refer for special toilet and dressing (palliative).

If you have to treat:

- irrigate with warm saline in a syringe,
- pack socket with 1 cm ribbon gauze in iodiform paste or pack a mixture of a paste of zinc oxide and oil of cloves,
- analgesics,
- mouth wash.

Note: Antibiotics are of no proven value.

The differential diagnosis for the dry tooth socket is descending infection.

A simple way of numbering teeth

Dentists utilise codes in which the teeth are numbered from 1 to 8 from the midline.

International notation

Each of the four quadrants are numbered:

Permanent teeth (n = 32; Fig. 10.3)

$$\text{R.}\dfrac{^1\,87654321\;|\;12345678\,^2}{_4\,87654321\;|\;12345678\,_3}\text{L.}$$

Deciduous teeth (n = 20)

There are five teeth in each quadrant, and the four quadrants are notated 5–8.

$$\text{R.}\dfrac{^5\,54321\;|\;12345\,^6}{_8\,54321\;|\;12345\,_7}\text{L.}$$

Examples

- 1.6 = upper right first molar,
- 3.2 = lower left lateral incisor,
- 6.3 = upper left deciduous canine.

Palmer's notation

In this notation a cross is drawn to represent quadrants, but the numerals are used as above for permanent teeth. Deciduous teeth are represented by the letters A–E.

The quadrants are noted by four right angles:

R. ⊣⊢ L.

Examples

- ⌊5 = upper left second premolar,
- C̄| = lower right deciduous cuspid.

Wisdom teeth

These are the third molars. They are usually normal teeth, but are prone to troublesome eruption and difficult extraction when impacted.

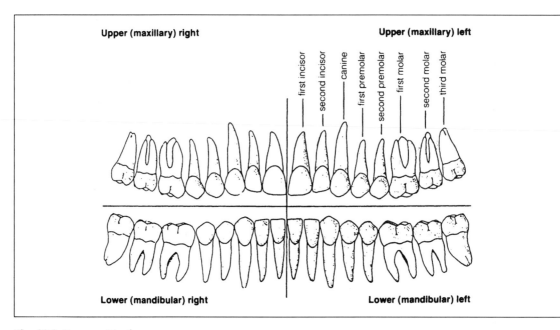

Upper (maxillary) right   **Upper (maxillary) left**

first incisor — second incisor — canine — first premolar — second premolar — first molar — second molar — third molar

Lower (mandibular) right   **Lower (mandibular) left**

Fig. 10.3 Permanent teeth

Aphthous ulcers (canker sores)

These acutely painful ulcers on the mobile oral mucosa are a common problem in general practice and puzzling in their cause and response to treatment. Their cause is unknown, but several factors indicate a localised abnormal immune reaction.
Minor ulcers: <1cm in diameter—last 10–14 days.
Major ulcers: >1 cm in diameter—last weeks and heal with scarring.

Associations to consider

Blood dyscrasias, denture pressure, Crohn's disease, pernicious anaemia, iron deficiency.

Precipitating factors

Stress and local trauma.

Treatment methods

These treatments should be used early when the ulcer is most painful. Several optional healing methods are presented.

Symptomatic relief

Apply topical lignocaine gel or paint, e.g. SM-33 adult paint formula or SM-33 gel (children) every 3 hours. If applied before meals, eating is facilitated.

Healing

One of the following methods can be chosen.

The teabag method

Consider applying a wet, squeezed out, black teabag directly to the ulcer regularly, such as 3–4 times daily. The tannic acid promotes healing.

Topical corticosteroid paste

Triamcinolone 0.1% (Kenalog in orobase) paste. Apply 8-hourly and at night.

Topical corticosteroid spray

Spray beclomethasone on to the ulcer 3 times daily.

Topical chloramphenicol

Use 10% chloramphenicol in propylene glycol. Apply with a cotton bud for 1 minute (after drying the ulcer) 6-hourly for 3–4 days.

Tetracycline suspension rinse for multiple ulcers

1. Empty the contents of a 250 mg tetracycline capsule into 20–30 mL of warm water and shake it.
2. Swirl this solution in the mouth for 5 minutes every 3 hours.

An alternative method is to apply the solution soaked in cotton wool wads to the ulcers for 5–10 minutes.

Note: This has a terrible taste but reportedly shortens the life of the ulcers considerably. We recommend spitting out the rinse, although some authorities suggest swallowing the suspension.

Topical sucralfate

Dissolve 1 g sucralfate in 20–30 mL of warm water. Use this as a mouth wash.

Geographical tongue

Treatment

Explanation and reassurance.

- No treatment if asymptomatic.
- Cepacaine gargles, 10 mL tds, if tender.
- Low dose spray of glucocorticoid (e.g. beclomethasone 50 mcg tds). Do not rinse after use.

Black or hairy tongue

Brush tongue with a toothbrush to remove stained papillae. Use pineapple as a keratolytic agent.

Method

1. Cut a thin slice of pineapple into eight segments.
2. Suck a segment on the back of the tongue for 40 seconds and then slowly chew it.
3. Repeat until all segments are completed.
4. Do this twice a day for 7–10 days. Repeat if symptoms recur.

Calculus in Wharton's duct

The commonest site for a salivary calculus is in the duct of the submandibular gland (Wharton's duct). Obstruction to the gland by the calculus causes the classic presentation of intermittent swelling of the gland whenever the patient attempts to eat. The following method applies if the clinician can easily palpate the calculus with the finger under the tongue.

Method

1. Localise the calculus in the duct by finger palpation.
2. Anaesthetise the area with a small bleb of LA or surface anaesthetic (preferable if available), e.g. 5% cocaine placed under the tongue.
3. Insert a stay suture around the duct immediately behind the calculus (Fig. 10.4), and use this to steady the stone by elevation.
4. Make an incision over the long axis of the duct (the calculus easily slips out).
5. Remove the stay suture and leave the wound unsutured.

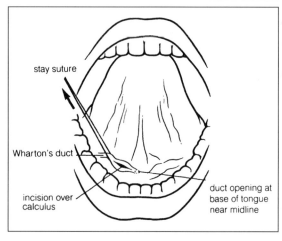

Fig. 10.4 Excision of calculus in Wharton's duct

A 'natural' method of snaring a calculus

1. Fast for about six hours.
2. Squeeze an unripe lemon and drink the juice.
3. Place a slice of lemon on the tongue. The calculus usually appears at the opening—it may then be possible to extract it using the preceding or following method.

Simple removal of calculus from Wharton's duct

If the calculus is visible at the opening of the duct it can be removed using the round end of a Jacob-Horne probe.

The round end of the probe is placed over the meatus and firmly pressed inwards.

Digital pressure is then applied from the opposite side of the frenulum. The calculus may 'pop out' quite readily.

Release of tongue tie (frenulotomy)

The ideal time to release a tongue tie (ankyloglossia) is in infancy, when it may cause breastfeeding problems and maternal nipple pain. However, the condition is often not noticed until later in life, when it causes such symptoms as speech defect (e.g. a lisp), dental problems with the lower teeth, inability to protrude the tongue, and accumulation of food in the floor of the mouth.

Treatment in infants (usually under 4 months)

1. Ideally, a frenulum spatula should be used.
2. When the spatula is in place the tongue is stretched upwards.

3. Use a scalpel blade or sterile iris scissors to slit the frenulum just above the floor of the mouth.

Treatment in adults or older children

1. Perform the procedure under local or general anaesthesia.
2. When the tongue is elevated use a no. 15 scalpel blade to incise the frenulum horizontally, taking care to avoid the Wharton's ducts.
3. Tongue traction will then convert the horizontal incision into a vertical one, which can be closed in a vertical plane with interrupted plain catgut sutures.

11 Ear, nose and throat

URTIs and sinus problems

Diagnosing sinus tenderness

Eliciting sinus tenderness is important in the diagnosis and follow-up of sinusitis.

Firm pressure over any facial bone, particularly in the patient with an upper respiratory infection, may cause pain. It is important to differentiate sinus tenderness from non-sinus bone tenderness.

Method

1. This is best done by palpating a non-sinus area first and last (Fig. 11.1), systematically exerting pressure over the temporal bones (T), then the frontal (F), ethmoid (E) and maxillary (M) sinuses, and finally zygomas (Z), or vice versa.
2. Differential tenderness both identifies and localises the main sites of infection.

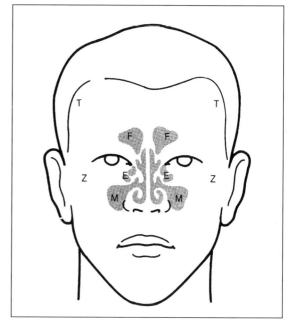

Fig. 11.1 T (temporal) and Z (zygoma) represent no sinus bony tenderness, for purposes of comparison (F=frontal sinuses; E=ethmoid sinuses; M=maxillary sinuses)

Diagnosis of unilateral sinusitis

A simple way to assess the presence or absence of fluid in the frontal sinus, and in the maxillary sinus (in particular), is the use of transillumination. It works best when one symptomatic side can be compared with an asymptomatic side.

It is necessary to have the patient in a darkened room and to use a small, narrow-beam torch.

Frontal sinuses

Shine the torch above the eye in the roof of the orbit and also directly over the frontal sinuses, and compare the illuminations.

Maxillary sinuses

Remove dentures (if any). Shine the light inside the mouth, on either side of the hard palate, pointed at the base of the orbit. A dull glow seen below the orbit indicates that the antrum is air-filled. Diminished illumination on the symptomatic side indicates sinusitis.

Inhalations for URTIs

Simple inhalations for upper respiratory tract infections (including upper airways obstruction from the oedema and secretions of rhinitis and sinusitis) can promote symptomatic relief and early resolution of the problem. The positive effect of making the patient responsible for active participation in management often helps to counterbalance the occasional disappointment when no antibiotic is prescribed.

The old method of towel over the head and inhalation bowl can be used, but it is better to direct the vapour at the nose.

Equipment

* Container. This can be an old disposable bowl, a wide-mouthed bottle or tin, or a plastic container.
* The inhalant. Several household over-the-counter preparations are suitable: e.g. friar's balsam (5 mL), Vicks Vapo-rub (one teaspoon) or menthol (5 mL).
* Cover. A paper bag (with its base cut out), a cone of paper (Fig. 11.2a) or a small cardboard carton (with the corner cut away; Fig. 11.2b).

Method

1. Add 5 mL or one teaspoon of the inhalant to 0.5 L (or 1 pint) of boiled water in the container.
2. Place the paper or carton over the container.
3. Get the patient to apply nose and mouth to the opening to breathe the vapour in deeply and slowly through the nose, and then out slowly through the mouth.
4. This should be performed for 5–10 minutes, 3 times a day, especially before retiring.

After inhalation, upper airway congestion can be relieved by autoinsufflation.

Hot water bottle method

A relatively safe and convenient way is to use a hot water bottle for inhalations. The top fits neatly over the mouth and nose.

Vacuum flask method

An old vacuum flask (thermos) is an ideal container to fill with very hot/boiling water and the inhalant. It is also portable.

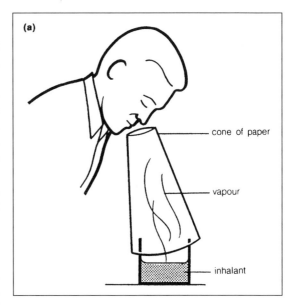

(a)

cone of paper

vapour

inhalant

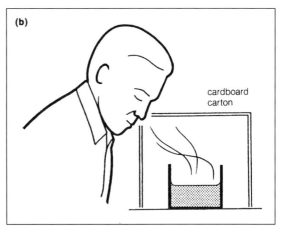

(b)

cardboard carton

Fig. 11.2 Inhalations using: **(a)** cone of paper; **(b)** cardboard carton

A practical inhalation method for busy workers

Dr Tony Dicker claims great success using a coffee cup for inhalations. By placing the inhalant, e.g. Vicks, on a teaspoon then adding boiling water, an inhalation bowl is made by placing the hands over the cup to suit the nose and mouth. People find this easy to use during meal/coffee breaks.

Nasal polyps

Nasal polyps are small 'bags' of fluid and mucus following engorgement of the mucosa of the sinuses usually due to allergic rhinitis. They pop out through the sinus openings into the nasal cavity (Fig. 11.3). They are best treated by medical polypectomy using topical nasal hydrocortisone solution or corticosteroid sprays for small polyps and oral corticosteroids for extensive polyps, e.g. prednisolone 50 mg per day for 5–7 days (avoid aspirin). Antibiotics may be needed for infection.

Surgery is usually reserved for failed medical treatment. Polyps can be simply removed under local anaesthetic by snaring the base or stalk with a loop of cutting wire. More severe cases may require sophisticated surgery.

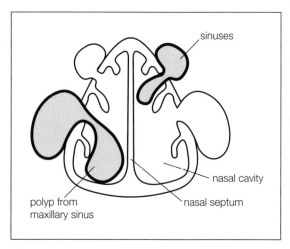

Fig. 11.3 Cross-section of nose demonstrating origin of nasal polyps

The ear and hearing

A rapid test of significant hearing loss

The age of the digital watch has meant a decline in the use of the 'ticking watch' test as a rough screening procedure for hearing loss.

In children and in adults with a reasonable amount of hair, an alternative method can be used.

Method

1. Grasp several scalp hairs close to the external auditory canal lightly between the thumb and index finger.
2. Rub lightly together (Fig. 11.4) to produce a relatively high-pitched 'crackling' sound.

If this sound cannot be heard, a moderate hearing loss is likely (usually about 40 dB or greater). If a hearing loss is detected, tuning fork assessment and other investigations will then be required.

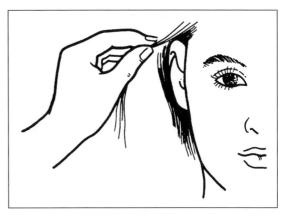

Fig. 11.4 Test for hearing loss in a child

The whispered voice test

The whispered voice test has been proved as an accurate screening test for hearing impairment. It is less accurate in children than in adults.

It is important to exhale quietly before whispering.

Method

1. Stand 60 cm behind the patient.
2. Mask the non-test ear by gently occluding the auditory canal and rubbing the tragus in a circular motion.
3. Exhale quietly before whispering a combination of numbers and letters (e.g. '5, M, 2, A').
4. If the patient responds correctly (i.e. repeats at least 3 out of 6 numbers and letters correctly), hearing is considered normal.
5. If the patient responds incorrectly, repeat the test using a different number-and-letter combination.
6. Test each ear individually, beginning with the better ear. Use a different number—letter combination each time.

Crumpled paper test

Another simple rapid test is to use the sound of paper. Gently rub two pieces of paper together about 1–2 cm from the ear and request the patient to indicate if they hear the sound. For infants, crush a piece of paper behind the ear and note their response.

Water- and soundproofing ears

Waterproofing ears with Blu-Tack

An excellent earplug can be made with Blu-Tack, which can be gently moulded to the external auditory canal. It is ideal for children if they need to keep an ear dry when swimming or showering, for example those with perforations, ventilating grommets and recurrent otitis externa ('swimmer's ear'). Ideally, a swimming cap should also cover the ear and diving should be advised against.

The Blu-Tack provides excellent waterproofing, stays in place and is reusable. Do not use in hot saunas, where it softens easily.

Children should be instructed not to keep poking the 'tack' into their ears with their fingers.

Be prepared to remove retained bits of Blu-Tack sometimes.

New type of ear plug

A new form of ear protection is the expanding ear plug. The plugs can be used during exposure to excessive noise and for middle ear protection while swimming, especially for children with ventilating tubes inserted in their ears.

Made of compressible foam, when cut in half the plug can be rolled into a cylindrical shape that fits neatly in a child's ear. Keeping a finger on the outer part of the ear canal allows the plug to expand and fill the canal. A small coating of petroleum jelly and a standard rubber bathing cap make them waterproof, but the child should not dive under water.

Parents who have tried to use a full-sized ear plug for a child have sometimes found that the bathing cap rubbed on the end of it, pulling it out of the ear— hence the reason for cutting them in half. (E.A.R. Plugs are available from most acoustic services for approximately $1.00 a pair. They are washed easily in warm, soapy water, and a pair will last between 6 and 12 months.)

Use of tissue 'spears' for otitis externa and media

The debris from otitis externa and the discharge from otitis externa or media can be mopped out with 'spears' fashioned from toilet paper or other tissue. They are widely used in indigenous children. In otitis externa this toileting can be followed by acetic acid 0.25% washout—then topical steroid and antibiotic ointment if necessary.

Preventing swimmer's otitis externa

Get patients to rinse ears out with fresh water (possibly using a 5 mL syringe) and then dry with a hair dryer on moderate heat.

Treatment and prevention of swimmer's ear

Use a drying topical medication, e.g. Aquaear or Ear Clear (acetic acid and isopropyl alcohol). An alternative less expensive preparation is a 'homebrew' mixture of acetic acid and methyl alcohol (methylated spirits), 3 parts to 2. Instil 2–3 drops daily during the swimming season.

Chronic suppurative otitis media and externa

Wash the canal with dilute povidone-iodine (Betadine) 5% solution using a 20 mL syringe with plastic tubing 1, 2 or 3 time daily. Dry mop with rolled toilet paper 'spears'. Teach this method to family members. If available, suction kits are useful.

Ear piercing

This simple method of ear piercing (for the insertion of 'sleepers') requires only an 18- or 19-gauge sterile needle. Local anaesthesia is optional. A freezing spray can be used.

Method

1. Carefully place marks on the ear lobe (this is better done by the patient or patient's parents).
2. Introduce the needle through the selected site (Fig. 11.5a). One can use a cork or piece of potato on the exit side.
3. Insert the pointed end of the sleeper into the bore of the needle, ensuring that it fits tightly, and withdraw the needle (Fig. 11.5b).

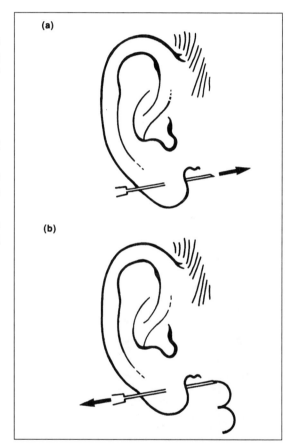

Fig. 11.5 Ear piercing method

Ear wax and syringing

Ear syringing is a simple and common procedure, but it should be performed with caution.

Contraindications

Syringing should not be performed in the acute stages of otitis media or when perforation of the tympanic membrane cannot be excluded. In these instances, wax should be cleared with a hook or curette under direct vision (Fig. 11.6a).

In otitis externa, syringing may be performed to remove debris from the canal. Meticulous drying after the procedure is mandatory.

(continues)

Wax softeners

Proprietary preparations may be used as an alternative to syringing or to assist removal, but dioctyl sodium sulphosuccinate should not be used if perforation is suspected. Sodium bicarbonate (available on prescription) or olive oil drops may also be used. Culinary vegetable oil can be used by the patient prior to visiting the office.

A study by Kamien led to the conclusion 'that the most effective, cheapest and least messy cerumenolytic is a 15% solution of sodium bicarbonate'. It can be readily made by dissolving ¼ teaspoon of sodium bicarbonate in 10 mL of water. Apply it with a dropper.

Another simple method is to fill the ear with liquid soap. Request the patient to 'pump' their tragus for a couple of minutes then attempt syringing.

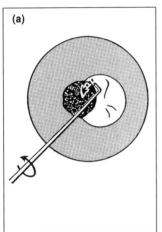
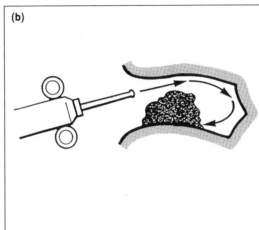
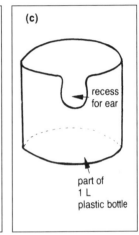
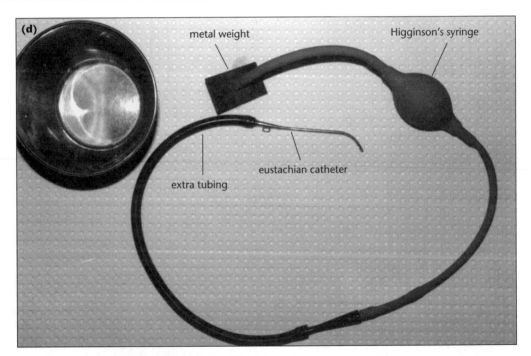

Fig. 11.6 Removal of wax: **(a)** a hook is rotated behind the wax to remove it; **(b)** syringing technique, in which water is directed around (not at) wax; **(c)** ear 'cup' to collect water; **(d)** the Higginson's syringe with special attachments

Ear syringing

Method 1

The syringe should have a properly fitting nozzle and an airtight plunger. Water at body temperature (37°C) is a satisfactory solution (vertigo, nausea and vomiting may be precipitated by excessively hot or cold fluid coming in contact with the tympanic membrane).

The nozzle of the syringe should rest just inside the auditory meatus and the syringe should be angled slightly upwards (Fig. 11.6b). Water directed along the roof of the external auditory canal cascades around and behind the plug of wax. Pulling the pinna upward and slightly backward straightens the canal, and may assist partial separation of the wax plug.

While a kidney dish is the traditional collecting vessel for the syringed fluid, an empty plastic ice cream 'bucket' is a practical alternative: the pliable sides mould easily into the shape of the neck. Another improvised ear 'cup' can be cut out from a used hospital 1 L plastic bottle. A small recess can be made for the ear (Fig.11.6c).

Method 2

This is a very effective system that provides a constant flow of water, maximum safety, and a free hand when syringing the ear.

The apparatus consists of:

- a Higginson's syringe,
- a heavy metal washer (acts as a weight),
- a metal eustachian catheter,
- additional tubing.

The washer maintains the rubber syringe in the basin of water during the ear syringing. The metal eustachian catheter provides an 'accurate' jet of water, which is aimed superiorly above the wax in the usual, recommended manner (Fig. 11.6b).

Post-syringing

If the patient complains of deafness due to water retention, instil acetic acid-alcohol drops (Aquaear or Ear Clear). This gives instant hearing. Some doctors routinely use these drops after syringing out the wax.

A 'gentle' ear syringe

A simple ear syringe can be improvised from a 20 mL or 50 mL syringe and a plastic 'butterfly' intravenous cannula. The apparatus is also useful for instilling ointment to treat otitis externa.

Method

Firmly attach the 'butterfly' cannula to the syringe and cut off the tubing, leaving it about 3–4 cm long (Fig. 11.7).

Use

This 'ear syringe' is flexible, safe, and easy to use, especially for children. The curve at the end of the tubing permits good positioning in the ear canal.

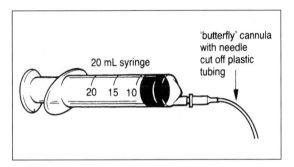

Fig. 11.7 A 'gentle' ear syringe

Note: Some doctors testify to the value of adding a small quantity of povidone-iodine solution to the water, especially if otitis externa is present. Others prefer hydrogen peroxide (100 mL bottles of 30 mg/mL are available in supermarkets) for ear toilet, especially with low-grade otitis externa.

Hair spray and hard wax

People who use hair sprays are prone to developing hard wax if it finds its way into the ear canal. Advise these people to cover their ears when they use the spray.

Recognising the 'unsafe' ear

Examination of an infected ear should include inspection of the attic region, the small area of drum between the lateral process of the malleus, and the roof of the external auditory canal immediately above it. A perforation here renders the ear 'unsafe' (Fig. 11.8a); other perforations, not involving the drum margin (Fig. 11.8b), are regarded as 'safe'.

The status of a perforation depends on the presence of accumulated squamous epithelium (termed cholesteatoma) in the middle ear, because this erodes bone. An attic perforation contains such material; safe perforations do not.

Cholesteatoma is visible through the hole as white flakes, unless it is obscured by discharge or a persistent overlying scab. Either type of perforation can lead to a chronic infective discharge, the nature of which varies with its origin. Mucus admixture is recognised by its stretch and recoil when this discharge is being cleaned from the external auditory canal. The types of discharge are compared in Table 11.1.

Table 11.1 Comparison of types of discharge

	Unsafe	Safe
Source	Cholesteatoma	Mucosa
Odour	Foul	Inoffensive
Amount	Usually scant, never profuse	Can be profuse
Nature	Purulent	Mucopurulent

Management

If an attic perforation is recognised or suspected, specialist referral is essential. Cholesteatoma cannot be eradicated by medical means: surgical removal is necessary to prevent a serious intratemporal or intracranial complication.

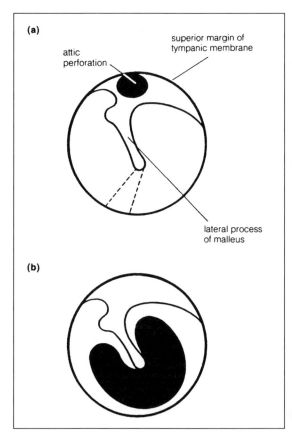

Fig. 11.8 Infected ear: **(a)** unsafe perforation; **(b)** safe perforation

Excision of ear lobe cysts

Small ear lobe cysts can be removed by simple excision with the aid of ring forceps (Meibomian clamps). Such forceps are especially useful when they can be applied over accessible areas, such as eyelids, lips, webbing, scrotum and ear lobes. They enable a firm hold over a small cyst and help to control haemostasis.

Method

1. For a small ear lobe cyst, apply the forceps over the ear and clamp so that the surface chosen for excision occupies the open ring.
2. Make an incision over the cyst with a small scalpel blade and dissect the cyst gently away from adherent tissue (Fig. 11.9).
3. Once it is relatively free, it may be possible to squeeze out the entire cyst by digital pressure on either side.

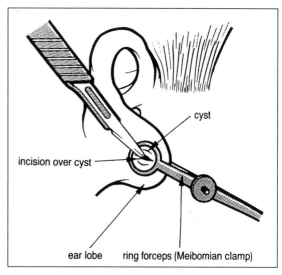

Fig. 11.9 Excision of ear lobe cysts

Infected ear lobe

The cause is most likely a contact allergy to nickel in the jewellery, complicated by a staphylococcus infection.

Management method

1. Discard the earrings.
2. Clean the site to eliminate residual traces of nickel.
3. Swab the site, then commence antibiotics (broad-spectrum antistaphylococcus).
4. Get the patient to clean the site daily, then apply the appropriate ointment.
5. Use a 'noble metal' stud to keep the tract patent.
6. Advise the use of only gold, silver or platinum studs in future.

Embedded earring stud

The embedded earring stud can be difficult to remove, but a simple technique using curved mosquito artery forceps can disimpact the stud easily. The typical stud consists of a post that slots into a butterfly clip.

Method

1. Insert the tips of the mosquito artery forceps into the two openings of the butterfly clip.
2. Open the forceps, thus gently springing apart the butterfly clip (Fig. 11.10). This manoeuvre removes the pressure on the post, and the stud can then be separated.

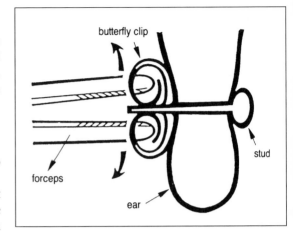

Fig. 11.10 Removal of embedded earring stud

Tropical ear

For severe painful otitis externa, which is common in tropical areas:

- prednisolone (orally) 15 mg statim, then 10 mg 8-hourly for six doses, followed by
- Merocel ear wick or ichthammol and glycerine wick
- topical Locacorten Vioform or Sofradex drops for 10 days.

Instilling otic ointment

Otic ointment can be instilled into the ear canal, starting from deep near the tympanic membrane, by using the 'gentle' ear syringe described on page 213 for ear syringing.

The nose
Treatments for epistaxis

Simple tamponade

In most instances, haemostasis can be obtained by pinching the 'soft' part of the nose between a finger and thumb for 5 minutes and applying ice packs to the bridge of the nose (Fig. 11.11).

Matchstick tamponade

Several practitioners claim excellent results using a matchstick ($^3/_4$ of its length) jammed up in a horizontal position under the upper lip to the roof of the gum reflection on the teeth. Leave it in place for several minutes. It compresses the superior labial arteries which also supply the nasal septum.

Note: Dental packing (hard cotton wool roll) would be ideal and preferable to a matchstick.

Simple cautery of Little's area
Local anaesthetic

Cophenylcaine forte nasal spray—leave 5 minutes.
  or
An equal equal mixture of 10% cocaine HCl and adrenaline 1:1000 (0.5 mL of each) soaked in a small piece of cotton wool about the size of a 5 cent piece. This pledget is gently compressed against the area and left for 2 minutes.

Cautery methods

The three methods of cautery are:

- electrocautery,
- trichloroacetic acid (pure),
- silver nitrate stick (preferred).

Fashion cotton wool onto the end of the silver nitrate stick to dry the treated site. Apply Vaseline twice daily to the cauterised area.

Use of dental broach for treatment of epistaxis

A dental broach can be modified to pick up a small but adequate amount of trichloroacetic acid (TCA) for nasal cautery.

Method

1 A small loop can be made in the broach by bending the wire around the tip of fine forceps.
2. The loop is placed in the TCA so that a small amount fits neatly in the loop.
3. The loop is then applied to the appropriate site on Little's area in the nasal septum (Fig. 11.12). The small amount of acid is delivered accurately and cauterises a specific area, without spillage to the healthy adjacent tissue.

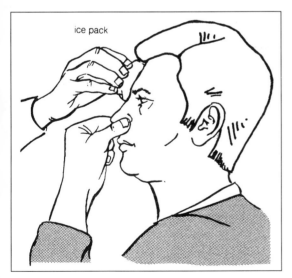

Fig. 11.11 Simple tamponade method for epistaxis

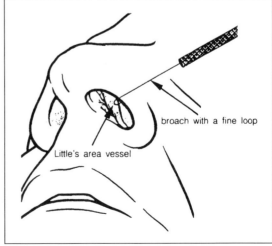

Fig. 11.12 Shows loop of broach applied to the site of bleeding

(continues)

Recurrent anterior epistaxis

For patients with recurrent epistaxis from Little's area, especially in the presence of localised rhinitis, several topical options are available:

- Nasalate cream tds for 7–10 days, or
- Aureomycin or Nemdyn otic ointment bd or tds for 10 days, or
- Rectinol ointment.

Rectal ointment containing local anaesthetic and a vasoconstrictor, e.g. Rectinol, is a very useful topical agent.

Persistent anterior bleed

Use Merocel (surgical sponge) nasal tampon or a Kaltostat pack or a vaginal tampon.

Severe posterior epistaxis

Occasionally, severe posterior nasal bleeding cannot be controlled by an anterior pack. Insertion of a nasopharyngeal pack via the oropharynx is technically difficult and distressing for the patient. A simple and effective method of applying postnasal pressure uses a Foley catheter.

Method

1. Anaesthetise the nasal passage.
2. Select a small Foley catheter (no. 12, 14 or 16) with a 30 mL balloon and self-sealing rubber stopper.
3. Lubricate the deflated catheter and pass it directly into the nasal passage along the floor of the nose until resistance is felt in the nasopharynx (the tip might be visible behind the soft palate).
4. Using a 20 mL syringe, partially inflate the balloon with 5–8 mL of saline or, preferably, air.
5. Gradually withdraw the catheter until resistance is felt; inject another 5 mL of saline or air.
6. Draw the catheter taut so that the balloon fits snugly in the nasopharynx against the choana (Fig. 11.13).
7. Pack the anterior chamber with ribbon gauze in the usual manner.

Note: The patient should be admitted to hospital. Administration of oxygen might be necessary for the elderly patient whose respiration is compromised.

The Epistat catheter A special catheter called the Epistat has been developed specifically for this method. It is ideal but relatively costly. It has two inflatable balloons, one to act as a stay posteriorly and a wider 'anterior' balloon. There is a central airway in the device. This catheter can be autoclaved for further use.

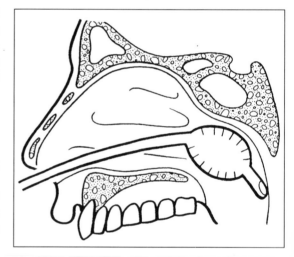

Fig. 11.13 Semi-inflated Foley catheter in nasopharynx and posterior nasal cavity

Instilling nose drops

To achieve the best results from nasal drops instil as follows:

- to insert into the left side, incline the head to the left,
- for the right side, incline the head to the right.

Offensive smell from the nose

Ensure no foreign body present.

Treatment

- mupirocin 2% nasal ointment
    instil 2–3 times a day
        or
- Kenacomb ointment
    instil 2–3 times a day

Stuffy, running nose

Treatment

- blow nose hard into disposable paper tissue or handkerchief until clear
- nasal decongestant for 2–3 days only
- steam inhalations with Friar's balsam or menthol

Miscellaneous ENT pearls

Hands-free headlight

The ideal hands-free light to examine the ears, nose and throat is the Vorath headlight kit.

A less expensive alternative is a caving headlamp, which can be obtained at a camping shop at a reasonable cost.

Self-propelled antral and nasal washout

This method works well for patients with persistent catarrh and sinus problems.

Equipment

You will need:

- a drinking straw,
- a tea cup,
- warm water with one teaspoon of salt and one teaspoon of sodium bicarbonate.

Method

1. Place the straw in the water and the other end in the nostril.
2. Holding the other nostril closed with a finger, the patient inhales the fluid rapidly into the nostril and then expectorates.

Hiccoughs (hiccups)

For simple brief episodes, try any of the following:

- Rebreathe air in a paper bag (as for hyperventilation).
- Hold the breath.
- Suck ice/swallow iced water.
- Swallow a teaspoon of table sugar (some practitioners add vinegar to the sugar; others, whisky or gin).
- Swallow 20 mL of spirits.
- Insert a catheter quickly in and out of the nose.
- Apply pressure on the eyeballs.

When persistent (assuming exclusion of the organic diseases):

- chlorpromazine orally or IV, or
- valproic acid.

Consider acupuncture, hypnosis or phrenic nerve block.

Nasal catheter for hiccoughs

Persistent hiccoughs can be arrested quickly by irritation of the nose with a soft rubber or plastic nasal catheter. The method is particularly useful for the post-operative patient.

A catheter is introduced into one of the nasal passages and withdrawn as soon as the patient shows irritation.

Worth a try?

Ask the patient what they ate for breakfast 2 days ago. The thoughtful pause that 'freezes' the diaphragm may work!

Snoring

Important strategies to prevent snoring include:

- avoid sleeping on the back,
- weight reduction to ideal weight,
- no alcohol in the evening.

Otherwise refer to a medical consultant in sleep disorders. Continuous positive airway pressure (CPAP) delivered through a special face mask may be prescribed.

Nasal device

A device suitable to prevent 'collapsing' of the front of the nose is 'Nozovent', which is a simple medical-grade plastic device that fits into the nose. The device, invented by a Swedish ENT surgeon, increases the diameter of the nostrils and prevents them from collapsing on inhalation. An Australian version is the Breathing Wonder®, which is inexpensive and freely available.

Tinnitus

Precautions

- Exclude drugs (including marijuana), vascular disease, depression, aneurysm and vascular tumours.
- Beware of lonely elderly people living alone (suicide risk).

Management

- educate and reassure the patient,
- relaxation techniques,
- background 'noise', e.g. music playing during night,
- tinnitus maskers,
- hearing aids.

Drug trials to consider (limited efficacy)

- betahistine (Serc) 8–16 mg daily (max 32 mg),
- carbamazepine (Tegretol),
- antidepressants,
- sodium valproate.

Acute severe tinnitus

Slow IV injection of 1% lignocaine (as for migraine—see page 263). Up to about 5 mL is very effective.

Swallowing with a sore throat

Rather than painful sipping of fluids, advise the patient to fill the mouth with as much fluid as possible and then swallow.

Glue ears

Autoinflation of ears via the eustachian tube can be achieved by a device called Otovent which consists of a balloon attached to a nose piece. The child with a glue ear holds the nose piece to the nostril and inflates the balloon to the size of a grapefruit while keeping the other nostril compressed with a finger and the mouth firmly closed. The balloon is then allowed to deflate while the child swallows. It is performed 2–3 times a day for 2–3 weeks.

Auriscope as an alternative to nasal specula

An auriscope with the widest possible attachment will allow an excellent view of the nasal cavity. The patient should mouth breathe during the inspection.

Chronic anosmia following URTI

For patients complaining of loss of the sense of smell following an upper respiratory infection, prescribe a nasal decongestant such as Spray-Tish Menthol for 5–7 days (maximum).

Ticklish throat

For an irritated persistent ticklish throat instruct the patient to make a trilling musical sound like an opera singer for 2–3 minutes.

12 The eyes

Basic kit for eye examination

Recommended by the Royal Victorian Eye and Ear Hospital, the kit comprises:

- eye-testing charts at 18 inches (46 cm) and 10 feet (305 cm),
- multiple pin holes,
- fluorescein sterile paper strips, e.g. Flourets,
- torch,
- magnification (necessary to examine cornea),
- isotonic saline solution to irrigate eyes,
- local anaesthetic (e.g. MINIMS unidose),
- sterile cotton buds,
- glass rod to double-evert eyelids in chemical burns,
- non-allergenic tape (e.g. Micropore).

Eye tip: The eye holds only one drop of liquid which usually remains in the eye for only a few seconds. The action can be prolonged by pinching on either side of the nose to occlude the lacrimal duct for 60 seconds.

Eversion of the eyelid

Paperclip method

No eye examination is complete without eversion of the upper eyelid to exclude hidden pathology, particularly a foreign body.

The method generally taught is to evert the lid over a matchstick, but this can be difficult. The use of a paperclip can simplify this examination.

1. By bending the long arm of the paperclip to make a right angle, you can create an instrument with a fine diameter, which is easy to withdraw and has a handle that keeps fingers out of the field of inspection (Fig. 12.1).
2. Care must be taken not to slide the end of the clip over the lid but to place it gently and precisely along the appropriate line (about 15 mm from the edge of the lid and parallel to it).
3. You must also make sure not to slide the end of the clip across the lid and scratch it on removal.

Care must also be taken with unco-operative children.

Cotton bud method

The use of a cotton bud is recommended for eyelid eversion. Its effectiveness depends on correct placement.

1. Ask the patient to put the chin up and to look down.
2. Gently grasp the eyelashes of the upper lid between the index finger and thumb of the non-dominant hand and pull gently downwards.
3. Apply the cotton bud 15 mm above the upper eyelid margin.
4. With gentle pressure, push the bud back while lifting the lashes upward.
5. Eversion of the lid can be maintained even after removal of the cotton bud.

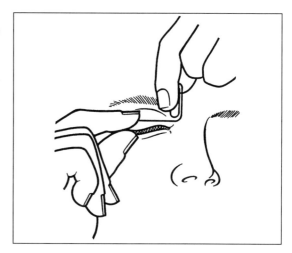

Fig. 12.1 Paperclip method for eyelid eversion

Blepharitis

Blepharitis is inflammation of the lid margins and is commonly associated with secondary ocular effects such as styes, chalazia and conjunctival or corneal ulceration. There are three main causes or types:

- seborrhoeic—associated with seborrhoeic dermatitis;
- rosacea—associated with facial seborrhoea;
- staphylococcal—due to *S. aureus*.

Precautions

Corneal ulceration, recurrent staphylococcal infections.

Management

- Eyelid hygiene is the mainstay of therapy. The crusts and other debris should be gently cleaned with a cotton wool bud dipped in clean, warm water or a 1:10 dilution of baby shampoo or a solution of sodium bicarbonate, once or twice daily.

An alternative is to apply a warm water or saline soak with gauze for 20 minutes followed by a rest for 60 minutes.

- Treat infection with an antibiotic ointment smeared on the lid margin (this may be necessary for several months), e.g. tetracycline 1% or bacitracin ointment to lid margins 3- to 6-hourly.
- For chronic blepharitis, short-term use of a corticosteroid ointment, e.g. hydrocortisone 0.5%, can be very effective.
- Ocular lubricants such as artificial tear preparations may greatly relieve symptoms of keratoconjunctivitis sicca (dry eyes), e.g. hypromellose 1%.
- Control scalp seborrhoea with regular medicated shampoos, e.g. ketoconazole.
- Systemic antibiotics may be required for lid abscess.
- Discontinue wearing contact lenses until the problem has cleared.

Flash burns

A common problem usually presenting at night is bilateral painful eyes from keratitis caused by ultraviolet 'flash burns' to both corneas some 5–10 hours previously. Sources of UV light such as sunlamps and snow reflection can cause a reaction.

Management

- Local anaesthetic (long-acting) drops, e.g. amethocaine 1% eye drops: once only application (do not allow the patient to take home more drops).
- Instil homatropine 2% drops statim.

- Analgesics, e.g. paracetamol, for 24 hours.
- Broad spectrum antibiotic eye ointment in lower fornix (to prevent infection).
- Firm eye padding for 24 hours, when eyes reviewed (avoid light).

The eye usually heals completely in 48 hours. If not, check for a foreign body. Use fluorescein if in doubt.

Note: Contact lens 'overwear syndrome' gives the same symptoms.

Wood's light and fluorescein

After fluorescein is instilled into the eye, look for a dendritic ulcer with a Wood's light.

Simple topical antiseptics for mild conjunctivitis

- Saline: prepare a saline solution by dissolving a dessert spoon of salt in 500 mL of boiled water then bathe the eye regularly (1–2 hourly) with cotton wool or gauze.

- Dilute povidone-iodine solution: dilute Betadine solution 1 in 10 parts water and use this to clean the eye.

Removing 'glitter' from the eye

Make up glitter can adhere to the conjunctiva and cornea. Its removal can be aided by ointment such as chloromycetin or hydrocortisone which binds it and 'flushes' it to the inner canthus where it can be removed by wiping with a tissue or gauze.

Dry eyes

Dry eyes can cause burning or stinging, itching, a gritty sensation, redness and a feeling of 'something in the eye'.

Simple test

Hold the eyelids wide apart for about 20 seconds—it will reproduce symptoms such as burning, stinging or dryness.

Treatment

For uncomplicated dry eyes it is usual to use artificial tear preparations which relieve the symptoms. In some people these may be needed for life.

There are 3 main types of artificial tears:

- Lubricating drops: these are instilled during the day, usually 1–2 drops about 4 times a day or as often as required.
  Examples: Liquifilm, Teardrops, Murine Tears, Isopto Tears, Tears Naturale, Methopt.
- Lubricating gels or ointments: these are instilled at bed time.
  Examples: Poly Vise, Duratears, Lacri-Lube OSP.
- Stimulant drops: these are given in the same ways as lubricating drops and are very effective.
  Examples: Thera Tears, Cellufresh.

Remember that bathing the eyes with clean water will help relieve dry eyes. Room humidifiers also help in rooms where there is dry heating.

Eyelash disorders

Irritation of the eye by lashes rubbing on it is usually caused by either entropion or ingrowing lashes.

Entropion

With entropion, the eyelashes of the lower lid are pushed to the side by the regular inturning. The condition can be demonstrated by asking the patient to close the eyes tightly and then open the eyes. The danger is ulcerative scarring of the cornea by the eyelashes, so it should be examined by staining with fluorescein.

Entropion in the frail elderly can be corrected by the use of a strip of hypoallergenic, non-woven surgical tape (1 cm × 3 cm). Attach one end to the lower lid just below the lashes, with tension sufficient to hold the lid everted, and the remainder to the face (Fig. 12.2). It should be changed as often as necessary and may be done by a relative, the doctor or a district nurse.

Ingrowing eyelashes (trichiasis)

In this condition the lid is in a normal position but the eyelashes may grow inward. Magnification may be necessary.

For only a few ingrowing lashes, epilation is the best method. Use fine-artery forceps, jeweller's forceps or, better still, eyebrow tweezers (available from chemists) to pluck out the offending eyelashes. The lashes tend to regrow, and regular epilation may be necessary.

If there are many ingrowing eyelashes, the best options are electrolysis of the hair roots or cryotherapy.

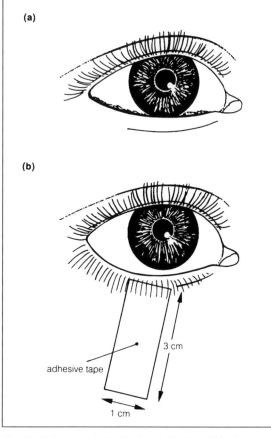

Fig. 12.2 Treatment of entropion: **(a)** before; **(b)** after

Removal of corneal foreign body

Use adequate magnification with a magnifying loupe, ideally those with an inbuilt light source. Use local anaesthetic (e.g. benoxinate HCl).

Recent and superficial

Attempt removal of the foreign body (FB) by using a sterile cotton bud, lightly moistened with a drop of local anaesthetic, to gently lift it off.

Embedded

Use a sterile, disposable needle (25- or 23-gauge) with a small syringe attached to steady the needle.

Hold the unit with a pen grip and keep the bevel upwards. Introduce the needle horizontally so that the tip lifts the edge of the FB (Fig. 12.3a).

The rust ring

The needle can lift loosely bound rust.

A sterile dental burr can be used. The burr, which is applied vertically, should be rotated gently once and then the cornea inspected after each rotation (Fig. 12.3b). This should not be attempted on deep rust or central FBs.

An 'automatic' safety burr can be used.

Follow-up

Instil antibiotic drops and pad the eye for 30 minutes only. Review at 24 hours. Inspect and stain the cornea with fluorescein. Continue to instil antibiotic drops 3 times a day for 3 days. (Drops are preferable to ointment.)

Precautions

- Do not give LA for pain relief.
- Refer deep rust stains to experts.
- Never forcibly rub the cornea.
- Do not use corticosteroids on the eye.
- Get patients to wait until LA wears off (about 20 minutes). They should drive home without an eye pad.

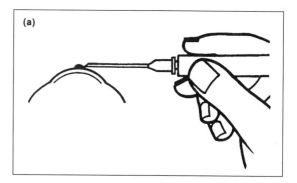

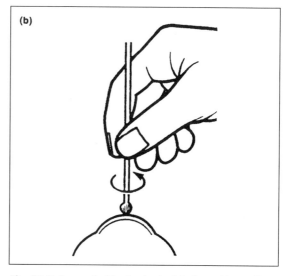

Fig. 12.3 Removal of foreign body: **(a)** disposable needle steadied with syringe using a horizontal approach; **(b)** dental burr rotated once, using a direct vertical approach

Excision of Meibomian cyst

The Meibomian cyst (tarsal cyst, chalazion) is simple to treat by incision of the cyst and curettage of its wall.

Equipment

You will need:
- a small syringe and needle,
- a chalazion clamp (blepharostat),
- a chalazion curette,
- a scalpel handle and no. 11 blade.

  Note: A disposable kit is now available.

Method

1. Instil LA drops (e.g. MINIMS oxybuprocaine, benoxinate HCl).
2. Inject about 1 mL of 2% lignocaine around the cyst through the skin (see Fig. 12.4a).
3. Apply the chalazion clamp, with the solid plate on the skin side.
4. Tighten the clamp just enough to stop the bleeding.
5. Evert the eyelid to expose the bulging cyst in the ring.
6. Make a vertical incision in the cyst (Fig. 12.4b) to avoid damage to other glands.
7. Vigorously scrape out cyst contents with the curette (Fig. 12.4c).
8. Apply a small quantity of chloramphenicol eye ointment.
9. Remove the clamp and then double-pad the eye, folding one pad over to ensure firm pressure.

Advise the patient to change the eye pad 24 hours later and to clean away the debris with warm water or saline. Apply the ointment daily until the conjunctiva has healed (3–5 days).

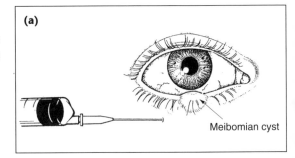

(a)

Meibomian cyst

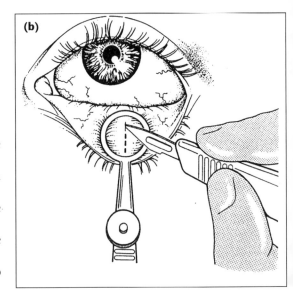

(b)

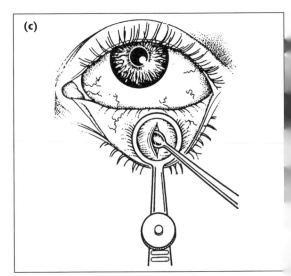

(c)

Fig. 12.4 Excision of Meibomian cyst: **(a)** the cyst; **(b)** incising with clamp in place; **(c)** curetting contents

Local anaesthetic for the eyelid

For minor surgical procedures of the eyelid, such as a Meibomian cyst, it is advisable to infiltrate local anaesthetic just under the skin of the eyelid around the lump.

Start from the outer aspect of the lid with the needle entry being about 10 mm below the eyelid margin for cysts of the lower lid.

Keep the needle tangential to the globe (Fig. 12.4a) and use about 1.5–2 mL of 1 or 2% lignocaine with adrenaline.

Non-surgical treatment for Meibomian cysts

Before proceeding to excision of a Meibomian cyst (chalazion), another method is worth attempting.

Method

- Twice daily 'hot spoon' the eye. (Pad a spoon with cotton wool and a bandage, dip in hot water and gradually bring it up to the eye—similar to steaming the painful eye) (Fig. 12.5).
- After 'hot spooning' for 5 minutes, instil 'golden eye ointment' (or soframycin eye ointment if use of mercury compounds is undesirable).
- Massage the ointment into the chalazion for 5 minutes.
- Using this method twice a day, it usually takes 2–4 weeks for the Meibomian cysts to resolve.

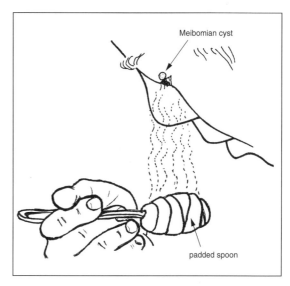

Fig. 12.5 Simple treatment for Meibomian cyst

Padding the eye

The materials used are single packs of sterile gauze eye pads and 25 mm non-allergenic (Micropore) tape. A single, flat eye pad is satisfactory for protection, but for healing, especially for the cornea, more care is required.

Method

1. Two pads are required for healing.
2. Fold the first eye pad so that the folded edge rests just below the eyebrow (Fig. 12.6).
3. The pad is then reinforced by a single, flat pad over the top.
4. Secure the pads firmly and apply 25 mm non-allergenic tape carefully to the skin.

Precaution: Never pad a discharging infected eye.

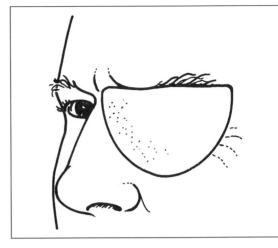

Fig. 12.6 Method of eye padding

Managing styes

A stye is an acute abscess of a lash follicle or associated glands, caused usually by *Staphylococcus aureus*.

Treat as for any acute abscess, by drainage when the abscess has pointed.

Method

1. Direct steam from a thermos onto the closed eye (see Fig. 12.8 on page 232), or use a hot compress. This helps the stye to discharge.
2. Perform lash epilation to allow drainage of pus. (Incise with a D11 blade if epilation does not work.)
3. Use chloramphenicol ointment if the infection is spreading locally.

Application of drops

The following instructions are advisable for patients:
1. Avoid contamination of the tip of the dropper bottle (fingers, eyelashes, etc.).
2. Lie down or sit with head over the back of a lounge chair.
3. Look up, spread the lower eyelid and instil the drop into the lateral conjunctival sac.
4. Close the eyes and press a finger against the lacrimal sac to stop quick drainage.

The pinhole test for blurred vision

The pinhole test (Fig. 12.7a) is a useful and under-utilised test in clinical practice.

It is important to use the test for any patient presenting with indistinct or blurred vision, whether it is sudden or gradual, painful or painless.

Theory

The pinhole reduces the size of the blur circle on the retina in the uncorrected eye.

A pinhole acts as a universal correcting lens and a 1 mm pinhole will improve acuity in refractive errors. If not, further investigation is mandatory as the defective vision is not due to a refractive error.

Using a multiple pinhole occluder

Multiple pinhole occluders are freely available (Fig. 12.7b). The patient is given the occluder and tests vision in one eye by covering the other eye and then examining an eye chart through any pinhole. The other eye is tested by reversing the procedure for the eyes.

If the blurred vision is normalised and no other abnormality is discovered on ophthalmic examination, the patient should be referred for a sight test. If the vision is unchanged, an organic cause should be suspected and appropriate referral arranged.

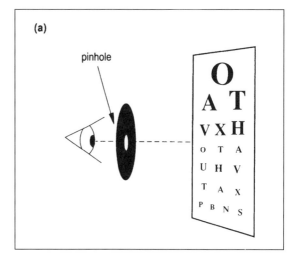

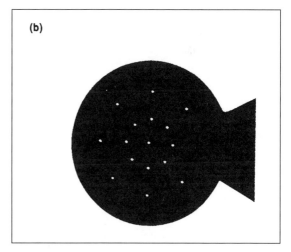

Fig. 12.7 **(a)** Pinhole test for blurred vision; **(b)** multiple pinhole occluder

Relief of ocular pain by heat

Heat, in the form of steam, applied to the closed eye is practical and very effective for the symptomatic relief of any ocular pain. Indications for the use of steam include styes, Meibomian cysts and iritis.

Method

1. Using a thermos of boiled water, allow steam to rise onto the painful eye.
2. The eye must be closed for this treatment (Fig. 12.8).
3. The steaming, which should be comfortable to the sore eye, is used for about 15 minutes.

Hot spoon bathing

Another method is to place a padded wooden spoon in very hot water and hold it close to the eye.

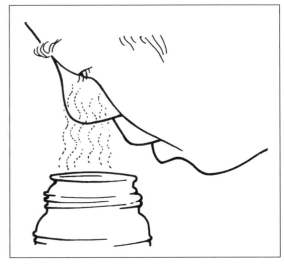

Fig. 12.8 Steaming the painful eye

Protective industrial spectacles

All workers at risk of eye injury should wear protective spectacles. One recommended set of economical spectacles with polycarbonate lenses is Alsafe 20-20 (made by New Zealand Safety Ltd).

Features

- One-piece wrap-around safety spectacles manufactured from high-impact-resistant polycarbonate material with scratch-resistant, coated lens.
- Available in clear, amber, green and infrared for harmful infrared and ultraviolet radiation.

Effective topical treatment of eye infections

The application of eye ointment or drops for such infections as conjunctivitis can be rendered ineffective by the presence of debris, such as mucopurulent exudate.

Method

One simple method is to use a warm solution of saline to bathe away any discharge from conjunctivae, eyelashes and lids. The solution of saline is obtained by dissolving a teaspoonful of kitchen salt in 500 mL of boiled water.

Hyphaema

This is usually caused by injury from a fist/finger or ball, e.g. squash ball.

Management

- First, exclude a penetrating injury.
- Avoid unnecessary movement: vibration will aggravate bleeding. (For this reason, do not use a helicopter if evacuation is necessary.)
- Avoid smoking and alcohol.
- Do not give aspirin (can induce bleeding).
- Prescribe complete bed rest for 5 days and review the patient daily.
- Apply padding over the injured eye for 4 days.
- Administer sedatives as required.
- Beware of 'floaters', 'flashes' and field defects.

Arrange follow-up ophthalmic consultation to exclude glaucoma and retinal detachment (within 1 month).

13 Tips on treating children

Making friends

- A good aphorism is: never examine the child until you have made the mother laugh.
- Establish rapport in the waiting area with children—show interest, use considerable eye contact and make favourable comments.
- Ask them what they like to be called.
- Have special stickers to put on the backs of their hands, T-shirts, etc.
- Take time to converse and/or play with them.
- Have interesting toys for them to handle while listening to their parents.
- Compliment the child on, for example, a clothing item or a toy or book they are carrying.
- Ask them about their teacher or friends.
- Try to examine them on their parent's lap.

Scalp lacerations

If lacerations are small but gaping, use the child's hair for hair as the suture. This, of course, only pertains to children with long hair. *Do not* use this method for large wounds.

Method

1. Make a twisted bunch of the child's own hair of appropriate size on each side of the wound. (The longer the hair, the better the result.)
2. Tie a reef knot and then an extra holding knot to minimise slipping (Fig. 13.1).
3. As you tie, ask an assistant to drip compound benzoin tincture solution (friar's balsam) or plastic skin on the hair knot.
4. As this congeals, the knot is further consolidated against slipping.

Leave the hair suture long. The parents can cut the knot about 5 days later when the wound is healed.

The whole procedure is painless until tetanus toxoid is given (if indicated).

Forehead lacerations

Despite the temptation, avoid using reinforced paper adhesive strips (Steri-strips) in children for open wounds. They will merely close the dermis and cause a thin, stretched scar. They can be used only for very superficial epidermal wounds and in conjunction with sutures.

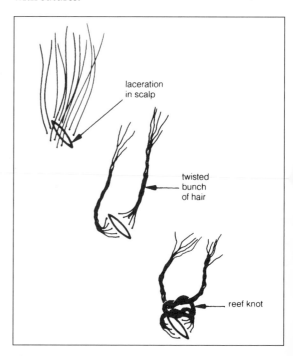

Fig. 13.1 Method of using hair to repair scalp lacerations

Glue for children's wounds

A tissue adhesive glue can be used successfully to close superficial, smooth and clean skin wounds, particularly in children.

Skin glues—an alternative to sutures

Cyanoacrylate tissue adhesions are available for wound closure. These glues act by polymerising with the thin water layer on the skin's surface to form a bond. Those available include Histoacryl, Dermabond and Epi-Glu. Some practitioners find that a similar type, such as Superglue, also serves the purpose but sterility and toxicity have to be considered and so this is not recommended.

Precautions

The glue should be used only for superficial, dry, clean and fresh skin wounds. It must not be applied for deep wounds or wounds under excessive tension. Contact with the cornea or conjunctiva must be avoided, as this can cause adhesions.

Method

- Ensure the wound is clean and dry and the wound edges are precisely opposed. No gaps are permissible with the glue method (Fig. 13.2).
- Apply a thin layer of glue directly to the tissue edges to be joined.
- Press the tissue surfaces together for 1 minute.
- Remove any excess glue immediately with a dry swab.
- Cover with a dressing for 3–4 days to prevent the child 'picking off' the glue.

Note: To facilitate application, permit reuse and avoid contamination, apply the glue with a new 25-gauge needle each time. If the needle creates a danger to a restless child, use flexible plastic tubing such as from a butterfly needle (without the needle).

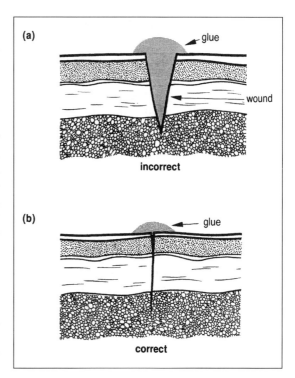

Fig. 13.2 Application of glue to a wound

Topical anaesthesia for children's lacerations

TAC solution has been reported to be very effective for topical anaesthesia prior to repair of children's lacerations (except digits, pinnae, tip of nose, penis or inside the mouth). The formula is:

- tetracaine (amethocaine) 0.5%,
- adrenaline 1:2000,
- cocaine 11.8%.

However, your pharmacist can make an equally effective, and less costly, AC mixture using adrenaline 1:2000 and cocaine 11.8%. A new mixture that overcomes concerns about cocaine toxicity is LET (lignocaine 4%, adrenaline 0.1%, tetracaine 0.5%) which is instilled into the wound for 20–30 minutes before suturing. A variation of LET as a freely available preparation is lignocaine and prilocaine mixture (EMLA cream), but it requires at least 60 minutes of skin contact.

Method

1. Thoroughly clean the wound (should be less than 5 cm).
2. Draw up 1–13 mL of AC solution and squirt it over a gauze pad placed in a sterile stainless steel bowl.
3. Place this pad over the wound for 5–10 minutes (use gentle pressure). An alternative is to instil 3 mL AC directly into the wound (especially if large and deep) and let stand for 5 minutes before applying the pad.

Repeat if anaesthesia is inadequate.

Note: Use this solution with caution. Death and convulsions with doses greater than 3 mL in infants have been reported.

Improvised topical 'anaesthesia'

Some practitioners use an ice block to freeze the lacerated site in children. The child is asked to hold the ice while a suture is rapidly inserted.

Liquid nitrogen topical 'anaesthesia'

A useful technique for a variety of topical anaesthesia, especially useful in older children, is to spray liquid nitrogen over the skin where a procedure such as incising an abscess is necessary.

Easier access to a child's arm

To achieve relaxation in an arm, for example to insert an intravenous line, distract the child by getting them to squeeze a special toy (as used in chidren's hospitals) with the hand of the opposite arm. This muscular activity of one arm leads to relaxation of the opposite arm.

Cleaning the child's 'snotty' nose

A child's blocked nose can be cleaned with sodium chloride (normal saline) including Narium mist spray. A simpler way to remove lumps of mucus is to use the firmer tissue 'spears' described on page 210.

Insert the 'spear' adjacent to and then behind the snot to dislodge it.

Another method is to use an all-rubber 30 mL ear syringe (usually stocked by pharmacies). Insert the lubricated tip in the infant's nostril and use the suction effect to clear the nares.

Test for lactose intolerance

Theory

If lactose intolerance is suspected in a child with diarrhoea, especially if fluid diarrhoea follows milk feeds, a simple test can be performed with a Clinitest tablet. This test detects reducing sugars such as lactose and glucose but not sucrose. Specific glucose oxidase reagents such as Testape and Glucostix detect glucose only and will not detect lactose or sucrose.

Method

1. Line a napkin with plastic and collect faecal fluid (Fig. 13.3a).

2. Pour some of the stool into a test tube and add two parts of water.
3. Place 15 drops into another test tube.
4. Add a Clinitest tablet and note the reaction.

Alternatively, put 5 drops of the faecal fluid directly into a test tube and add 10 drops of water.

Interpretation

A reading of 0.75–2 indicates lactose intolerance. A reading of 0 or 0.25 is probably negative (Fig. 13.3b).

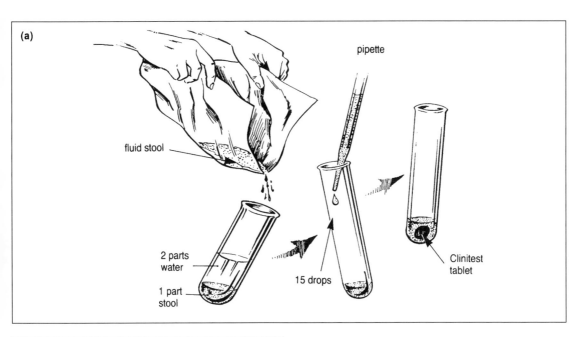

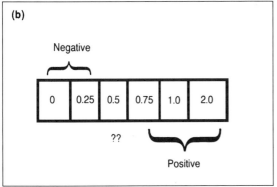

Fig. 13.3 Test for lactose intolerance: **(a)** test method; **(b)** interpreting reading

Breath-holding attacks

Diagnosis

- Precipitating event (minor emotional or physical).
- Children emit a long loud cry, then hold their breath.
- They become pale and then blue.
- If severe, may result in unconsciousness or a fit.
- Lasts between 10–60 seconds.
- Age group usually 6 months to 6 years (peak 2–3 years).

Management

- Reassure the parents that attacks are self-limiting and are not associated with epilepsy or mental retardation.
- Advise parents to maintain discipline and to resist spoiling the child.
- Try to avoid incidents known to frustrate the child or to precipitate a tantrum.

'Biting the bullet' strategy

A novel method of achieving the co-operation of some children for an uncomfortable procedure such as giving injections or injecting local anaesthetic for suturing is to distract them by asking them to 'bite the bullet' at the appropriate time. Boys of primary school age in particular seem very attracted to this novelty, as they equate it with being brave and tough.

Rather than use a dead (gunpowder removed) .38 or .45 calibre bullet, which is too hard, a 'toy' bullet made out of a plastic or rubber compound would be ideal.

Method

1. Explain the method to the child and parents.
2. Place the 'bullet' between the child's teeth and ask a parent or assistant to hold the end of the bullet firmly.
3. Ask the child to bite the bullet as you perform the painful part of the procedure.

Biting on a chocolate with a hard coating and a soft centre is another novel tip.

Using dummies to ease pain

A study reported in the *British Medical Journal* (1999, 319, pp. 1393–7) recommended that all newborn babies undergoing minor procedures (e.g. venepuncture, IV injections, lumbar puncture) should be given a dummy to ease the pain.

Deep breath with blowing distraction

A distraction technique for giving children injections, e.g. routine immunisations, is to get them to take a deep breath followed by a series of rapid blowing (similar to childbirth exercises).

How to open the mouth

Some children refuse to open their mouths to have an examination of their throat. Getting the spatula between clenched teeth is not easy. Hold their nose closed by gently pinching the nostrils together and they will reflexively open their mouth.

Another tip is to ask the child to take a deep breath while you inspect the pharynx with your torch.

Instilling nose drops

A trick to get a toddler to inhale nose drops is to instill a drop or two at the nasal openings and cover the child's mouth. The reverse of the previous tip.

Traumatic forehead lump

If a child develops a forehead lump, such as after a fall onto the edge of the table, apply a cold flannel, then a thick smear of honey. Repeat twice a day for 3 days.

Splints for minor greenstick-type fractures

Non-displaced fractures of the arm can be splinted using one or two plastic tongue depressors under the bandage as an alternative to a plaster backslab.

Removing plaster casts from children

To facilitate removal of plaster, especially a plaster cylinder from a child, request that the patient soaks the plaster in warm water prior to seeing you. The patient should soak it in the water for about 15 minutes or longer on the evening or morning prior to his or her visit. Alternatively, the plaster can be soaked in water at the surgery, but it is preferable for it to be performed at home in a large bucket or container (the bath is suitable) (Fig. 13.4a). The POP bandage can then be easily teased out and unrolled (Fig. 13.4b), or cut with a knife or scalpel. This method saves time and the unpleasant experience of a plaster cutter or saws.

Note: Making the initial plaster: a fun thing is to add a food dye to children's plaster when smoothing it out, or the dye can be put in the bucket of water.

Cutting plaster with an electric saw

Children will be more reassured if a wooden tongue depressor or similar object is inserted under the plaster in the sawing line.

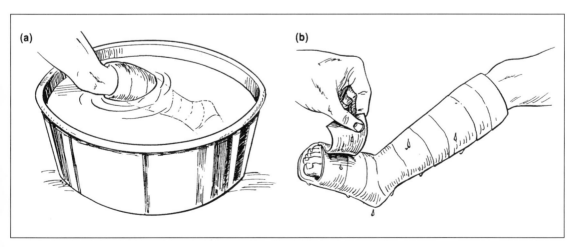

Fig. 13.4 Removal of plaster cast: **(a)** soak in warm water to soften; **(b)** unroll bandage

Distracting children

Children are sometimes difficult to examine but can be readily distracted, a characteristic the general practitioner can use effectively in carrying out the all-important examinations.

In the consulting room, a small duck with a rattle inside it can be used for palpating the abdomen of young children. This seems more acceptable to them, as it becomes a game and you obtain the same information as if you had palpated with your hand.

Another method of examining the abdomen in an upset child is to use a soft toy to play a game on the abdomen and then slip your other hand under the toy for closer assessment.

Alternatively, use the diaphragm of your stethoscope (preferably one with a small soft toy attached) to apply pressure, starting lightly and then pressing harder while watching the child's reaction. Rebound tenderness can also be tested.

Perhaps the best abdominal palpation method is to use the child's hand under yours to palpate.

Another way of diverting a child's attention, especially if giving an injection, is to blow up a balloon in front of them and let the air out slowly through a narrow opening to make a high-pitched 'squealing' sound—or let it go and 'shoot' around the room.

When examining the ears of young children sitting on their mothers' laps, difficulty is encountered when the child follows the auroscope light and moves his or her head. A small rabbit or other animal on the desk which, at the press of a button under the desk, will play a drum, distracts the child sitting to the right and enables you to get a good look into the left ear.

Similarly, over the examination couch, a clockwork revolving musical toy will distract the child for examination of the ear. It is also a distraction for the examination of children on the couch, and can become a most useful instrument.

An excellent method to distract upset or uncooperative children is to blow bubbles for them. Have a bubble blowing kit on hand for this.

Instilling eye drops in co-operative children

Method

1. Gently hold the lower lid down.
2. Get the child to look up and instil the necessary drops.
3. Ensure that the tip of the bottle does not touch the eye (Fig. 13.5a).

If the child is unable to keep the eyes open:

1. Lay the child on his or her back.
2. When the eyes are 'screwed up', instil the drops into the depression formed above the inner canthus (Fig. 13.5b).
3. When the child opens the eyes (preferably slowly), the drops soon gravitate into the eye.

Note: This is suitable for antibiotic drops, but unsuitable for drops acting through the autonomic nervous system.

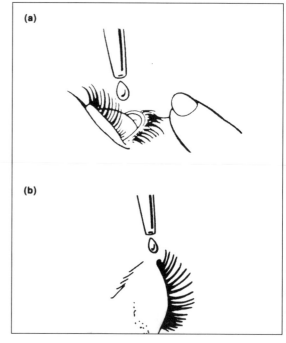

Fig. 13.5 Instilling eye drops in co-operative children

Administration of fluids

Oral Sabin vaccine

Some older children refuse to take the vaccine from a spoon.

Method

1. Introduce the vaccine with a syringe. The vaccine will draw up readily into a 1 mL syringe (three drops equals 0.2 mL: the usual dose is two drops).
2. Squirt the solution well back into the oropharynx and to one side.

This avoids choking and prevents the child spitting out the vaccine, a common problem with taking it from a spoon. Many children enjoy the 'waterpistol' connotation.

Improving fluid intake in a small child

Place a child who is refusing oral fluids in a bath with a face washer in such a way that the child is encouraged to suck the wet washer. Some children will do this even when they refuse to take fluids in the conventional manner.

This method will help to reduce fever, if present.

Spatula sketches for children

Many young patients have quickly forgotten any inspection of their throats while observing the preparation of a 'present' in the form of a drawing on the wooden spatula used in one practitioner's examination.

After the examination they are informed of their special present, and you can then proceed to draw on the unused end of the spatula. The drawings take about 15 seconds.

Figure 13.6 illustrates three sketches from one repertoire: a penguin (with optional bow tie), a caterpillar and a racing car.

Tip: Use an ink pad with special stamps, e.g. Disney characters, Bananas in Pyjamas, to stamp onto the spatulas.

Another idea is to make a human face on the spatula then make a split of about 1–2 cm at the top of the spatula. Insert wisps of cotton wool or tissue to create the impression of hair.

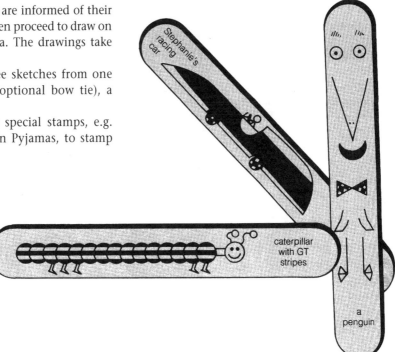

Fig. 13.6 Spatula sketches

Swallowed foreign objects

Hard objects swallowed by children are common emergencies in general practice.

A golden rule

The natural passage of most objects entering the stomach can be expected. This includes:

- coins,
- buttons,
- sharp objects,
- open safety pins,
- glass (e.g. ends of thermometers).

    Special cases are:

- very large coins (e.g. 50 cent pieces): watch carefully,

- hair clips (usually cannot pass duodenum if under 7 years).

Management

- Manage conservatively.
- Investigate unusual gagging, coughing and retching with X-rays of the head, neck, thorax and abdomen (check nasopharynx and respiratory tract).
- Watch for passage of the foreign body in stool (usually 3 days).
- If not passed, order an X-ray in 1 week.
- If a blunt foreign body has been stationary for 1 month without symptoms, remove at laparotomy.

The 'draw a dream' technique

A useful interview technique for children with behavioural disorders is to ask them to 'draw a dream', especially if bad dreams are a feature of their problem. It is an excellent avenue to help children effectively communicate their understanding of the stressful events in their lives.

Professor Tonge believes that 'it is the royal road to the child's mental processes and the family doctor is ideally placed to use the technique'.

Method

1. Make a simple drawing of someone in bed and add a large cartoon balloon (Fig. 13.7).
2. If the child's name is John, for example, say as you draw the dream balloon, 'Here is a boy named John having a bad dream; perhaps it is even you. I wonder if you could draw that dream for me'.
3. Then ask the child to help you interpret the significance of the drawing.

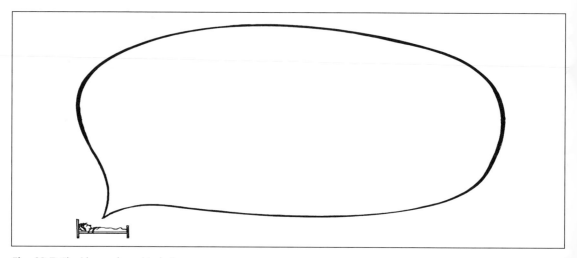

Fig. 13.7 The 'draw a dream' technique

Assessing anxious children and school refusal

Assessment of the degree and nature of the child's anxiety and possible contributing factors to school refusal is an essential first step in management and provides a base line against which to monitor progress. The following three useful measures of school refusal assist in the assessment of such children.

Fear thermometer

The fear thermometer (Fig. 13.8) is an easily adminis-tered measure that provides a global rating of the child's fear about school attendance. In relation to their worst day in the past few weeks of school, the child is asked: 'How afraid were you of going to school on that day?' They are asked to nominate their level of fear, from 0 'not scared' to 100 'very scared', on the pictorial thermometer. This global rating may reflect fear related to (a) separation from significant others; or (b) a dreadful aspect of the school setting.

Self-statement questionnaire

The self-statement questionnaire (Fig. 13.9) allows for a more detailed understanding of the sorts of things that may be contributing to school refusal. It taps the child's thoughts about seven aspects of school attendance (including such things as the other children at school, and the process of actually going to school in the morning). In addition, it allows the child to nominate any other issues that may lead to a reluctance to attend.

    The clinician can use the information elicited during administration of the questionnaire to help in the development of a treatment program that addresses the specific anxiety-provoking thoughts of the child.

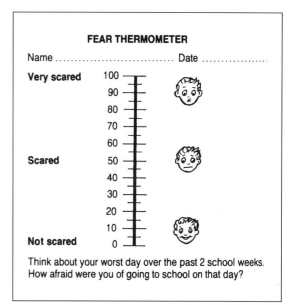

Fig. 13.8 The fear thermometer

Date: _____
Child: _____
Interviewer: _____

Tell me what thoughts you have about . . .

(a) going off to school _____

(b) being separated from mum and/or dad _____

(c) school work _____

(d) how clever you are _____

(e) other kids at school _____

(f) teachers _____

(g) the principal _____

(h) (anything the child would like to nominate regarding why he/she doesn't want to go to school) _____

Fig. 13.9 Self-statements: Child form

Suprapubic aspiration of urine

This is the most accurate way of collecting urine in children less than 2 years old. It is very suitable in the toxic and ill child.

Contraindications

- Age greater than 2 (unless the bladder is palpable).
- Coagulopathy.

Preparation

- Best performed when the child has not voided for at least 1 hour. Give the child a drink, e.g. bottle over the preceding hour or so.
- Select a 23-gauge needle attached to a 5 mL syringe.
- Local anaesthetic is not necessary.

Position of patient

- The patient's legs should be straight or bent in the frog-leg position.

Method

1. Check the bladder position by gentle percussion.
2. Prepare the skin in the suprapubic area with povidone-iodine solution.
3. Insert the needle attached to the syringe directly through the abdomen wall in the midline 1–2 cm above the symphysis pubis (this usually corresponds to the skin crease above the pubis) (Fig. 13.10).
4. Insert it to a depth of about 2–3cm in infants or deeper according to the child's age.
5. Apply steady suction until urine is obtained.
6. Aspirate the urine while slowly withdrawing the needle.
7. Take the needle from the syringe and express the sample into a sterile microurine container.
8. Forward the urine for microscopy and culture.

Note: If unsuccessful, the bladder is probably empty so try at another time.

Tip: Hold the tip of the penis in males to prevent voiding but have a sterile bottle on standby for a clean catch should voiding occur.

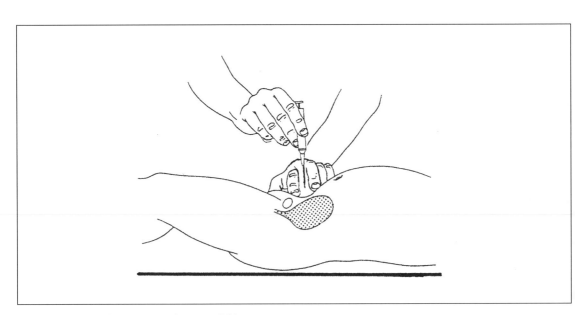

Fig. 13.10 Suprapubic aspiration of urine in child

Cannulating veins

To raise a vein for cannulation in chubby children, consider the methods on page 281 but remember that a neat vein can be raised over the fourth metacarpal on the dorsum of the hand.

Surgery in children

Table 13.1 Optimal times for surgery/intervention in children's disorders

Disorder	Surgery/intervention
Squint (fixed or alternating)	12–24 months absolutely before 7 years
Deafness (children are born with hearing)	screen at or before 8 months hearing aids required by 12 months
Inguinoscrotal lumps	
• Undescended testes	best assessed before 6 months surgery best at 6–18 months
• Umbilical hernia	leave to age 4 surgery at 4 if persistent (tend to strangulate after 4) never tape down!

• Inguinal hernia	general rule is ASAP, especially infants and irreducible hernias
	reducible herniae: the '6–2' rule
	    birth–6 weeks: surgery within 2 days
	    6 weeks–6 months: surgery within 2 weeks
	    over 6 months: surgery within 2 months

• Femoral hernia	ASAP
• Torsion of testicle	surgery within 4 hours (absolutely within 6 hours)
• Hydrocele	leave to 12 months then review (often resolve)
• Varicocele	leave and review
Leg and foot development problems	
• Developmental dysplasia of hip	most treated successfully by abductor bracing with a Pavlic harness
• Bowed legs (genu varum)	normal up to 3 years usually improve with age: refer if ICS > 6 cm
• Knock knees	normal 3–8 years then refer if IMS > 8 cm
• Flat feet	no treatment unless stiff and painful
• Internal tibial torsion	refer 6 months after presentation if not resolved
• Medial tibial torsion	leave for 8 years then refer if not resolved
• Metatarsus varus	refer 3 months after presentation if not resolved

14 The skin

Rules for prescribing creams and ointments

How much cream?

On average, 30 g of cream will cover the body surface area of an adult. Ointments, despite being of a thicker consistency, do not penetrate into the deeper skin layers so readily, and the requirements are slightly less. Pastes are applied thickly, and the requirements are at least 3–4 times as great as for creams.

The 'rule of nines', used routinely to determine the percentage of body surface area affected by burns (Fig. 14.1), may be used also to calculate the amount of a topical preparation that needs to be prescribed.

For example:

- If 9% of the body surface area is affected by eczema, approximately 3 g of cream is required to cover it.

- Nine grams of cream is used per day if prescribed 3 times daily.
- A 50 g tube will last 5 or 6 days.

One gram of cream will cover an area approximately 10 cm × 10 cm (4" × 4"), and this formula may be used for smaller lesions.

Some general rules

1. Use creams or lotions for acute rashes.
2. Use ointments for chronic scaling rashes.
3. A thin smear only is necessary.
4. On average, 30 g:

   - will cover an adult body once,
   - will cover hands twice daily for 2 weeks,
   - will cover a patchy rash twice daily for 1 week.

5. On average, 200 g will cover a quite severe rash twice daily for 2 weeks.

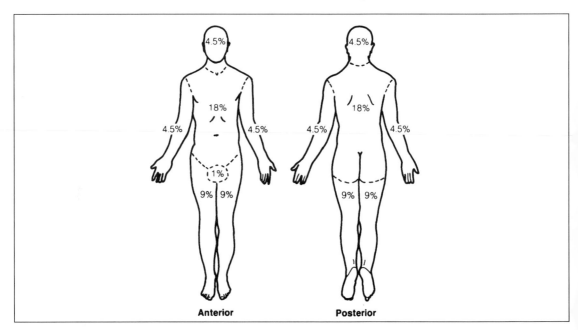

Fig. 14.1 'Rule of nines' for body surface area

Topical corticosteroids for sunburn

When a patient with severe sunburn presents early, the application of 1% hydrocortisone ointment or cream can reduce significantly the eventual severity of the burn. This has been proved experimentally by covering one-half of the burnt area with hydrocortisone and comparing the outcome with the untreated area.

The application can be repeated 2–3 hours after the initial application and then the next morning. The earlier the treatment is applied the better, as it may not be useful after 24 hours.

Hydrocortisone should be used for unblistered erythematous skin, and not used on broken skin.

Skin exposure to the sun

There is evidence that we need sufficient exposure to sunlight to produce a gentle pinking of the face and hands to provide a substantial dose of Vitamin D. This is a preventive for osteoporosis. Hats and sunscreens prevent the natural synthesis of Vitamin D in the body.

There should be a balance between receiving enough sunlight exposure to prevent Vitamin D deficiency on one hand and receiving too much, causing skin cancer, on the other (see Table 14.1).

Table 14.1 Recommended sunlight exposure to the head and hands per day (minutes)

Australian city	Summer	Winter
Darwin	5	5
Brisbane	5	5
Perth	5	12
Sydney	5	15
Adelaide	6	20
Melbourne	8	25
Hobart	10	65

Ocular protection from UV light

The best protection from the harmful effects of strong UV light is from wraparound UV-absorbing sunglasses (Australian Standard 100%).

Acne

Some topical treatment regimens

Mild to moderate acne

1. Apply isotretinoin 0.05% gel or tretinoin 0.05% cream each night (especially if comedones).
2. After 2 weeks, add benzoyl peroxide 2.5% or 5% gel or clindamycin once daily (in the morning). That is, after 2 weeks, maintenance treatment is:

   - isotretinoin 0.05% gel at night,
   - benzoyl peroxide 2.5% or 5%
       or
     clindamycin topical
   } mane

3. Maintain for 3 months and review.

An alternative regimen, if recalcitrant

Use clindamycin HCl in alcohol. Apply to each comedone with fingertips twice daily.

- A ready clindamycin preparation is Clindatech.
- Clindamycin is particularly useful for pregnant women and those who cannot tolerate antibiotics or exfoliants.

Oral antibiotics

Use if acne is resistant to topical agents. Tetracycline 1 g per day or doxycycline 100 mg per day or minocycline 50–100 mg bd for 4 weeks (or up to 10 weeks if slow response), then reduce according to response (e.g. doxycycline 50 mg for 6 weeks).

Facial scars

Injections of collagen can be used for the depressed facial scars from cystic acne.

Nappy rash

- Keep the area dry.
- Change wet or soiled napkins often—disposable ones are good.
- Wash area gently with warm water and pat dry (do not rub).
- Avoid excessive bathing and soap.
- Avoid powders and plastic pants.
- Use emollients to keep skin lubricated, e.g. zinc oxide and castor oil cream.

- Standard treatment for persistent or widespread rash is 1% hydrocortisone with nystatin or clotrimazole cream (qid after changes)—you can get separate steroid and antifungal creams and mix before application. Avoid stronger steroid preparations. Consider continuing the antifungal cream for another 7 days.

If seborrhoeic dermatitis: 1% hydrocortisone and ketoconazole ointment.

Tip: If rash is resistant and ulcerated, add Orabase ointment bd or tds. Another tip is to add petroleum jelly to the above medication in equal parts—this can be used for a 'normal' nappy rash since it promotes longer action.

Atopic dermatitis (eczema)

Medication

Mild atopic dermatitis

- Soap substitutes, such as aqueous cream or emulsifying ointment.
- Emollients (choose from):
  —aqueous cream,
  —emulsifying ointment with 1% glycerol
  —sorbolene with 10% glycerol, e.g. Hydraderm,
  —bath oils, e.g. Alpha-Keri.
- 1% hydrocortisone (if not responding to above).

Moderate atopic dermatitis

- As for mild eczema.
- Topical corticosteroids (twice daily):
  —vital for active areas,
  —moderate strength, e.g. fluorinated, to trunk and limbs,
  —weaker strength, e.g. 1% hydrocortisone, to face and flexures.
- Oral antihistamines at night for itch.

Severe dermatitis

- As for mild and moderate eczema.
- Potent topical corticosteroids to worst areas (consider occlusive dressings).
- Consider hospitalisation.
- Systemic corticosteroids (may be necessary).

Weeping dermatitis (an acute phase)

This often has crusts due to exudate. Burrow's solution diluted to 1:20 or 1:10 can be used to soak the affected areas.

Tip for children

If severe eczema is not responding to topical treatment, try evening primrose oil.

General tips

- Rehydration is the single most important treatment strategy. Avoid soaps.
- Topical steroids:
  —potent steroids safe for short periods,
  —intermittent rather than continuous use,
  —replace with emollients when clear.

Psoriasis

General adjunctive therapy

- Tarbaths, e.g. Pinetarsol or Polytar,
- Sunlight (in moderation).

For chronic stable plaques on limbs or trunks

Combined method

- dithranol 0.1%
  salicylic acid 3% ⎫ in white soft paraffin
  LPC tar 10% ⎭
  Leave overnight (warn about dithranol stains—use old pyjamas and sheets). Review in 3 weeks, then gradually increase strength of dithranol to 0.25%, then 0.5%, then 1%.
  Can cut down frequency to 2–3 times per week. Shower in morning, and then apply topical fluorinated corticosteroid.

Note: Dithranol tends to 'burn' skin.

- Don't use dithranol on face, genitalia or flexures.
- A higher strength (0.25% to start) can be used for short contact therapy (30 minutes before shower).

New method (adults only)

- Calcipotriol ointment—apply bd. Tends to irritate face and flexures; wash hands after use.

For milder stabilised plaques

- Egopsoryl TA—apply bd or tds, or
- topical fluorinated corticosteroids.

For resistant plaques

- Topical fluorinated corticosteroids (II–III class) with occlusion.
- Intralesional injection of triamcinolone mixed (50:50) with LA or normal saline (see Fig. 3.17 on page 66).

For failed topical therapy

Refer for PUVA or other effective therapy.

Skin scrapings for dermatophyte diagnosis

Equipment

You will need:

- a scalpel blade,
- glass slide and cover slip,
- 20% potassium hydroxide (preferably in dimethyl sulfoxide),
- a microscope.

Method

1. Scrape skin from the active edge.
2. Scoop the scrapings onto the glass microscope slide.
3. Cover the sample with a drop of potassium hydroxide.
4. Cover this with a cover slip and press down gently.
5. Warm the slide and wait at least 5 minutes for 'clearing'.

Microscopic examination

1. Examine at first under low power with reduced light.

2. When fungal hyphae are located, change to high power.
3. Use the fine focus to highlight the hyphae (Fig. 14.2).

Note: Some practice is necessary to recognise hyphae.

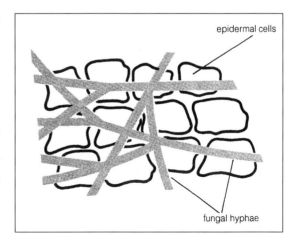

Fig. 14.2 Diagrammatic representation of microscopic appearance of fungal hyphae

Spider naevi

The most effective treatment of spider naevi for cosmetic reasons is to insert the fine tip of the electro-cautery or the hyfrecator (diathermy) needle into the central papule and cauterise the vascular lesion.

No local anaesthetic is required.

Wood's light examination

Wood's light examination is an important diagnostic aid for skin problems in general practice. It has other uses, such as examination of the eye after fluorescein staining. (New, low-cost, small ultraviolet light units called 'the black light' are available, e.g. the Radio Shack UV scanner or fluorescent lantern.)

Method

Simply hold the ultraviolet light unit above the area for investigation in a dark room.

Limitations of Wood's light in diagnosis

Not all cases of tinea capitis fluoresce, because some species that cause the condition do not produce porphyrins as a byproduct. See Table 14.2 for a list of the skin conditions that do fluoresce.

Porphyrins wash off with soap and water, and a negative result may occur in a patient who has shampooed the hair within 20 hours of presentation. Consequently, a negative Wood's light reading may be misleading. The appropriate way of confirming the clinical diagnosis is to send specimens of hair and skin for microscopy and culture.

Note: Wood's light examination can also be used for eye diagnosis after instilling fluorescein.

Table 14.2 Skin conditions that produce fluorescence in Wood's light

Tinea capitis	green
Erythrasma	coral pink
Tinea versicolor	pink
Pseudomonas pyocyanea	yellowish green
Porphyria	red (urine)
Squamous cell carcinoma	bright red

Applying topicals with a 'dish mop'

The self-application of creams or ointments to relatively inaccessible areas such as the back, especially in the elderly, can be difficult. One method is to acquire an old-fashioned dish mop, give it a 'crew cut' and use this to apply the preparations.

Chilblains

Precautions

- Think Raynaud's.
- Protect from trauma and secondary infection.
- Do not rub or massage injured tissues.
- Do not apply heat or ice.

Physical treatment

- Elevate affected part.
- Warm gradually to room temperature.

Drug Rx

- Apply glyceryl trinitrate vasodilator spray or ointment or patch, e.g. Nitro-Bid ointment (use plastic gloves and wash hands for ointment).

Other Rx

- Rum at night
- Nifedipine 20 mg bd

Herpes simplex: treatment options

Herpes labialis (classical cold sores)

The objective is to limit the size and intensity of the lesions.

Topical treatment

At the first sensation of the development of a cold sore:

- apply an ice cube to the site for up to 5 minutes every 60 minutes (for first 12 hours)
- topical applications include:
  —idoxuridine 0.5% preparations (Herplex D liquifilm, Stoxil topical, Virasolve) applied hourly, or
  —povidone-iodine 10% cold sore paint: apply on swab sticks 4 times a day until disappearance, or
  —10% silver nitrate solution: apply the solution carefully with a cotton bud to the base of the lesions (deroof vesicles with a sterile needle if necessary). May be repeated, or
  —acyclovir 5% cream, 5 times daily for 4 days.

Oral treatment

Acyclovir or famciclovir or valaciclovir for 7–10 days or until resolution (reserve for immuno-compromised patients and severe cases).

Zinc treatment

This empirically based treatment is favoured by some therapists. Zinc sulfate 220 mg tds, half an hour before meals, and large amounts of coffee during the day.

Topical zinc treatment

Zinc sulfate solution 0.025–0.05%, apply 5 times a day for cutaneous lesions and 0.01–0.025% for mucosal lesions.

Prevention

If exposure to the sun precipitates the cold sore, use a 15+ sun protection lip balm, ointment or solarstick. Zinc sulfate solution can be applied once a week for recurrences. Oral acyclovir 200–400 mg bd or similar agent (6 months) can be used for severe and frequent recurrences (> six per year).

Genital herpes: Antimicrobial therapy

Topical treatment

The proven most effective topical therapy is topical acyclovir (not the ophthalmic preparation).

Alternatives:

- 10% silver nitrate solution applied with a cotton bud to the raw base of the lesions, rotating the bud over them to provide gentle debridement. Repeat once or twice. This promotes healing and helps prevent spreading, or
- 3% chromic acid, or
- 10% povidone-iodine (Betadine) cold sore paint on swab sticks for several days.

Pain relief can be provided in some patients with topical lignocaine.

Saline baths and analgesics are advisable.

Oral treatment

Acyclovir for the first episode of primary genital herpes (preferably within 24 hours of onset).

Dosage: 200 mg 5 times a day for 7–10 days or until resolution of infection.

Famciclovir or valaciclovir can be given bd for 5–10 days.

This appears to reduce the duration of the lesions from 14 days to 5–7 days. These drugs are not usually used for recurrent episodes, which last only 5–7 days. Very frequent recurrences (six or more attacks in 6 months) benefit from low-doses of these agents for 6 months (200 mg 2–3 times per day).

Herpes zoster (shingles)

Topical treatment

For the rash, use a drying lotion such as menthol in flexible collodion. Acyclovir ointment can be used but it tends to sting.

Oral medication

1. Analgesics, e.g. paracetamol, codeine or aspirin.
2. Guanine analogue antiviral therapy for:

   - all immuno-compromised patients
   - any patient, provided rash present <72 hours (especially those over 60 years)
   - ophthalmic zoster (evidence to reduce—reduces scarring and pain but not neuralgia)
   - severe acute pain

Drugs and dosage

- acyclovir 800 mg 5 times daily for 7 days
                           or
- famciclovir 250 mg 8 hourly for 7 days
                           or
- valaciclovir 1000 mg 8 hourly for 7 days

Post-herpetic neuralgia

Some treatment options are:

1. *Topical capsaicin (Capsig) cream.* Apply the cream to the affected area 3–4 times a day.
2. TENS as often as necessary, e.g. 16 hours/day for, 2 weeks, plus antidepressants.

3. *Excision of painful skin scar.* If the neuralgia of 4 months or more is localised to a favourable area of skin, a most effective treatment is to excise the affected area, bearing in mind that the scar tends to follow a linear strip of skin. This method is clearly unsuitable for a large area.

Method

1. Mark out the painful area of the skin.
2. Incise it with its subcutaneous fat, using an elongated elliptical excision (Fig. 14.3).
3. Close the wound with a subcuticular suture or interrupted sutures.

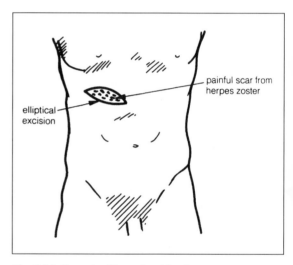

Fig. 14.3 Example of type of excision for severe post-herpetic neuralgia

---

Unusual causes of contact dermatitis

Reactions to the following have been reported:

- spirit preparation;
- paper-based 'hypoallergenic' tape.

15 Varicose veins

Percutaneous ligation for the isolated vein

This method can be used for the cosmetically unacceptable, isolated varicose vein in the leg, as an alternative to sclerotherapy. A 3/0 polyglycolic acid (Dexon) suture is simply inserted through the skin to encircle and ligate the vein.

Equipment

You will need:

- 3/0 polyglycolic acid suture,
- cutting-edge needle,
- needle holder and scissors,
- local anaesthetic agent.

Method

1. Infiltrate LA around the site or sites of the vein to be ligated:

   - small veins (up to 5–10 cm), a single suture,
   - larger veins, multiple sutures, 5–10 cm apart.

2. Using a cutting-edge needle, pass the suture under the vein (Fig. 15.1a).
3. Bring the suture through the skin and then simply tie it tightly to occlude the vein by constriction (Fig. 15.1b). The treated vein thromboses and atrophies after a short period.
4. Review the patient in 4 weeks and remove the suture.

Precautions

Avoid areas near the dorsalis pedis artery and the common peroneal nerve, or other significant arteries, veins or nerves.

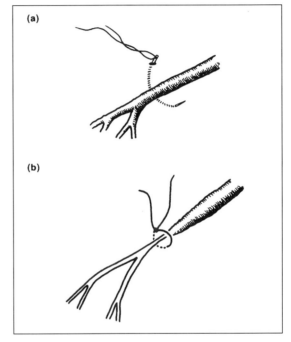

Fig. 15.1 Percutaneous ligation for isolated varicose vein

Avulsion of the isolated varicose vein

This method can be used to treat the cosmetically unacceptable isolated varicose vein in the leg. It is possible to avulse the vein using local anaesthesia along the length of the varicose vein.

Equipment

You will need:

- local anaesthetic,
- no. 15 scalpel blade with scalpel handle,
- 6 small Halsted artery forceps ('mosquitoes'),
- self-adhesive closure strips 1.2 cm (Steri-strips), or nylon suture with cutting edge needle,
- non-stick gauze dressing with wool and crepe bandage.

Method

1. Infiltrate LA along the length of varicose vein to be avulsed (up to 20 mL of 1% lignocaine can be used):

- small vein (up to 5–10 cm): a single incision (5–10 mm) along or across the midpoint of the vein;
- larger veins: multiple incisions 5–10 cm apart, depending on the length of the varicose vein avulsed at first incision (Fig. 15.2a).

2. Locate and identify the vein using an artery forceps, ensuring that it is not a nerve. The vein is then divided between two forceps (Fig. 15.2b).

3. Avulse the vein on either side by applying further forceps while pulling on the vein (Fig. 15.2c). Provided the length of the varicose vein has been infiltrated with LA, there should be no pain. Apply pressure for 2–3 minutes to stop bleeding once the vein has been avulsed.

4. Achieve skin closure by using either self-adhesive closure strips or suture. The suture can be removed in approximately 10–14 days.

5. Apply non-stick gauze dressing to the wound, followed by a wool and crepe bandage. The dressing can be left for 3 days and then removed.

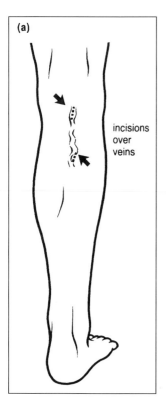
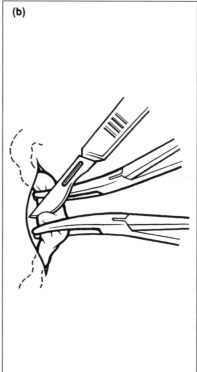
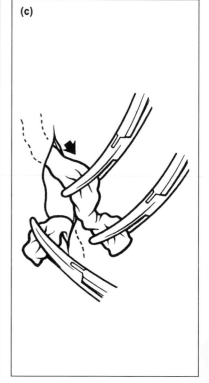

(a) incisions over veins

(b)

(c)

Fig. 15.2 Avulsion of the isolated varicose vein

If multiple avulsions have been carried out, it may be necessary to reapply a crepe bandage for another 2–3 days.

6. The patient should be free to do limited walking after the operation, and usually unrestricted walking after 24 hours.

Special precautions

Beware of nerves and arteries, avoiding areas involving the foot and the region of the lateral popliteal nerve where it curves around the neck of the fibula.

Treatment of superficial thrombophlebitis

When a large varicose vein becomes thrombosed, a tender, raised nodular cord is formed along the line of the vein. There is thrombosis in the superficial vein with no connection to deeper veins.

Clinical features

1. The skin is reddened and the tender nodular cord is palpable (Fig. 15.3a).
2. There is pain.
3. Localised oedema is present.
4. There is no generalised swelling of the limb or the ankle.

Management method

Propagation of thrombus can usually be prevented by uniform pressure over the cord.

1. The whole of the tender cord should be covered by an adhesive pad or a thin strip of foam (Fig. 15.3b) and then a firm crepe bandage applied.
2. The bandage and the pad are left on for 7–10 days.
3. Prescribe a non-steroidal anti-inflammatory drug for about 7 days. No anticoagulants are required.

A specialist opinion should be sought for superficial thrombophlebitis above the knee, as this disorder may require ligation at the saphenofemoral junction.

Finally, one must always bear in mind the association between thrombophlebitis and deep-seated carcinoma elsewhere in the body.

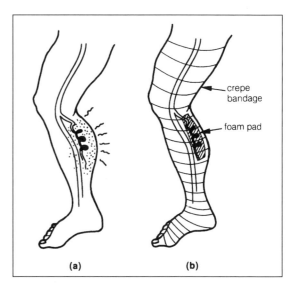

Fig. 15.3 Superficial thrombophlebitis

Ruptured varicose vein

Advice for this potentially dangerous (because of heavy blood loss) problem is often sought over the telephone. Advise local pressure (not proximal) and elevation. Both a proximal and a distal percutaneous suture (see Fig. 15.1a, b on page 253) may be necessary.

Venous ulcers

The area typically affected by varicose eczema and ulceration is shown in Figure 15.4. The secret of treating ulcers due to chronic venous insufficiency is the proper treatment of the physical factors, especially compression. Removal of fluid from a swollen leg is also mandatory. Debridement of leg ulcers using topical anaesthesia (e.g. EMLA cream applied 30 minutes beforehand) is considered to hasten ulcer healing.

Treatment method

1. Clean the ulcer with N saline. If slough, apply Intra Site Gel.
2. Apply paraffin gauze, then pack the defect with sponge rubber (Fig. 15.5).
3. Apply a compression bandage below the knee (e.g. graduated compression stockings, Eloflex bandage, Unna's type boot).
   Alternatively, an occlusive medicated paste bandage (e.g. Viscopaste or Icthaband) can be applied for 7 days from the base of the toe to just below the knee.
4. Consider using a Tubigrip stockinette cover.
5. Prescribe diuretics if oedema is present.
6. Insist on as much elevation of the leg as is possible.

Note: Dressings should be changed when they become loose or fall off, or when discharge seeps through. Patients may get ulcers wet and have baths.

Leg ulcers—unorthodox methods

For uncomplicated ulcers, such as non-infected post-traumatic and venous ulcers, various simple preparations have been claimed by many prac-titioners to promote healing. These include:

- honey,
- sugar,
- sugar and povidone-iodine (Betadine) paste,
- Intal powder.

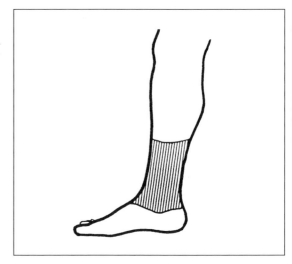

Fig. 15.4 Area typically affected by varicose eczema and ulceration (the 'gaiter' area)

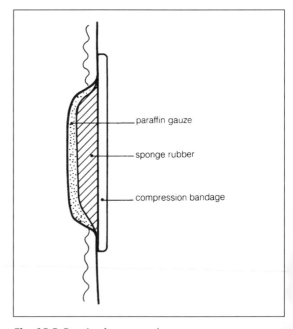

Fig. 15.5 Dressing for venous ulcer

Applying a compression stocking

To facilitate the sliding of a compression stocking over an ulcer on the leg place a plastic shopping bag firmly over the foot and then slide the stocking over this. Once on, the plastic bag is pulled down and out.

16 Emergency procedures

Urgent intravenous cutdown

In emergencies, especially those due to acute blood loss, intravenous cannulation for the infusion of fluids or transfusion of blood can be difficult. For the short-term situation, a surgical cutdown into the long saphenous vein at the ankle or the cephalic vein at the wrist is life-saving. Ideally, the long saphenous vein should be used in children.

Surface anatomy

Long saphenous vein The vein lies at the anterior tip of the medial malleolus. The best site for incision is centred about 2 cm above and 2 cm anterior to the most prominent medial bony eminence (Fig. 16.1a).

Cephalic vein The cephalic vein 'bisects' the bony eminences of the distal end of the radius as it winds around the radius from the dorsum of the hand to the anterior surface of the forearm. The incision site is about 2–3 cm above the tip of the radial styloid (Fig. 16.1b).

Equipment

You will need:

- scalpel and blade (disposable),
- small curved artery forceps,
- aneurysm needle (optional),
- vein scissors,
- absorbable catgut,
- vein elevator,
- intravenous catheter.

(continues)

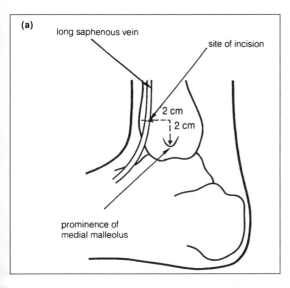

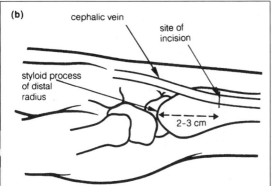

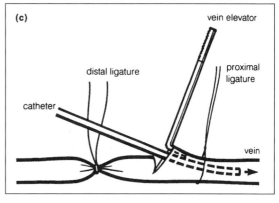

Fig. 16.1 Urgent intravenous cutdown: **(a)** site of incision over long saphenous vein (medial perspective); **(b)** site of incision over cephalic vein at wrist (radial or lateral perspective); **(c)** method of introduction of catheter into vein

Method of cutdown

After fitting gloves and using a skin preparation:

1. Make a 1.5–2 cm transverse skin incision over the vein.
2. Locate the vein by blunt dissection. (Do not confuse the vein with the pearly white tendons.)
3. Loop an aneurysm needle or fine curved artery forceps under and around the vein.
4. Place a ligature around the distal vein and use this to steady the vein.
5. Place a loose-knotted ligature over the proximal end of the vein.
6. Incise the vein transversely with a small lancet or scissors or by a carefully controlled stab with a scalpel.
7. Use a vein elevator (if available) for the best possible access to the vein.
8. Insert the catheter (Fig. 16.1c).
9. Gently tie the proximal vein to the catheter.
10. After connecting to the intravenous set and checking the flow of fluid, close the wound with a suitable suture material.

Intraosseous infusion

In an emergency situation where intravenous access in a collapsed person (especially children) is difficult, parenteral fluid can be infused into the bone marrow (an intravascular space). Intraosseous infusion is preferred to a cutdown in children under 5 years. It is useful to practise the technique on a chicken bone.

Site of infusion:

- adults and children over 5: distal end of tibia (2–3 cm above medial malleolus)
- children under 5: proximal end of tibia
- the distal femur: 2–3 cm above condyles in midline is an alternative (angle needle upwards).

Avoid growth plates, midshafts (which can fracture) and the sternum.

Method for proximal tibia (Fig. 16.2)

Note: Strict asepsis is essential (skin preparation and sterile gloves).

1. Inject local anaesthetic (if necessary).
2. Choose a 16-gauge intraosseous needle (Dieck-mann modification) or a 16–18-gauge lumbar puncture needle (less expensive).
3. Hold it at right angles to the anteromedial surface of the proximal tibia about 2 cm below the tibial tuberosity (Fig. 16.2). Point the needle slightly downwards, away from the joint space.
4. Carefully twist the needle to penetrate the bone cortex; it enters bone marrow with a sensation of giving way (considerable pressure usually required).
5. Remove the trocar, aspirate a small amount of marrow or test with an 'easy' injection of 5 mL saline to ensure its position.
6. Hold the needle in place with a small POP splint.
7. Fluid can be infused with a normal IV infusion—rapidly or slowly. If the initial flow rate is slow, flush out with 5–10 mL of saline.
8. The infusion rate can be markedly increased by using a pressure bag at 300 mmHg pressure.

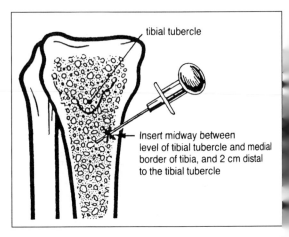

Fig. 16.2 Intraosseous infusion

Acute paraphimosis

In paraphimosis the penile foreskin is retracted, swollen and painful. Manual reduction should be attempted first. This can be done without anaesthesia, but a penile block with local anaesthetic (never use adrenaline in LA) can easily be injected in a ring around the base of the penis.

Method 1

Manual reduction can be performed by trying to advance the prepuce over the engorged glans with the index fingers while compressing the glans with the thumb (Fig. 16.3a).

Method 2

1. Take hold of the oedematous part of the glans in the fist of one hand and squeeze firmly. A gauze swab or warm towelette will help to achieve a firm grip (Fig. 16.3b).
2. Exert continuous pressure until the oedema passes under the constricting collar to the shaft of the penis.
3. The foreskin can then usually be pulled over the glans.

Method 3

If manual reduction methods fail, a dorsal slit incision should be made in the constricting collar of skin proximal to the glans under local or light general anaesthesia (Fig. 16.3c). The incision allows the foreskin to be advanced and reduces the swelling. Follow-up circumcision should be performed.

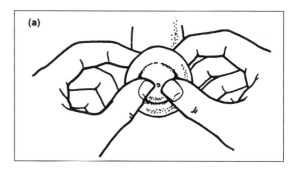

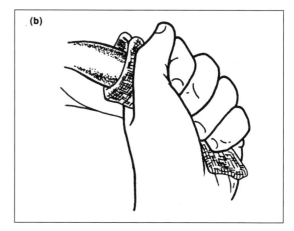

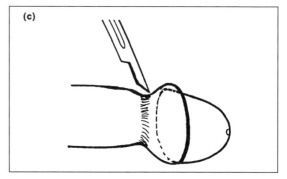

Fig. 16.3 Acute paraphimosis: **(a)** manual reduction; **(b)** squeezing with swab; **(c)** dorsal slit incision in the constricting collar of skin

Diagnosing the hysterical 'unconscious' patient

One of the most puzzling problems in emergency medicine is how to diagnose the unconscious patient caused by a conversion reaction. These patients really experience their symptoms (as opposed to the pretending patient) and resist most normal stimuli, including painful stimuli.

Method

1. Hold the patient's eye or eyes open with your fingers and note the reaction to light.
2. Now hold a mirror over the eye and watch closely for pupillary reaction (Fig. 16.4). The pupil should constrict with accommodation from the patient looking at his or her own image.

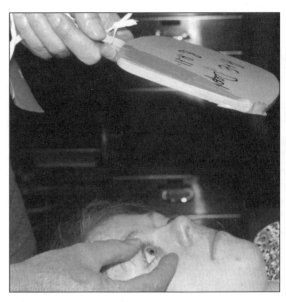

Fig 16.4 Testing for pupillary reaction

Electric shock

Household shocks tend to cause cardiac arrest due to ventricular fibrillation (Fig. 16.5).

Principles of management

- Make the site safe: switch off the electricity. Use dry wool to insulate the rescuers.
- 'Treat the clinically dead'.
- Attend to the ABC of resuscitation.
- Give a praecordial thump in a witnessed arrest.
- Consider a cervical collar (? cervical fracture).
- Provide basic cardiopulmonary resuscitation, including defibrillation (as required).
- Give a lignocaine infusion (100 mg IV) after cardiac arrest.
- Investigate and consider:
  —careful examination of all limbs,
  —X-ray of limbs or spine as appropriate,
  —check for myoglobinuria and renal failure,
  —give tetanus and clostridial prophylaxis.
- Get expert help—intensive care unit, burns unit.

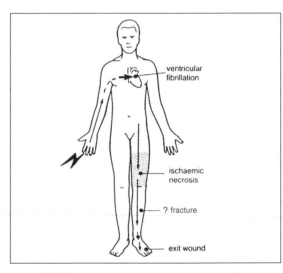

Fig. 16.5 Effect of electric shock passing through the body

Head injury and conscious state

It is important to have a system to assess a patient's cerebral status.

Simplified system

A useful simplified method of recording the conscious state is to use a five-level system rating:

1. awake,
2. confused,
3. responds to shake and shout,
4. responds to pain,
5. unresponsive coma.

Glasgow coma scale (Table 16.1)

The Glascow coma scale (GCS) is frequently used as an objective guide to the conscious state.
If the GCS score is:

- 8 or less: severe head injury
- 9–10: serious
- 11–12: moderate
- 13–15: minor

Arrange urgent referral if the score is less than 12. If the score is 12–15, keep under observation for at least 6 hours.

Table 16.1 Glasgow coma scale

	Score
Eye opening (E)	
• Spontaneous opening	4
• To verbal command	3
• To pain	2
• No response	1
Motor response (M)	
• Obeys verbal command	6
Response to painful stimuli	
• Localises pain	5
• Withdraws from pain stimuli	4
• Abnormal flexion	3
• Extensor response	2
• No response	1
Verbal response (V)	
• Orientated and converses	5
• Disorientated and converses	4
• Inappropriate words	3
• Incomprehensible sounds	2
• No response	1
Coma score E + M + V	
Minimum 3	
Maximum 15	

Sexual assault

What you should do for the patient is to first offer and provide privacy, confidentiality and emotional support.

Three important things to say initially to any victim

- 'You are safe now.'
- 'We are sorry this happened to you.'
- 'It was not your fault.'

Initial advice to the victim

- *If victim reporting to police*

  1. Notify the police at once.
  2. Take along a witness to the alleged assault (if there was a witness).
  3. Do not wash or tidy yourself or change your clothing.
  4. Do not take any alcohol or drugs.
  5. Don't drink or wash out your mouth if there was oral assault.
  6. Take a change of warm clothing.

- *If not reporting to police or unsure*

  Contact any of the following:

  1. a friend or other responsible person,
  2. 'Lifeline' or 'Lifelink' or similar service,
  3. a doctor,
  4. a counselling service.

Obtaining information

1. Obtain consent to record and release information.
2. Take a careful history and copious relevant notes.

3. Keep a record, have a protocol.
4. Obtain a kit for examination.
5. Have someone present during the examination (especially in the case of male doctors examining women).
6. Air-dry swabs (media destroy spermatozoa).
7. Hand specimens to the police immediately.
8. Work with (not for) the police.

Making reports

Remember that as a doctor you are impartial. Never make inappropriate judgments to authorities (e.g. 'This patient was raped' or 'Incest was committed').

Rather, say: 'There is evidence (or no evidence) to support penetration of the vagina/anus.' or 'There is evidence of trauma to _____.'

Handy tips

- Remember that some experienced perpetrators carry lubricants or amylnitrate to dilate the anal sphincter.
- Urine examination in female children may show sperm. (If the child is uncharacteristically passing urine at night, get the mother to collect a specimen.)
- Vaginal and rectal swabs should be air-dried.
- For suspected abuse of children, you cannot work in isolation: refer to a sexual assault centre or share the complex problem.
- When the victim is undressing for examination, get them to stand on a white sheet. This helps to identify small foreign objects that fall to the floor.

Migraine: Intravenous lignocaine

Intravenous lignocaine has been used for many years for the treatment of acute migraine headache.

Lignocaine (1% solution intravenously) can give rapid relief to many people with classic or common migraine. It does not work for tension headache, hypertensive headache or narcotic addiction headache.

Indications

A history consistent with either classic or common migraine.

Contraindications

- Known hypersensitivity to local anaesthetics.
- Patients with pacemakers or who are taking anti-arrhythmic medication.
- Patients with marked bradycardia of whatever cause.

Dosage

- A maximum dose of 1 mg of lignocaine per kilogram should not be exceeded.
- A 1% solution of lignocaine contains 52.5 mg of lignocaine in 5 mL (approx. 10 mg per mL). Thus, a 70 kg adult would have a maximum dose of 7 mL. (*Note:* A bolus of 5 mL of Xylocaine is given to patients with acute myocardial infarction.)

Method

1. Place the patient in the supine position.
2. Take blood pressure and leave the cuff on as a tourniquet.
3. Insert a 23-gauge butterfly needle in a vein on the dorsum of the hand.
4. Draw up the maximum calculated dose in a 10 mL syringe. (Do not leave excess in the syringe, as it may be injected unintentionally.)
5. *Quietly* explain to the patient what is happening as you inject the lignocaine. (Patients can expect to feel a 'pounding' sensation in their ears, a tingling of the lips and extremities, a floating sensation and a feeling of acute anxiety in their stomach.) Continue to focus their attention on their headache, and ask them to tell you when the pain disappears.
6. The injection should be given at a steady rate over about 90 seconds. If given too rapidly it will tend to cause more noticeable symptoms; if given too slowly it may not resolve the headache.
7. Once the migrainous part of the headache has gone, the patient may still complain of nausea. If so, give 5–10 mg of metoclopramide intravenously into the needle in situ.
8. Soluble aspirin can be given for any residual 'tension' headache of the neck or occiput.
9. Generally the patient can resume normal activities in 30 minutes.

Other migraine tips

At first symptoms:
- aspirin or paracetamol + anti-emetic, e.g.
  —soluble aspirin 600–900 mg (o) and
  —metoclopramide 10 mg (o)
  For established migraine:
- IV metoclopramide 10 mg, then 10–15 minutes later give 2–3 soluble aspirin and/or codeine tablets
                    or
- IM metoclopramide 10 mg, then 20 minutes later IM dihydroergotamine 0.5–1 mg
                    or
- lignocaine 4% topical solution—as spray 2.5 mL per nares
                    or

- serotonin receptor agonist:
  —sumatriptan (o), SC injection or nasal spray,
                    or
  —zolmitriptan (o), repeat in 2 hours if necessary,
                    or
  —naratriptan (o), repeat in 4 hours if necessary.
    If very severe (and other preparations are unsuccessful):
- IV metoclopramide 10 mg, then 5 minutes later IV dihydroergotamine 0.5 mg, slowly.

Note: Avoid pethidine.

The IV fluid load method

Many practitioners claim to obtain rapid relief of migraine by giving 1 litre of intravenous fluid over 1 hour, supplemented by oral paracetamol.

Hyperventilation

Improvised methods to help alleviate the distress of anxiety-provoked hyperventilation include:

- Breathe in and out of a paper bag.
- Breathe in and out slowly and deeply into cupped hands.
- Suck ice blocks slowly (a good distractor).

Pneumothorax

Pneumothoraces can be graded according to the degree of collapse:

- small: up to 15% (of pleural cavity)
- moderate: 15–60%
- large: > 60%

A small pneumothorax is usually treated conservatively and undergoes spontaneous resolution.

Simple aspiration can be used for a small to moderate pneumothorax—usually 15–20%.

Traumatic and tension pneumothoraces represent potential life-threatening disorders.

Tension pneumothorax requires immediate management.

Intercostal catheter

A life-saving procedure for a tension pneumothorax is the insertion of an intercostal catheter (a 14-gauge intravenous cannula is ideal) or even a needle as small as 19-gauge (if necessary) into the second intercostal space in the midclavicular line along the upper edge of the rib. The site should be at least two finger-breadths from the edge of the sternum, so that damage to the internal mammary artery is avoided. The catheter is connected to an underwater seal.

An alternative site which is preferable in females for cosmetic reasons is in the mid-axillary line of the fourth or fifth intercostal space (Fig. 16.6).

Simple aspiration for pneumothorax

For patients presenting with pneumothorax, the traditional method of insertion of an intercostal catheter connected to underwater seal drainage may be avoided with simpler measures. Patients with a small pneumothorax (less than 15% lung collapse) can be managed conservatively. Larger uncomplicated cases can be managed by simple aspiration using a 16-gauge polyethylene intravenous catheter.

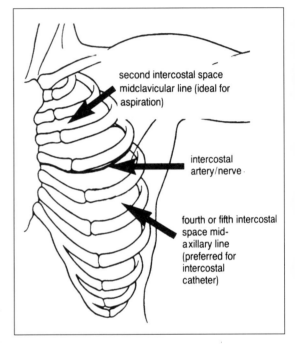

second intercostal space midclavicular line (ideal for aspiration)

intercostal artery/nerve

fourth or fifth intercostal space mid-axillary line (preferred for intercostal catheter)

Fig. 16.6 Positioning of intercostal catheter

Method

1. The patient lies propped up to 30°–40°.
2. Infiltrate LA in the skin over the second intercostal space in the midclavicular line on the affected site.
3. Insert a 16-gauge polyethylene intravenous catheter into the pleural space under strict asepsis.
4. Aspirate air into a 20 mL syringe to confirm entry into this space, and then remove the stilette.
5. Connect a flexible extension tube to this catheter, and then connect this tube to a three-way tap and a 50 mL syringe.
6. Aspirate and expel air via the three-way tap until resistance indicates lung re-expansion.

Obtain a follow-up X-ray. Repeat aspiration may be necessary, but most patients do not require inpatient admission.

Cricothyroidostomy

This procedure may be life-saving when endotracheal intubation is either contraindicated or impossible. It may have to be improvised or performed with commercially available kits such as the Surgitech rapitrac kit or the Portex minitrach II kit. Cricothyroidostomy can be performed using a standard endotracheal tube, from which the excess portion may be excised after insertion.

Method for adults

1. The patient should be supine, with the head, neck and chin fully extended (Fig. 16.7a).
2. Operate from behind the patient's head.
3. Palpate the groove between the cricoid and thyroid cartilage.
4. Make a short (2 cm) transverse incision (or longitudinal) through the skin and cricothyroid membrane (Fig. 16.7b).

   • Ensure the incision is not made above the thyroid cartilage.
   • Local anaesthesia (1–2 mL of 1% lignocaine) will be necessary in some patients.

5. Use an introducer to guide the cannula into the trachea.
6. Insert an endotracheal or tracheostomy tube if available.

(continues)

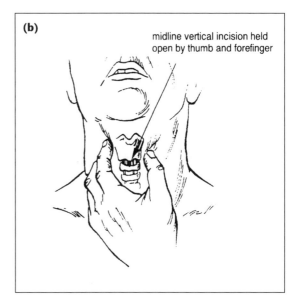

(b)

midline vertical incision held open by thumb and forefinger

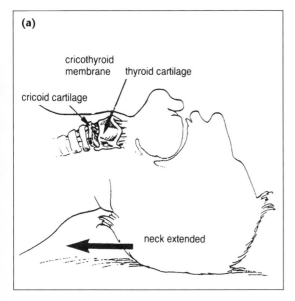

(a)

cricothyroid membrane   thyroid cartilage

cricoid cartilage

neck extended

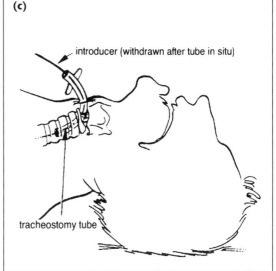

(c)

introducer (withdrawn after tube in situ)

tracheostomy tube

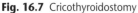

Fig. 16.7 Cricothyroidostomy

Method for children

1. Do not perform a stab wound in children because of poor healing.
2. Use a 14–15-gauge intravenous cannula.
3. Pierce the cricothyroid membrane at an angle of 45°. Free aspiration of air confirms correct placement.
4. Fit a 3 mm endotracheal tube connector into the end of the cannula or a 7 mm connector into a 2 mL or 5 mL syringe barrel connected to the cannula.

5. Attach the connector to the oxygen circuit; this system will allow oxygenation for about 30 minutes but carbon dioxide retention will occur.

Improvisation tips

- Any piece of plastic tubing, or even the 'shell' of a ballpoint pen, will suffice as a makeshift airway.
- A 2 mL or 5 mL syringe barrel will suffice as a connector between the cannula and the oxygen source.

Carotid sinus massage

Carotid sinus massage causes vagal stimulation and its effect on supra ventricular tachycardia is all or nothing. It has no effect on ventricular tachycardia. It slows the sinus rate and breaks the SVT by blocking AV nodal conduction.

Method

1. Locate the carotid pulse in front of the sterno-mastoid muscle just below the angle of the jaw (Fig. 16.8).
2. Ensure that no bruit is present.
3. Rub the carotid with a circular motion for 5–10 seconds.
4. Rub each carotid in turn if the SVT is not 'broken'.

In general, right carotid pressure tends to slow the sinus rate, and left carotid pressure tends to impair AV nodal conduction.

Precautions

In the elderly, there is a risk of embolism or brady-cardia.

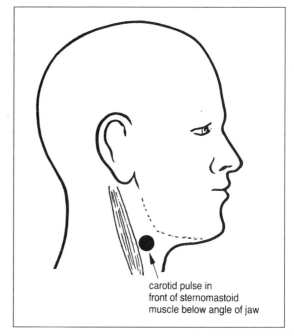

carotid pulse in front of sternomastoid muscle below angle of jaw

Fig. 16.8 Carotid sinus massage

Bite wounds

Snake bites

Most bites do not result in envenomation, which tends to occur in snake handlers or in circumstances where the snake has a clear bite of the skin.

First aid

1. Keep the patient as still as possible.
2. Do not wash, cut or manipulate the wound, or apply ice or use a tourniquet.
3. Immediately bandage the bite site firmly (not too tight). A crepe bandage is ideal: it should extend above the bite site for 15 cm, e.g. if bitten around the ankle, the bandage should cover the leg to the knee.
4. Splint the limb to immobilise it: a firm stick or slab of wood would be ideal.
5. Transport to a medical facility for definite treatment. Do not give alcoholic beverages or stimulants.
6. If possible, the dead snake should be brought along.

Note: A venom detection kit can be used to examine a swab of the bitten area or a fresh urine specimen (the best) or blood.

The bandage can be removed when the patient is safely under medical observation. Observe for symptoms such as vomiting, abdominal pain, excessive perspiration, severe headache and blurred vision.

Treatment of envenomation

1. Set up a slow IV infusion of N saline.
2. Give IV antihistamine cover (15 minutes beforehand) and 0.3 mL of adrenaline 1:1000 SC (0.1 mL for a child).
3. Dilute the specific antivenom (1:10 in N saline) and infuse slowly over 30 minutes via the tubing of the saline solution.
4. Have adrenaline on standby.
5. Monitor vital signs.

Spider bites

First aid

Sydney funnel-web: as for snake bites.
Other spiders: apply ice pack, do not bandage.

Treatment of envenomation

- Sydney funnel-web:
  —specific antivenom,
  —resuscitation and other supportive measures.
- Red back spider:
  —give antihistamines,
  —antivenom IM (IV if severe) 15 minutes later.

Human bites and clenched fist injuries

Human bites, including clenched fist injuries, often become infected by organisms such as *Staphylococcus aureus*, Streptococcus species and beta-lactamase producing anaerobic bacteria.

Principles of treatment

- Clean and debride the wound carefully, e.g. aqueous antiseptic solution or hydrogen peroxide.
- Give prophylactic penicillin if a severe or deep bite.
- Avoid suturing if possible.
- Tetanus toxoid.
- Consider rare possibility of HIV, hepatitis B or C, or infections.

For wound infection

- Take swab.
- Procaine penicillin 1 g IM, plus Augmentin 500 mg, 8-hourly for 5 days.

For severe penetrating injuries, e.g. joints, tendons

- IV antibiotics for 7 days.

Dog bites (non-rabid)

Animal bites are also prone to infection by the same organisms as for humans, plus *Pasteurella multocida*.

(continues)

Principles of treatment

- Clean and debride the wound with aqueous antiseptic, allowing it to soak for 10–20 minutes.
- Aim for open healing—avoid suturing if possible (except in 'privileged' sites with an excellent blood supply, such as the face and scalp).
- Apply non-adherent, absorbent dressings (paraffin gauze and Melolin) to absorb the discharge from the wound.
- Tetanus prophylaxis: immunoglobulin or tetanus toxoid.
- Give prophylactic penicillin for a severe or deep bite: 1.5 million units of procaine penicillin IM statim, then orally for 5 days. Tetracycline or flucloxacillin are alternatives.
- Inform the patient that slow healing and scarring are possible.

Cat bites

Cat bites have the most potential for suppurative infection. The same principles apply as for management of human or dog bites, but use flucloxacillin. It is important to clean a deep and penetrating wound. Another problem is cat-scratch disease, presumably caused by a Gram-negative bacterium.

Sandfly bites

For some reason, possibly the nature of body odour, the use of oral thiamine may prevent sandfly bites.

Dose: Thiamine 100 mg orally, daily.

Stings

Bee stings

First aid

1. Scrape the sting off sideways with a fingernail or knife blade. Do not squeeze it with the fingertips.
2. Apply 20% aluminium sulfate solution (Stingose).
3. Apply ice to the site.
4. Rest and elevate the limb that has been stung.

If anaphylaxis occurs, treat as appropriate.

Centipede and scorpion bites

The main symptom is pain, which can be very severe and prolonged.

First aid

1. Apply local heat, e.g. hot water with ammonia (household bleach).
2. Clean site.
3. Local anaesthetic, e.g. 1–2 mL of 1% lignocaine infiltrated around the site.
4. Check tetanus immunisation status.

Other bites and stings

This includes bites from ants, wasps and jellyfish.

First aid

1. Wash the site with large quantities of cool water.
2. Apply vinegar (liberal amount) or 20% aluminium sulfate solution (Stingose) to the wound for about 30 seconds.
3. Apply ice for several minutes.
4. Use soothing anti-itch cream or 5% lignocaine cream or ointment if very painful.

Medication is not usually necessary, although for a jellyfish sting the direct application of Antistine-Privine drops onto the sting (after washing the site) is effective.

Box jellyfish or sea wasp (*Chironex fleckeri*)

Treatment

- The victim should be removed from the water to prevent drowning.
- Inactivate the tentacles by pouring vinegar over them for 30 seconds (do not use alcohol)—use up to 2 L of vinegar at a time.
- Check respiration and the pulse.
- Start immediate cardiopulmonary resuscitation (if necessary).
- Give box jellyfish antivenom by IV injection.
- Provide pain relief if required (ice, lignocaine and analgesics).

Stinging fish

The sharp spines of the stinging fish have venom glands which can produce severe pain if they spike or even graze the skin. The best known of these is the stonefish. The toxin is usually heat sensitive.

Treatment

- Bathe or immerse the affected part in very warm to hot (not scalding) water—this may give instant relief.
- If pain persists, give a local injection/infiltration of lignocaine 1% or even a regional block. If still persisting, try pyroxidine 50 mg intralesional injection.
- A specific antivenom is available for the sting of the stonefish.

Coral cuts

Treatment

- Carefully debride the wound.
- If infected, phenoxymethyl penicillin 500 mg (o), 6-hourly.

17 Miscellaneous

Measurement of temperature

Temperature can be measured by several methods, including the mercury thermometer, the liquid crystal thermometer and the electronic probe thermometer. The *mercury thermometer*, however, is probably still the most widely used and effective temperature-measuring instrument. Table 17.1 gives a basic guide to interpreting the temperature values obtained.

Table 17.1 Interpretation of temperature measurement

Normal values		
Mouth		36.8°C
Axilla		36.4°C
Rectum		37.3°C
Ear		37.3°C
Pyrexia		
Mouth	>37.2 early morning	>37.8°C at other times of day

Basic rules of usage

1. Before use, shake down to 35°–36°C.
2. After use:
   - shake down and store in antiseptic,
   - do not run under hot water,
   - wipe rectal thermometers with alcohol and store separately.
3. Recording time is 3 minutes orally, 1–2 minutes rectally.

Oral use

1. Place under the tongue at the junction of the base of the tongue and the floor of the mouth to one side of the frenulum—the 'heat pocket'.
2. Ensure that the mouth is kept shut.
3. Remove dentures.

Note: Unsuitable for children 4 years and under, especially if irritable.

Rectal use

An excellent route for babies and young children under the age of 4.

Method

1. Lubricate the stub with petroleum jelly.
2. Insert for 2–3 cm (1 inch).
3. Keep the thermometer between the flexed fingers with the hand resting on the buttocks (Fig. 17.1).

Don't:
- dig thermometer in too hard,
- hold it too rigidly,
- allow the child to move around.

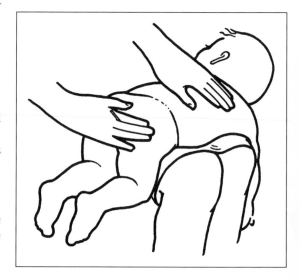

Fig. 17.1 Rectal temperature measurement

Axillary use

Very unreliable, and generally should be avoided but it is practical for young chidren and gives a helpful guide. If used it should be placed high in the axilla for 3 minutes.

Groin use

This route is not ideal but is more reliable than the axilla. It closely approximates oral temperature.

In infants, the thigh should be flexed against the abdomen.

Vaginal use

Mainly used as an adjunct to the assessment of ovulation during the menstrual cycle. Should be placed deeply in the vagina for 5 minutes before leaving the bed in the morning.

Aural (ear drum) use

The temperature can be measured in 3 seconds with a new infrared device placed in the ear canal (e-2 therm.). There is much debate about its efficacy but it appears to be worthwhile as it is a simple method.

Accidental breakage in mouth

If children bite off the end of a mercury thermometer there is no need for alarm, as the small amount of mercury is non-toxic and the piece of glass will usually pass in the stool.

Obtaining reflexes

Ankle-jerk technique

The method, illustrated in Figure 17.2a, provides a good opportunity to see and feel for a doubtful reflex. It is readily performed on a patient lying prone to allow examination of the back.

Method

1. Lift the foot slightly off the examination couch and hold it so that the Achilles tendon is under slight tension.
2. With the plessor held in the other hand, tap the tendon.

Alternatively, have the patient kneel on a chair with the feet freely suspended over the edge (Fig. 17.2b). Ask him or her to grasp the back of the chair firmly; this adds an element of reinforcement, which tends to increase the reflex. Tap the Achilles tendon in the usual way.

Unco-operative children

Children under 10 years of age have a disturbing tendency to tense their arms and legs at the wrong moment. Give them a squash ball or similar rubber object and instruct them to squeeze the ball as hard as possible on the count of 3.

Test the required reflex during this distraction.

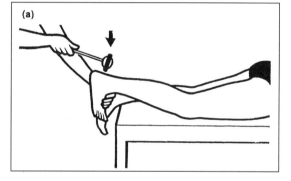

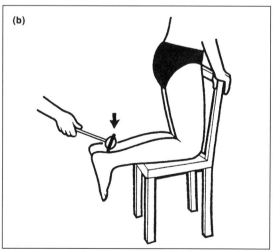

Fig. 17.2 Testing a doubtful reflex: **(a)** while the patient lies prone; **(b)** while the patient kneels on a chair

Tapping ascites

Abdominal paracentesis is often required as a therapeutic procedure to drain ascitic fluid in patients with terminal malignancy. The method is very simple. Select a site where there is shifting dullness and under which there are no solid organs (including an enlarged spleen). The ideal site is in the left iliac fossa (the LHS equivalent of McBurney's point) and lateral to the line of the inferior epigastric artery (Fig. 17.3).

Method

1. Ask the patient to lie supine.
2. Swab the skin with antiseptic.
3. Insert a 19-gauge intravenous cannula on a 20 mL syringe.
4. When ascitic fluid is obtained, remove the stilette and syringe and connect the plastic indwelling catheter via intravenous tubing to a drainage bag, so that drainage occurs by gravity.
5. The rate of flow can be regulated by the control on the IV tubing.

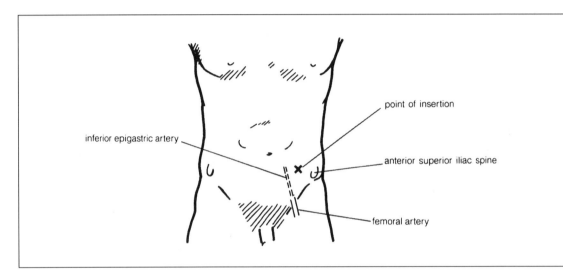

Fig. 17.3 Ideal site to tap ascites

Restless legs syndrome

Also known as Ekbom's syndrome, this consists of poorly localised aching in the legs (a crawling sensation) and spontaneous, continuous leg movements. Organic causes that need to be excluded include the neuropathies caused by diabetes, uraemia, hypothyroidism and anaemia. However, it is generally a functional disorder affecting the elderly, and results in marked insomnia.

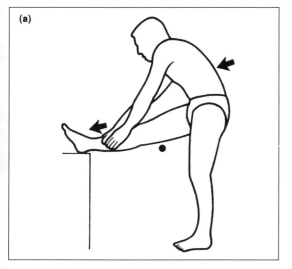

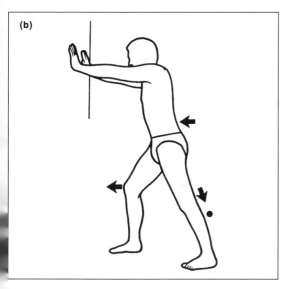

Management

- *Diet.* Eliminate caffeine and follow a healthy diet.
- *Medications (last resort).* These include hypnotics, tricyclic antidepressants, clonazepam, carbamazepine and propranolol. First choice is clonazepam 1 mg, 1 hour before retiring.
- *Exercises.* These involve stretching of the hamstrings and posterior leg muscles for at least 5 minutes before retiring (Fig. 17.4). Exercise (a) demonstrates hamstring stretching; (b) illustrates calf muscle stretching; (c) stretches all posterior muscles of the lower limb, especially the hamstrings. The patient lies on his or her back and uses a 1.2 m (4 foot) length of rope or flat tape to lift the leg. This exercise should be repeated to produce effective stretching.

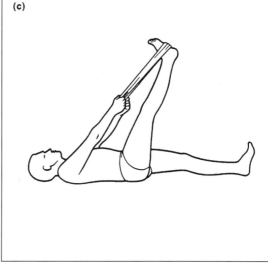

Fig. 17.4 Exercises for: **(a)** hamstring stretching; **(b)** calf muscle stretching; and **(c)** stretching of all posterior muscles of the lower limb

Nightmares

For severe persistent nightmares, give a trial of phenytoin (in recommended dosage) for 4 weeks and review.

Nocturnal cramps

Physiological muscle-stretching and relaxation techniques may be effective in the prevention of nocturnal cramps.

Exercise 1

1. Get the patient to stand bare-footed approximately 1 m (3 foot) from a wall, leaning forwards with the back straight and outstretched hands against the wall.
2. Then get them to lift the heels off the floor and then force the heels to the floor to produce tension in the calf muscles.
3. They should then hold for 30 seconds and repeat 5–6 times.

An alternative is to keep the heels on the floor and climb the hands up the wall. Patients should do these exercises 2–3 times a day for 1 week, then each night before retiring (Fig. 17.5).

Exercise 2

This can follow Exercise 1 before retiring.

The patient should rest in a chair with the feet out horizontally to the floor, with support from a cushion under the tendoachilles, for 10 minutes.

Drug treatment

- quinine sulfate 300 mg nocte, or
- biperiden 2–4 mg nocte.

Quinine drinks

Consider quinine-containing drinks, e.g. tonic water or bitter lemon, last thing at night.

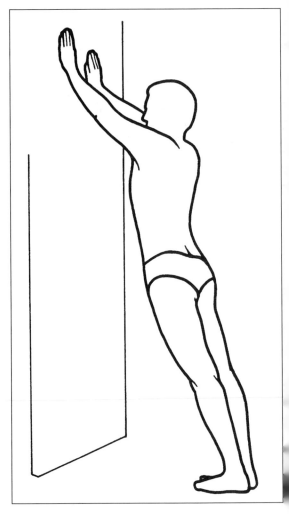

Fig. 17.5 Exercise for leg cramps

Special uses for vasodilators

Venepuncture

Venepuncture, whether for blood collection, the introduction of intravenous drugs or cannulation, can be very difficult in some patients whose veins are not dilated.

Methods

- Rub glyceryl trinitrate ointment (e.g. Nitro-Bid, Nitrolate) over the vein that you wish to puncture.
  or
- Give the patient one-half of an Anginine tablet sublingually, provided there are no contra-indications to glyceryl trinitrate use. The veins will soon appear.

Painful heels

Some patients, particularly elderly diabetics with small-vessel disease, develop painful heels. Glyceryl trinitrate ointment or transdermal pads applied to the painful area can provide considerable relief.

The transdermal pads (e.g. Nitradisc, Transderm-Nitro) are applied once daily and the ointment applied twice daily in a small amount under tape.

Chilblains

Apply glyceryl trinitrate ointment over the painful chilblains as necessary. Advise use of plastic gloves or immediate washing of hands (to avoid headache).

Other tips for chilblains include taking rum at night or nifedipine for prevention.

Nocturnal bladder dysfunction

The woman with the urethral syndrome or bladder dysfunction who constantly wakes during the night with an urge to micturate, yet only produces a small dribble of urine, can be helped by the following.

Method

Instruct the patient to perform a pelvic lift exercise when she awakes. In this exercise:

1. She balances on her upper back.
2. She then lifts her pelvis, supported by her flexed knees, and holds this position for about 30 seconds.
3. During this time she can squeeze the pelvic floor inward.
4. The exercise is repeated a couple of times.

Facilitating a view of the cervix

Fists under the buttocks

If having difficulty viewing a cervix for smear taking, ask the patient to rest her hands, preferably as fists, under her buttocks. If necessary she can lift her buttocks slightly higher with her fists.

A small, firm cushion could be placed under the buttocks as an alternative.

If you are still having trouble have the patient cough.

Note: Remember to warm the metal speculum in warm water and test the comfort of the temperature on the patient's thigh.

Condom on the speculum

If you are troubled by the vaginal walls collapsing into the gap between the two blades of the bivalved speculum you can slip a condom over the blades and then cut the tip off the condom. The condom then supports the vaginal walls.

Priapism

Various methods can be attempted to alleviate the acute or subacute onset of priapism, especially that which is drug induced:

• ice-cubes, inserted rectally,
• pseudoephedrine, especially for alprostadil (Caverjet injection or Muse) induced priapism.

If drug-induced priapism lasts longer than 2 hours, give the patient 2 pseudoephedrine tablets—repeat at 3½ hours if necessary.

If all fails and specialist help is remote, aspiration and irrigation should be attempted and is best performed in the first 6–8 hours (exclude polycythemia and leukaemia via an urgent blood film).

Under local anaesthetic and using a 16-gauge needle, aspirate thick blood from the ipsilateral corpora cavernosa through the glans penis. 20 mL of blood is drawn out at a time and the penis is then flushed with saline.

If resolution is incomplete, use a very slow injection of 10 mL of saline containing 1 mg aramine, followed by massage.

Premature ejaculation

It is worth a trial of a SSRI antidepressant agent e.g. fluoxetine (Prozac) 20 mg daily.

Indomethacin for renal/ureteric colic

After a patient has received an intramuscular injection of pethidine or morphine for the severe pain of renal colic, further pain can be alleviated by indomethacin. Suppositories are most satisfactory, but should be limited to two a day.

Some practitioners have submitted an anecdotal tip of getting the sufferer of ureteric colic to jump up and down vigorously on the leg of the affected side.

An effective alternative treatment is an IM injection of 75 mg diclofenac (if available), then diclofenac 50 mg (o) tds for 1 week.

ECG recording

It is useful to note that the ECG leads work effectively through stockings, including pantyhose.

Record-keeping for after-hours calls

When called at weekends or at night to make a home visit, general practitioners are often faced with the choice of going to the surgery for the records or writing the new notes in a notebook or on scraps of paper.

If the patient record is not required for immediate management, a practical suggestion is to carry sheets of self-adhesive, plain paper on which to take notes to include in the practice record later. This paper is available in gloss or matt finish.

Write the patient's name in the top left-hand corner of the space and record notes in your usual style within a confined space. If you have to see two or three patients, leave a clear space between the notes for each.

On return to the surgery, cut the notes of each patient into individual blocks, strip off the backing and apply to the appropriate section of the patient's practice file.

Self-adhesive paper may be bought in widths of approximately 170 mm and in various lengths from most stationery stores (Millfix or Quick-Stick, for example, are two suitable brands.)

Sticking labels in the patient's history

After administering vaccine that has a sticky label on it, such as Infanrix, remove the label and place it in the patient's notes.

Aspiration of pleural effusion

Use a recent chest X-ray to aid the clinical examination in order to select the best site for aspiration. This site is usually on the posterior chest wall medial to the angle of the scapula, in the intercostal space below the upper limit of dullness to percussion. Avoid going too low.

Method

1. Explain the procedure to the patient, who sits on a chair facing the bed and leaning slightly forwards with the arms folded in front resting on a pillow on the bed.
2. Using a sterile procedure with gloves and gown, swab the skin with antiseptic.
3. Infiltrate the overlying skin with 1% lignocaine with adrenaline (25-gauge needle) and change to a 21-gauge needle and two-way tap with Leur connectors. Slowly infiltrate the chest wall down to pleura. Fluid appears in the syringe on aspiration after the pleura is penetrated.
4. Aspirate the fluid and by turning the tap, direct the fluid into the collecting container. This is repeated until all the fluid is tapped.
   Caution: Ensure that air does not enter the pleural space at any stage.
5. Upon withdrawing the catheter, immediately apply a collodian dressing.

A simpler technique

This technique is useful for tapping recurrent malignant effusions and can be performed at home. Insert a size 18 intravenous cannula. Withdraw the stilette and connect the plastic cannula to an intravenous tubing set with the end draining into a drainage bag by gravity.

Subcutaneous fluid infusions

Subcutaneous fluids are useful when:

- Relatively small amounts of crystalloid are needed (15 mL/kg per 12 hours).
- Intravenous access is not required for systemic therapy.

This method of administering fluid has been used for more than 30 years. It can be sited and supervised by the nursing staff.

Complications are rare and usually relate to local oedema, which settles spontaneously once the infusion has been ceased.

Practical aspects

- Access to the subcutaneous space is via a 21-gauge butterfly needle, which is replaced daily.
- One ampoule of hyaluronidase (hyalase) is given prior to infusion and before subsequent bags of crystalloid. (This is necessary when skin elasticity is high, as in children.)
- Crystalloid solution (normal saline or 4% dextrose and $^1/_5$ normal saline) with infusion set is then connected to the butterfly needle.
- The infusion is usually run at a maximum of 15 mL per kg over 4–12 hours per 24 hours. (This enables the patient to move about.)
- Most regions are suitable. The more convenient are the abdomen, the anterior thigh and the shoulder.
- The drip rate can be reduced if any discomfort is produced.

Continuous subcutaneous infusion of morphine

When the oral and/or rectal routes are not possible or ineffective, a subcutaneous infusion of morphine (for terminal pain) with a syringe pump can be used.

It is also useful for symptom control when there is a need for a combination of drugs, e.g. for pain, nausea and agitation. It may avoid bolus peak effects (sedation, nausea or vomiting) or trough effects (breakthrough pain) with intermittent parenteral morphine injections.

Practical aspects

- Access to the deep subcutaneous space is via a 21-gauge butterfly needle which is replaced regularly (1, 2, 3 or 4 days).
- Most regions are suitable. The more convenient are the abdomen, the anterior thigh, and the anterior upper arm. (Usually the anterior abdominal wall is used.)
- The infusion can be managed at home.
- About one-half to two-thirds of the 24-hour oral morphine requirement is placed in the syringe.
- The syringe is placed into the pump driver, which is set for 24-hour delivery.
- Areas of oedema are not suitable.

Uses of a fine cataract knife

The fine size 52 L eye knife known as a Beaver eye knife (Fig. 17.6) or Eent-Super Sharps can be used for several minor procedures involving minimal surgical invasiveness.

Examples include:

- neurofasciotomy for painful trigger spots in back pain,
- lateral and medial epicondylitis (tennis elbow),
- lateral sphincterotomy (see page 70).

Neurofasciotomy of back

This procedure is a well-known treatment for very painful localised chronic back problems, especially in the soft paraspinal tissue of the lumbosacral spine.

Method

1. Identify the painful trigger spot or spots by deep palpation. They usually lie 2–3 cm from the midline (level of spinous processes).
2. This site (or sites) is infiltrated deeply and widely with 10–15 mL of 1% lignocaine with adrenaline.

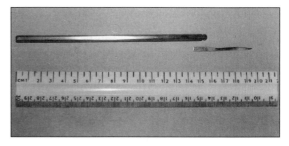

Fig. 17.6 The fine cataract knife

3. Make a stab incision with the eye knife which is inserted to the hilt of the blade and directed towards the underlying facet joint.
4. Sweep the blade upwards (cranially) and downwards (caudally) through an arc of about 150° to achieve sagittal division of the fascia which includes branches of the posterior rami of the segmental nerves (Fig. 17.7).
5. Take care not to snap the fine blade when performing this sweeping action. Withdraw the blade and control haemorrhage by digital pressure.
6. Apply a sterile pressure dressing and cover with adhesive plaster. *(continues)*

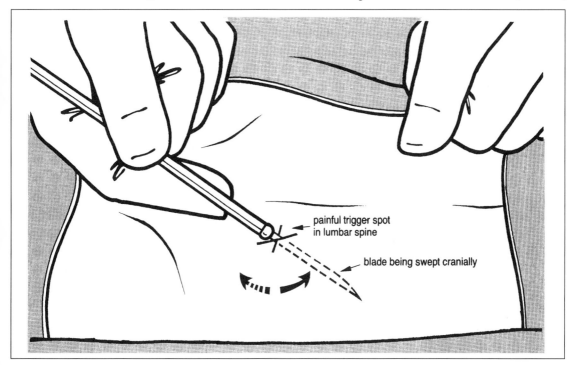

painful trigger spot in lumbar spine

blade being swept cranially

Fig. 17.7 Neurofasciotomy of lower back trigger point

Epicondylitis (tennis elbow)

A simple tenotomy procedure can be used for the tenoperiosteal variety of medial or lateral epicondylitis which has become chronic and resistant to conservative treatment. This percutaneous method can be used when major surgical intervention is being considered.

Method

1. Localise the exact tender site (corresponding to painful scar tissue) by palpation and mark it with a permanent marking pen.
2. Infiltrate the site (down to the periosteum) with 1% or 2% lignocaine with adrenaline.
3. Insert the eye knife through the skin until it reaches bone.

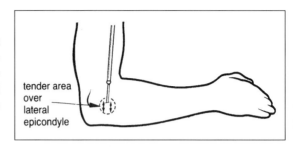

tender area over lateral epicondyle

Fig. 17.8 Releasing painful scar tissue of lateral epicondylitis (sharp edge moves in direction of arrow)

4. Then scrape the scar tissue off the bone, moving the knife to and fro in a horizontal (transverse) plane until all the painful area is covered (Fig. 17.8).

Alternative scalpels for this procedure include tenotomes and a size 11 scalpel blade.

Cool cabbages for hot breasts

Cabbage leaves have been used in some cultures for hundreds of years in the treatment of sprains, infections and some breast problems. Recently, they have become popular in many maternity hospitals for managing breast engorgement. There appears to be an unknown substance that is absorbed from the cabbage leaf through the mother's skin, resulting in decreased oedema and improved milk flow.

Uses

Local breast engorgement:

- blocked ducts or mastitis.

Generalised breast engorgement:

- when milk supply is greater than demand
  —early postpartum
  —sudden weaning

- when lactation suppression is required
  —after a baby dies
  —after mid-trimester abortion.

Method

1. Wash the cabbage leaves well (beware risk of contamination with dirt or pesticides) and dry. Store the cabbage in a refrigerator.
2. Cut stalks from leaves (to prevent pressure on breast) and apply the leaves to the breast, avoiding the nipple area. (Cut out openings for the nipples.)
3. Remove after 2 hours (or earlier if the leaves are limp) and assess the need for further leaves.
4. Cease using leaves when engorgement settles, as prolonged use can reduce the milk supply.
5. Do not use if the patient has a history of allergy to cabbage.

Many women using this home remedy have found cool cabbage leaves soothing when their breasts are engorged. Cabbage leaves have a role as an adjunct to the management of breastfeeding problems. It is still essential to correctly position the baby on the breast and not restrict the baby's access to the breast.

Makeshift spacing chambers for asthmatics

An improvised temporary 'aerochamber' can be made by one of two methods:
1. Plunge the end of the puffer through the bottom of a paper or polystyrene (preferable) cup.

2. Cut the end (base) off a plastic soft drink bottle and insert the end of the puffer into the mouth of the bottle.

Coping with tablets

Breaking tablets in half

When a tablet is manufactured with a line down the middle it may be easily broken, especially if it is a big tablet with a deep scored line.

Method

1. Place the tablet on a flat surface with the line uppermost.
2. Place one finger on each side of the tablet and press down firmly (Fig. 17.9).
3. The tablet will split easily.

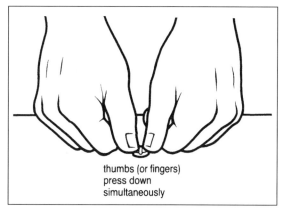
thumbs (or fingers) press down simultaneously

Fig. 17.9 Coping with tablets

Swallowing tablets

This method is recommended for those who may have trouble swallowing tablets.

Method 1

Try swallowing the tablet with the head bent forward.

Method 2

Simply place the tablet on the tongue and drink water through a straw with the head slightly flexed forwards. The stream of water 'hoses' the tablet down the throat.

Venepuncture and intravenous cannulation

Basic venepuncture

Purpose

Collection of blood, including large volume collection for transfusion. The ideal site is the basilic vein (Fig. 17.10). Use local anaesthetic for large volume blood collection.

Method

1. Explain the method to the patient. Ensure the patient is warm and comfortable.
2. Dilate the vein by means of a tourniquet applied to occlude venous return.
3. Place a padded block under the arm to keep it straight.
4. After using a sterile swab to prepare the site, place the needle with attached syringe on the skin. Using downwards oblique pressure, puncture the vein firmly, ensuring the needle lies well within the vein. Remove the tourniquet.

(continues)

Tips to aid dilation of veins

There are several ways in which peripheral veins can be dilated to facilitate venepuncture. The following are some of the methods used.

Vasodilation methods

- Apply a warm flannel for 60 seconds, or
- Rub glyceryl trinitrate ointment over the vein, or
- Give the patient half a glyceryl trinitrate tablet (if no contraindications).

Sphygmomanometer methods

- Dilate the vein by means of the sphygmo-manometer to keep BP at about 80–90 mmHg (veins will stand out).

or

- Using the sphygmomanometer, inflate it to a pressure around 30 mmHg above systolic arterial pressure for 1–2 minutes while the patient opens and closes their hand. Thereafter it is deflated to around 80 mmHg and the resulting reactive hyperaemia is effective in filling even the shyest of veins. According to Wishaw this is the method par excellence.

Venesection tourniquet method

Apply the tourniquet tightly and then release. After a reactive hyperaemia occurs reapply it and the veins should stand out well.

Cannulation

Use sterile gloves for this procedure.

Best site

- Choose a suitable prominent vein in the non-dominant forearm (not over a joint), e.g. dorsum of hand, cephalic vein just above wrist (dorso-lateral position).
- Use elbow veins as last resort.

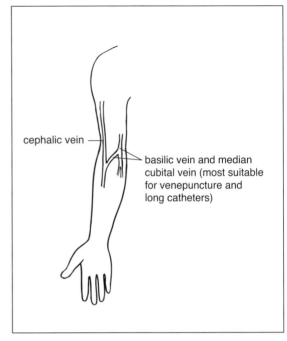

cephalic vein

basilic vein and median cubital vein (most suitable for venepuncture and long catheters)

Fig. 17.10 Main veins of arm for venepuncture

- Choose a relatively fixed vein, e.g. where it penetrates the fascia.
- Choose a vein running parallel to the long axis of the arm.

Method

1. Apply a small bleb, e.g. 0.5 mL of local anaesthetic, over or adjacent to the vein (keep very superficial) and wait 5 minutes, or apply EMLA cream at least 60–90 minutes beforehand.
2. Insert the needle and catheter unit through the skin beyond the shoulder of the plastic part.
3. Pierce the vein and ensure that the unit lies flat as it is guided along the vein lumen for a short distance.
4. When blood enters the chamber, put a finger over the vein to stop backflow. Remove the tourniquet and guide the plastic catheter into the vein.

Lumbar puncture

Main indications

- Diagnostic purposes, e.g. meningitis, MS, Guillain-Barre syndrome, SAH, CNS syphilis.
- Introducing contrast media.
- Introducing chemotherapeutic agents.

In children:

- Febrile, sick infant with no focus of infection.
- Fever with meningism.
- Prolonged seizure with fever.

Contraindications

Absolute: Local skin infection.
Relative: Raised intracranial pressure.
　　　　　Depressed conscious state.

Essentials of lumbar puncture 1: Preparation

1. Explain the procedure to the patient.
2. The patient should be in the lateral recumbent position, with the back maximally flexed and vertical to the table (Fig. 17.11).
3. The patient should be well immobilised.
4. Adopt the sterile procedure (mask, gloves, antiseptic prep.).
5. Apply 1% lignocaine to skin and subcutaneous tissue (not necessary in infants).

Surface anatomy

Imaginary line between tops of iliac crests lies at spinous process of L_4 or between L_4 and L_5. Insert the needle at L_4–L_5 or L_3–L_4.

Essentials of lumbar puncture 2: Procedure

1. Use a 20–21-gauge LP needle (9 cm) for an average adult; 22-gauge × 4 cm for infants, × 5 cm for 4–10 years, × 6 cm for older children.
2. Insert the needle at right angles to the skin.
3. Slowly advance slightly cephalad (aim for the umbilicus), otherwise perfectly parallel.
4. Advance 1 millimetre at a time. You will feel a 'give' when the dura is pierced (about 4–7 cm in adults, 2–3 cm in children).
5. Withdraw the stylus, and wait 30 seconds for CSF flow. Rotating the needle through 90–180° may allow CSF to flow.
6. If CFS is blood stained, get three samples.
7. Remove the needle with one quick motion.

Recordings

- CSF pressure with manometer (N < 180 mm).
- CSF biochemistry, microbiology, immunology (oligoclonal bands).

Note: Don't aspirate CSF.

Post care

Careful observation and bed rest.

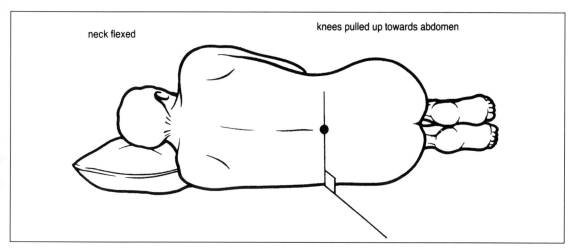

Fig. 17.11 Lumbar puncture: the patient is placed in the foetal position with the back perpendicular to the bed. A line between the posterior superior iliac spines will intersect the midline at approximately the interspinous space between L_4 and L_5

Urethral catheterisation of males

Preliminary questions

1. What is the aim of this procedure and can it be achieved without urethral catheterisation?
2. How long must the catheter remain in situ?
3. Do I have the skill to perform the procedure safely?

Equipment

You will need:

- prepackaged set including swabs,
- aqueous (not alcoholic) skin antiseptic,
- one or two pairs of forceps,
- sterile kidney dish to collect urine,
- suitable catheter—usually medium size,
- sterile lubricant, e.g. lignocaine jelly in syringe,
- sterile syringe,
- suitable catheter drainage bag,
- catheter dressing,
- sterile gown and mask.

Technique essentials

1. Explain the procedure to the patient, who is best placed in the heel-to-heel position.
2. Sterile preparation/clean glans penis.
3. Fit nozzle to the syringe of lignocaine jelly and insert gently into the penile meatus—inject the jelly slowly: compress the glans and leave 5 minutes.
4. Grasp the catheter a few centimetres from its tip with forceps (the funnel end rests in the kidney dish).
5. Hold the penis straight with one hand and gently insert and slowly advance the catheter. Do not rush or use force (Fig. 17.12).
6. When the catheter reaches the penoscrotal junction (it now rests against the external sphincter), pull the penis downwards between the patient's thighs.
7. Continue insertion through the sphincter or prostatic urethra until the entire length is inserted, even if urine emerges before then.
8. *Non-retaining catheter:* Ensure urine is flowing, then withdraw a few centimetres. Eventually press on the abdomen to ensure the bladder is empty.
   Retaining catheter: Inflate balloon (usually 5 mL of water) and gently withdraw until the balloon impinges on the bladder neck.
   Note: Ensure the catheter is in the bladder before inflating the balloon.
9. Replace the retracted prepuce over the glans (to prevent paraphimosis).

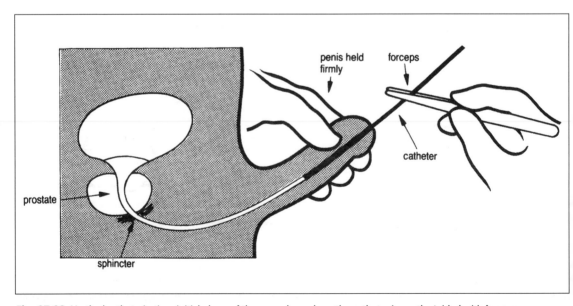

Fig. 17.12 Urethral catheterisation: initial phase of the procedure where the catheter is gently guided with forceps

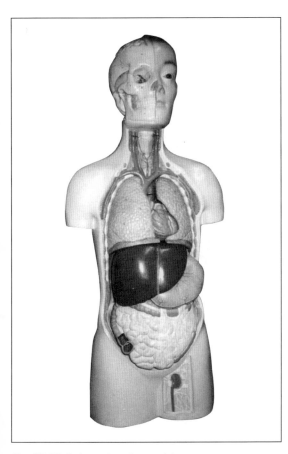

Fig. 17.13 Patient education model

Patient education techniques in the consulting room

Organ removal torso model

A colourful model of the human body (head to groin) can be obtained to install in the surgery. The organs can be systematically removed and explained to the patient (Fig. 17.13).

Whiteboard

A small whiteboard can be installed, either portable or fixed to the wall, in the consulting room. A Sandford Expo kit can be installed alongside the board. It consists of a set of coloured whiteboard markers which clip onto slots in the kit, and an eraser. This is ideal for explanatory sketches.

Computer education

Your patient can be briefly taken through a patient education information program (for example, J. Murtagh's *Patient Education*, 4th edn, McGraw-Hill Australia, Sydney, 2004) on the computer screen and then take home a printout. This can be individualised by including the patient's name on the top of the general sheet.

This visual education can be enhanced by the use of graphics which some practitioners who have developed skills in computing are now using with amazing effectiveness.

Improvised suppository inserter

Some people find it difficult or unaesthetic to insert a suppository digitally. An interesting method is to rearrange a disposable plastic syringe so that it is converted into a plunger for ease of insertion of the suppository.

Rearranging the syringe

- Remove the plunger.
- Cut the end off the barrel (at the narrow end).
- Place the plunger through the opposite end at this new opening.

Inserting the suppository

- Place the suppository in the syringe barrel (Fig. 17.14).
- Firmly place the flange up against the anus.
- Press the plunger rapidly.

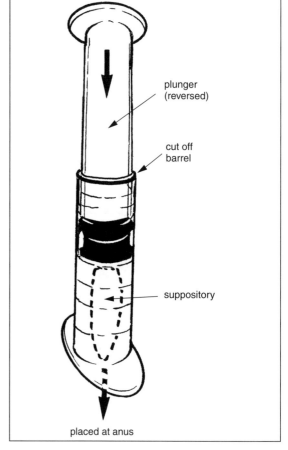

Fig. 17.14 Position of suppository

The many uses of petroleum jelly (Vaseline)

- To kill lice, e.g. pubic lice or those on the eyelashes, apply petroleum jelly twice daily for 8 days, then pluck off any remaining nits.
- Apply to dry and cracked skin (also useful to prevent cracking), e.g. on heels.
- Apply for the protection of normal skin surrounding lesions such as warts and seborrhoeic keratoses before the application of corrosive substances, e.g. chromic acid or liquid nitrogen.
- Use as a lubricant for rectal examination.
- Use as a lubricant and sealant for the plunger on the metal ear syringe.
- For nappy rash use it in equal parts with a mixture of hydrocortisone and antifungal creams to promote length of action of the medication.
- Dr Clarrie Dietman (personal communication) claims great success using petroleum jelly as a first-line treatment for allergic rhinitis. He recommends insertion of a liberal amount high into each nostril twice daily for as long as necessary. It has to be considered as a trial. It is important to advise patients to blow each nostril separately, before and after, to avoid middle-ear and parasinus complications.

Sea sickness

There are several 'mariner's tips' to prevent sea sickness, especially involving the use of ginger.

- Take a ginger preparation, e.g. drink ginger ale or ginger beer.
- Place a plug in one ear.
- Look to the horizon.

Honey as a wound healer

At the 2002 Australian Wound Management Conference in Adelaide, researchers emphasised the healing powers of honey, especially Manuka honey, for conditions such as infected wounds, burns, ulcers and possibly acne. Honey has anti-bacterial activity but its healing power is adversely affected by arterial insufficiency. Professor Molan of New Zealand claimed that leg ulcers healed within three months.

The usual method is to apply 20 mL of honey (25–30 g) on a 10 cm × 10 cm absorbent dressing pad daily, reducing to twice weekly.

Snapping the top off a glass ampoule

Breaking off the top of those stubborn ampoules can cause injury. To reduce the risk of this, it is best to use a small file; however, even these may not be effective. If you are using your hands to complete the snap, try using a gauze swab, the alcohol swab package or an appropriate-sized plaster auriscope earpiece.

Bibliography

Brown, J.S., *Minor Surgery. A Text and Atlas*, Chapman and Hall, London, 1986.

Chan, C., & G. Salam, 'Splinter removal' *American Family Physician*, 2003, 67, pp. 2557–62.

Chapeski, A., 'Simple Care for the Ingrown Toenail', *Australian Family Physician*, 1998, 27, 4, p. 299.

Claesson, M., & R. Short, 'Lancet with Less Pain', *Lancet*, 1990, December 22–9, pp. 1566–7.

Cook, J., B. Sankaran, & A. Wasunna, *General Surgery at the District Hospital*, World Health Organization, Geneva, 1986.

Corrigan, B. & G.D. Maitland, *Practical Orthopaedic Medicine*, Butterworths, Sydney, 1986.

Eriksson, E., *Illustrated Handbook in Local Anaesthesia*, Munksgaard, Copenhagen, 1969.

Forrest, A.P.M., D.C. Carter & I.B. MacLeod, *Principles and Practice of Surgery*, Churchill Livingstone, Edinburgh, 1985.

Györy, A.E., 'A duct tape-free wart remedy', *Complementary Medicine*, September/October 2003, p. 4.

Hayes, J.A. & J.G.W. Burdon, 'The Management of Spontaneous Pneumothorax by Simple Aspiration', *Australian Family Physician*, 1988, 17, pp. 458–62.

Hoppenfield, S., *Physical Examination of the Spine and Extremities*, Prentice-Hall, Englewood Cliffs, NJ, 1976, pp. 172–30.

Kamien, M., 'Which Cerumanolytic?', *Australian Family Physician*, 1999, 28, p. 817.

Kenna, C. & J.E. Murtagh, *Back Pain and Spinal Manipulation*, 2nd edn, Butterworths Heinemann, Oxford, 1997.

La Villa, G., 'Methylprednisolone Acetate in Local Therapy of Ganglion', *Clinical Therapeutics*, 1968, 47, pp. 455–7.

Marwood, J., 'Sebaceous Cyst Excision', *General Practitioner*, 1994, 2, pp. 4–5.

McGregor, I., *Fundamental Techniques of Plastic Surgery*, Churchill Livingstone, Edinburgh, 1989.

McLaren, P., 'Dilating Peripheral Veins', *Anaesthesia and Intensive Care*, 1994, 22, p. 318.

Molan, P.C., 'Treatment of wounds and burns with honey', *Current Therapeutics*, September 2001, pp. 33–9.

Orlay, G., 'Non-malignant rectal and anal conditions', *Australian Doctor*, 16 April 2004, pp. I–IV.

Penfield, W. & E. Boldrey, 'Somatic Motor and Sensory Representation in the Cerebral Cortex of Man as Studied by Electrical Stimulation', *Brain*, 1937, 60, pp. 389–443.

Peterson, L. & P. Renstrom, *Sports Injuries and their Prevention and Treatment*, Methuen, Sydney, 1986.

Quail, G., 'Regional Nerve Blocks', *Australian Family Physician*, 1996, 25, pp. 391–6.

Sheon, R.P., R.W. Moscowitz & V.M. Goldberg, *Soft Tissue Rheumatic Pain*, 2nd edn, Lea & Febiger, Philadelphia, 1987.

Snell, G.F., *Primary Care Clinics in Office Practice: Office Surgery*, Saunders, Philadelphia, 1986, p. 25.

Tonge, B., 'I'm upset, you're upset and so are my mum and dad', *Australian Family Physician*, 1983, 12, pp. 497–9.

van der Walt, J.H., 'Dilating Peripheral Veins—Another Suggestion', *Anaesthesia and Intensive Care*, 1994, 22, p. 624.

Warren, G., 'Controlling callus', *Medicine Today*, 2003, 4, 4, p. 95–7.

White, A.D.N., 'Dislocated Shoulder—A Simple Method of Reduction', *Medical Journal of Australia*, 1976, 2, pp. 726–7.

Wishaw, K.L., 'Dilating Veins, a Simple Approach', Letter to editor, *Anaesthesia and Intensive Care*, 1995, 23, p. 123.

Zagorski, M., 'Analgesia-free Reduction of Anterior Dislocation of the Shoulder Joint', *Aust. J. Rural Health*, 1995, 3, pp. 53–5.

Acknowledgments

I would like to acknowledge the many general practitioners throughout Australia who have contributed to this book, mainly in response to the invitation through the pages of *Australian Family Physician,* to forward their various practice tips to share with colleagues. Many of these tips have appeared over the past decade as a regular series in the official publication of the Royal Australian College of General Practitioners. The RACGP has supported my efforts and this project over a long period, and continues to promote the concept of good-quality care and assurance in general practice. I am indebted to the RACGP for giving permission to publish the material that has appeared in the journal.

My colleagues in the Department of Community Medicine at Monash University have provided invaluable assistance: Professor Neil Carson encouraged the concept some 20 years ago, and more recently my senior lecturers provided considerable input into skin repair and plastic surgery (Dr Michael Burke) and expertise with orodental problems and facial nerve blocks (Dr Geoff Quail). Special thanks go also to Dr John Colvin, Co-Director of Medical Education at the Victorian Eye and Ear Hospital, for advice on eye disorders; Dr Ed Brentnall, Director of Accident and Emergency Department, Box Hill Hospital; the editorial staff of *Australian Family Physician*; Mr Chris Sorrell, graphic designer with *Australian Family Physician*; and in particular to Dr Clive Kenna, co-author of *Back Pain and Spinal Manipulation* (Butterworths), for his considerable assistance with musculoskeletal medicine, especially on spinal disorders.

Medical practitioners who contributed to this book are: Lisa Amir, Tony Andrew, Philip Arber, Neville Babbage, Peter Barker, Royce Baxter, Andrew Beischer, Ashley Berry, Peter Bourke, Peter Bowles, Tony Boyd, James Breheny, Ed Brentnall, Charles Bridges-Webb, John Buckley, Michael Burke, Marg Campbell, Hugh Carpenter, Peter Carroll, Ray Carroll, Neil Carson, Robert Carson, John Colvin, Peter Crooke, Graham Cumming, Joan Curtis, Hal Day, Tony Dicker, Clarrie Dietman, Mary Doyle, Graeme Edwards, Humphrey Esser, Iain Esslemont, Howard Farrow, Peter Fox, Michael Freeman, John Gambrill, John Garner, Jack Gerschman, Peter Graham, Neil Grayson, Attila Györy, John Hanrahan, Geoff Hansen, Warren Hastings, Clive Heath, Tim Hegarty, Chris Hogan, Damian Ireland, Anton Iseli, Rob James, Fred Jensen, Stuart Johnson, Dorothy Jones, Roderick Jones, Dennis Joyce, Max Kamien, Trevor Kay, Tim Kenealy, Clive Kenna, Peter Kennedy, Hilton Koppe, Rod Kruger, Sanaa Labib, Chris Lampel, Bray Lewis, Ralph Lewis, Greg Malcher, Karen Martens, Jim Marwood, John Masterton, Sally McDonald, Peter McKain, A. Breck McKay, Peter Mellor, Thomas Middlemiss, Philip Millard, Les Miller, Geoff Mitchell, David Moore, Michael Moynihan, Alister Neil, Rowland Noakes, Colin Officer, Helene Owzinsky, Michael Page, Dominic Pak, Geoff Pearce, Alexander Pollack, Vernon Powell, Cameron Profitt, Andrew Protassow, Geoff Quail, Farooq Qureshi, Anthony Radford, Peter Radford, Suresh Rananavare, Jan Reddy, Sandy Reid, David Ross, Harvey Rotstein, Jackie Rounsevell, Carl Rubis, Sharnee Rutherford, Avni Sali, Paul Scott, Adrian Sheen, Jack Shepherd, Peter Stone, Helen Sutcliffe, Royston Taylor, Alex Thomson, Jim Thomson, John Togno, Bruce Tonge, John Trollor, Ian Tulloch, Talina Vizard, Vilas Wavde, David White, David Wilson, Ian Wilson, John Wong, Ian Wood, Freda Wraight, David Young, Mark Zagorski.

In reference to part of the text and figures in spinal disorders, permission from the copyright owners, Butterworths, of *Back Pain and Spinal Manipulation* (1989), by C. Kenna and J. Murtagh, is gratefully acknowledged.

Acknowledgment is given to the World Health Organization, publishers of J. Cook et al., *General Surgery at the District Hospital* (1986), for permission to use Figures 1.6, 1.15a, 2.22, 2.25, 2.26, 2.27, 7.13,

9.50, 9.57, 12.2 and 16.3b, and to Dr Leveat Efe for permission to use Figures 1.35, 1.36, 3.10c,d, 3.21a,b, 7.1, 9.74, 13.3a,b, 13.4 and 16.7a,b,c.

Permission to use many drawings from *Australian Family Physician* is also gratefully acknowledged.

Finally, my thanks to Nicki Constable, Kris Berntsen and Caroline Menara for secretarial help in the preparation of this material.

Index